John Dickinson is Emeritus Professor of Medicine at the University of London and visiting Professor at the Wolfson Institute for Preventive Medicine. He is the author of numerous books and articles including *21 Medical Mysteries* published by The Book Guild in 2000 and *Neurogenic Hypertension: A Synthesis and Review* (Chapman & Hall, 1991) which was described as 'an invaluable review of a difficult field' which should be read as 'a model of its kind'. He has been Chairman of the British Medical Research Society, Vice-President of the Royal College of Physicians and Vice-Chairman of the Council of the British Heart Foundation (reflecting his particular interest in hypertension and its many related conditions). He is married with four children, two of whom are doctors. Apart from clinical physiology, his other passions are playing the organ and competing at squash. He is a lifelong city motorcyclist.

By the same author:

Electrophysiological Technique

Clinical Pathology Data (2 editions and Italian translation)

Neurogenic Hypertension (1965)

A Computer Model of Human Respiration

Neurogenic Hypertension: A Synthesis and Review (1991)

21 Medical Mysteries

Software for Educational Computing
(jointly with K Ahmed and D Ingram)

Clinical Physiology (5 editions)
(jointly edited, with EJM Cambell, JDH Slater, CRW Edwards and EK Sikora)

MEDICAL MYSTERIES

The Testament of a Clinical Scientist

John Dickinson

Book Guild Publishing
Sussex, England

First published in Great Britain in 2005 by
The Book Guild Ltd
25 High Street
Lewes, East Sussex
BN7 2LU

Typesetting in Times by
Acorn Bookwork Ltd, Salisbury, Wiltshire

Printed in Great Britain by
Athenaeum Press Ltd, Gateshead

A catalogue record for this book is available from
The British Library.

ISBN 1 85776 976 7

CONTENTS

PREFACE AND ACKNOWLEDGEMENTS

A few years ago I published a short book entitled *21 Medical Mysteries*. This was well enough received to stimulate me to revise, expand, annotate and bring up to date my original topics, adding another 21 to embrace a lot more subjects and choosing those which are both important and being actively researched. I have been able to cover a large amount of what can be classified as 'general internal medicine', describing current theories about causes. A down-to-earth perspective comes from my personal experience of looking after patients with complaints relating to every one of my 42 chosen subjects. Part of this book is thus autobiographical, written by a physician who has been lucky to have worked all his life in exciting medical environments with stimulating mentors and colleagues.

To make the book easier for non-scientists to read I have tried to demystify obscure medical terms by giving their (usually Greek) origins. When some new unfamiliar word or concept is introduced for the first time I have defined or explained it. Later usages are cross-referenced back to the first occurrence. I hope that scientifically literate readers will not be too irritated by my use of homely words like womb, or mentioning pounds, pints, feet and inches before giving the proper international units, or introducing each topic in a very elementary way. All this is to allow people without much scientific training or knowledge to share some of the excitement I have felt in medicine and medical research. All technical terms are explained. Most of the book can easily be understood by non-medical and non-scientific readers, but I have cut no corners to bring the reader bang up-to-date with the latest discoveries and insights. Technical material is put in small type, so that it can easily be skipped over. Contentious issues are clarified with numbered endnotes.

ACKNOWLEDGEMENTS

This book could not have been written without the superb facilities I have enjoyed in the last few years at the Wolfson Institute of Preventive Medicine, which is now part of London University's medical faculty at Queen Mary. In particular, Neville Young (Database Manager) and Dallas Allen (Academic Administrator) have given me a great deal of practical help and advice.

I am most grateful to many kind friends and colleagues who have read and helped with individual chapters: Eric Beck, Ben Benjamin, the late Moran Campbell, Tim Cox, Paul Dieppe, the late Israel Doniach, David Galton, Richard Godfrey, Ashley Grossman, Jim Lawrence, Andrew Lees, Irene Leigh, David Leslie, Ewa Paleolog, Chris Redman, Andy Rees, Ben Sacks, Maxine Sacks, Pamela Shaw, the late John Swales, Howard Thomas, Dan Tunstall Pedoe, Nick Wald, Tony Weetman, Gareth Williams, the late Derek Willoughby and David Wingate. Two of our children (Mark and Caroline) have helped with several chapters. All have made useful suggestions. Pierre Bouloux very kindly read the proofs and corrected many of my errors of fact or emphasis. I am also grateful to Ian MacDonald for letting me reproduce the magnetic resonance brain scans in Chapter 3, to John Kanis for his illustrations of Paget lesions in Chapter 29, and to Kathy Driver, Nelly Pecheva and their colleagues in the Medical Illustration Department at Barts for preparing the other illustrations.

JOHN DICKINSON
Wolfson Institute of Preventive Medicine,
Queen Mary, University of London.

INTRODUCTION

Medical research has never been more exciting than it is today. We now know the molecular chemical structure of DNA (deoxyribose nucleic acid) and the way in which DNA can embody genes, replicate itself and provide a template for the synthesis of proteins. These discoveries have provided the most spectacular advances in biology since the origin of species was revealed in the nineteenth century.

Molecular biology has shown us how human diseases can result from minor faults in DNA. At the other end of the size scale, new techniques now allow us to probe the human body in new ways. Unfortunately many medical mysteries seem to occupy a middle ground between molecular chemistry and gross anatomy. We find a faulty gene which seems to cause a disease like schizophrenia or high blood pressure, but then find that someone who has the same faulty gene is entirely normal. Or we find a condition like endometriosis or Parkinson's disease which seem to have rather little to do with genes and for which we have to try to identify environmental causes, with few clues to guide us.

The triumphant march of molecular biology has already led to many advances in our understanding of disease mechanisms. Cancer, which once seemed utterly mysterious, is gradually being explained in molecular terms, notably by a sequence of disadvantageous mutations in body cells. Some of these may have been genetic and thus present before birth, some may have been caused by chemical or radiation damage, some by cancer-inducing ('oncogenic') viruses, and some by selective damage to genes involved in DNA repair. The understanding of cancer is advancing at tremendous speed. But there remain many important medical problems which cannot be explained by single gene defects. Indeed there are very few which can be so explained. The medical mysteries which I shall describe in this book are mostly complex, being partly due to environmental factors and partly due to the ill effects of many genes rather than of a single one.

The book contains a plentiful supply of numerical data. A rough general rule says that science begins when quantities begin to be measured. I have tried for each of my topics first to describe the condition, disease or phenomenon as accurately and succinctly as possible, to set the stage for discussing its mysteries and for suggesting possible

1

solutions to some of them. One trap is to mislead by oversimplifying. It is difficult to avoid this. On each subject discussed here there have been hundreds – more often thousands – of relevant papers published in learned journals. I have tried in each case first to describe the condition, disease or problem as accurately as possible. Then I have summarised the main facts about it, to set the stage for discussing its mysteries.

Not all my topics can be classified as 'diseases'. The chapter on clubbing of the fingers is an intellectual exercise and a medical detective story. Many people would not classify 'chronic fatigue syndrome' (so-called 'ME'), 'irritable bowel syndrome' or even 'essential hypertension' as diseases at all. But all of them are certainly medical mysteries.

When I was first a medical student, I wanted to find out what the mysteries were, so that I could choose the most interesting and important ones to work on when I had the chance. At that time we seemed to understand a lot. There had been marvellous advances in treatment, such as antibiotics, anti-cancer drugs and steroids. Each year since then has brought new understanding. Each has also thrown up new puzzles. Research fields get wider, and more exciting, with time. My choice of subjects in this book should not be taken to mean that I am not interested in the many medical mysteries I have not discussed, but simply that I have tried to choose the more important and potentially soluble problems to write about – the ones about which I had something original to say.

All the first-class scientists I have met have had one characteristic in common: they are interested in everything. One never knows whether work in one field might not open up a completely different field. Experienced clinicians reading this book will find their own subjects dealt with in an elementary and naive fashion, but I hope that they will find some less familiar medical mysteries interesting and stimulating. I have also tried to envisage an intelligent non-scientist skimming through the book, omitting most of the technical stuff, but perhaps suddenly coming across something interesting. The technical matter and the Notes at the end of the book will then allow the reader to follow right through to the latest discoveries about mechanisms.

I hope that this book will convey some of the pleasures and excitement of scientific research – in this case research into the causes of human diseases. Although the supreme excitement may be reserved for the first discoverer, it is almost as fascinating to watch from the sidelines as nature's secrets are successively revealed. In the last fifty years there have been huge strides forward in genetics, in immunology, in epidemiology and in clinical pharmacology. There have also been innumerable smaller steps by which medical mysteries are being unravelled.

Organisation of chapters

In each chapter I have tried to summarise briefly what is known about the inheritance ('genetics') of each condition, phenomenon or disease. In most cases I shall also use the general heading 'Epidemiology', to describe not only the study of disease epidemics, but also disease associations of all kinds other than those associated with genes – though strictly speaking the study of environmental factors causing disease should be classed as 'ecology'.

The book can obviously be dipped into at random. I have tried to make it palatable to be read straight through, though many sittings will be needed to avoid indigestion. For every subject I have sometimes had to slip into technical detail, to avoid insulting established clinical scientists by pretending that my medical mysteries are unduly simple. Technical material is printed in small type so that general readers can more easily skip over it. My last chapter, describing motor neurone disease – a common, mysterious and fatal condition – assumes in the reader considerably more background scientific knowledge than is assumed for the rest of the book. I have included it to illustrate the enormous number of different lines of evidence which sometimes have to be examined by scientists trying (so far unsuccessfully in this case) to solve a particularly intractable medical mystery. The study of motor neurone disease nicely exemplifies a universal rule of science: the more we know about a subject, the more we appreciate its complexities and realise what we don't know. But when a breakthrough comes, there is no excitement to match it.

1

EMPHYSEMA AND CHRONIC BRONCHITIS

Longstanding *irreversible* obstruction of the airways of the lungs is referred to by doctors as Chronic Obstructive Pulmonary Disease (COPD) or Chronic Obstructive Airways Disease (COAD). It is usually associated with 'emphysema' (Greek: *en* = in; *physema* = a blowing). The small terminal air spaces of the lungs are enlarged, with patchy destruction of their walls. COPD is also strongly associated with 'chronic bronchitis', i.e. longstanding or recurrent cough with excess sticky phlegm (sputum) production.

The single large windpipe or trunk (the trachea) starts in the neck at the larynx, which makes the so-called 'Adam's apple' in the front of the neck. Hard cartilage protects the delicate vocal cords within. The trachea descends into the chest where it divides into two main airways (bronchi) which lie behind the heart. Each main bronchus divides into smaller and smaller airways (bronchioles), terminating eventually in thousands of tiny air sacs (alveoli). Inhaled air in the alveoli can diffuse into and thus make intimate contact with the blood stream. The whole structure resembles an inverted tree (Fig. 1).

The consequences of chronic airways obstruction

The prime function of the lungs is to extract oxygen from the air so that later it can combine with (i.e. 'oxidise' or burn up) foodstuffs to produce energy. At rest, an average-sized man needs about half a pint (250 cubic centimetres) of oxygen every minute, a woman slightly less. During exercise this requirement may increase ten- or even fifteen-fold. Since oxygen makes up only about one fifth of the air we breathe – the rest is mostly nitrogen – and the lungs can only extract about a quarter of the oxygen contained in the air, an adult needs a certain minimum amount of ventilation: that is, the volume of air going in and out of the lungs in a given time. An average adult needs to breathe at least 7 pints (4 litres) of air in and out each minute. With ventilation much less than this someone would soon die just from lack of oxygen.

The supply of oxygen can be increased artificially by adding extra

5

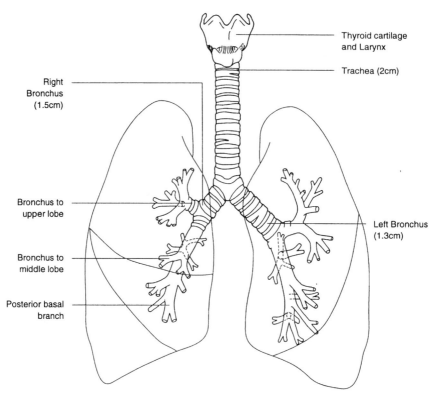

Right
Bronchus
(1.5cm)

Thyroid cartilage
and Larynx

Trachea (2cm)

Bronchus to
upper lobe

Left Bronchus
(1.3cm)

Bronchus to
middle lobe

Posterior basal
branch

Figure 1 The main airways of the lungs, seen from the front, indicating the approximate internal diameters of the trachea and main bronchi. The two lungs are shown in outline. The left lung (on the right of the diagram) is slightly smaller than the right, because the heart occupies some of the left chest cavity.

oxygen to the air. But lack of oxygen is not the only problem faced by people who are not breathing enough. There is also a need to get the waste gas (carbon dioxide) out of the body. In terms of volume, the amount of carbon dioxide produced by the oxidation of food is about 80% of the amount of oxygen consumed – about $\frac{1}{5}$ litre (200 cc) per minute. When carbon dioxide dissolves in water it forms a weak acid (carbonic acid). The breakdown of food typically generates so much carbon dioxide that in the absence of ventilation the body would become fatally acid in an hour or two even if there was plenty of oxygen available. In days before the dangers of giving oxygen 'ad lib' to people with severe exacerbations of COPD were appreciated, many people died of carbon dioxide poisoning even though their blood and their bodies contained plenty of oxygen.

This posed a real problem when treating people whose severe longstanding airways obstruction was being made worse by an intercurrent lung infection. Such people needed more oxygen, but the amount was critical. The 21% concentration of oxygen already present in the air we all breathe was not enough to keep these people alive, but 100%, 50% or even 30% oxygen enrichment could lead to fatal poisoning by carbon dioxide accumulation. When I was working at the Middlesex Hospital in the same laboratory as Moran Campbell, fifty years ago, I watched him trying to improve peoples' ventilation by giving chemical stimulants to breathing, such as nikethamide and salicylate. This was not successful. The effects soon wore off. In the end it was necessary in most patients to put a tube down into the lungs and artificially ventilate them with a pump to tide them over their infection. But Campbell made enquiries and found that a small jet of oxygen at high pressure infused into a venturi or pitot tube could entrain ten or more times its volume of surrounding air. Thus the 'Ventimask' and its progeny were born. These devices allowed the effective inspired air to be enriched by a controlled percentage (e.g. 3%, 5% or 7%) of oxygen. Appropriately enriched air flowed fast into a comfortable loose-fitting mask. This marvellously simple idea has been spectacularly successful. Face masks which allow this type of controlled oxygen enrichment are in use all over the world. Campbell himself, and London University, neither patented these devices nor ever sought to make money from them.

The functional disorder in chronic obstructive pulmonary disease

Breathing in ('inspiration') is done by expanding the size of the chest cavity, mainly by contracting the muscles of the diaphragm. The diaphragm (Greek: *diaphragma* = partition wall) is a sheet of muscle shaped like an umbrella, separating the lung compartments on each side of the heart from the abdominal cavity below. When the diaphragm contracts and moves downwards (making the umbrella shape flatter) the pressure inside the chest cavity is reduced and all the elastic airways of the lungs are pulled open. Airways obstruction is minimised.

Breathing out ('expiration') is a different matter. Healthy people at rest do not need to make any muscular effort at all to breathe out. Normal lungs behave like a child's balloon. If the diaphragm is not contracting and there is no airways obstruction, the elasticity of the lungs will almost empty them of air in a second or two. But if the air passages are obstructed the lungs may not deflate enough, or fast enough, while a subject is trying to breathe out. The residual air left in the lungs at the end of expiration will increase. The next breath in will start from a larger lung volume. It might seem that this process could lead to more and more air being left in the lungs at the end of each expiration until there was no room in the rib cage for further expansion. Although this situation can arise in a fatal asthma attack, or in the terminal stage of chronic airways obstruction, an equilibrium position is normally reached. As the lungs get bigger, the elastic recoil force available to empty the lungs increases. This is then enough to make the amount of air breathed out the same as the amount breathed in, though at the expense of an increase in the amount of air left in the lungs at the end of breathing out. When this reaches some arbitrary value – perhaps a few hundred extra cubic centimetres of air – an individual is described as having 'emphysema'. The diagnosis can be made and the severity of disease measured by physiological studies of lung function and lung volume. Severe emphysema can also be diagnosed from a chest X-ray because the shadow of the diaphragm at full inspiration becomes flat and horizontal, instead of remaining convex upwards.

A simple and widely used measure of fixed airways obstruction in emphysema is the 'Forced Expiratory Volume in one second' (FEV_1). Figure 2A illustrates the pattern of peak flow of a healthy young man breathing out as fast as he can after taking the maximum possible breath in. The vertical scale on the left represents lung volume. The time scale along the bottom goes from left to right. In the first second breathing out he has been able to expel 80% of the air in his lungs. By contrast, Figure 2B shows a typical time/volume curve (spirogram) of an individual with severe chronic airways obstruction and emphysema. He has only been able to expel 30% of the volume of air in his lungs in one second, despite using all his expiratory muscles. The flow pattern of someone in an attack of asthma (next chapter) would be very similar. Someone with normal lungs should have a FEV_1 which is at least 75% of the 'Vital Capacity' (the difference between the amount of air a subject can breathe in with maximal effort and the amount he can force out, again using maximal effort). An even simpler test makes use of the peak flow meter.[1] This measures the maximum speed of airflow in litres per minute that someone can achieve when forcibly breathing out as fast as possible.

An observant clinician can recognise at the bedside some of the instinctive manoeuvres which people with emphysema learn to help them breathe out. The most characteristic is to purse the lips. If the larger airways have already been partly closed by their elastic recoil and by active contraction of the muscles of expiration, pursing the lips

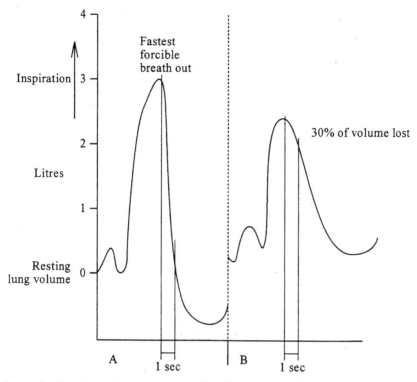

Figure 2 Tracings of spirometer records of forced expiration by (A) a normal healthy young adult and (B) by someone with severe chronic airways obstruction and emphysema. The vertical scale measures volume, in litres. The first large upstroke in each case represents the change in volume of the lungs during breathing in (inspiration) as fully as possible. The timing marks show a one second interval. The downstroke that follows shows the rate of change of volume during the most forceful breathing out (expiration) that each subject could achieve. Note that the volume at the end of breathing out (the 'residual air') is greater in the obstructed than in the normal subject, and the Forced Expired Volume in 1 second (the FEV_1) is much less. In the normal subject it is about 80% of 'vital capacity'; in the subject with emphysema it is only about 30% of the vital capacity.

increases the pressure inside the chest during breathing out and widens the airways inside the chest, allowing air to flow out faster. Severely disabled subjects have to use additional muscles of respiration not only to breathe out actively when there is airways obstruction, but even to breathe in fast enough. Almost all the muscles of the rib cage, shoulders, neck, back and abdomen may need to be brought into use to overcome obstructed breathing.

Sufferers from chronic airways obstruction were memorably differentiated into two contrasted categories by Tony Dornhorst,[2] according to their symptoms and signs. There is the normally-built 'pink puffer' who is red in the face, who complains of shortness of breath even on mild exercise, but who has no swelling of the legs and who manages to maintain near normal concentrations of oxygen and carbon dioxide in his blood. On the other hand, the 'blue bloater' is overweight, sluggish in movement, blue in the face and with legs swollen by excess tissue fluid. His blood is deficient in oxygen and it has an abnormally high concentration of carbon dioxide. We do not know exactly why some people with similar degrees of lung damage seem to react in these different ways, but recurrent lung infections tend to produce blue bloaters while genetic lung diseases (see below) tend to produce pink puffers.

The role of elastin

Breathing out, being normally a passive process, is critically dependent on the elastic recoil of the airways and of lung tissue. In turn this is provided by the protein 'elastin'. This is synthesised during lung development, towards the end of fetal life, as a precursor protein, tropoelastin. This forms a self-assembling polymer (Greek: *poly* = many; *meros* = part). This is an ordered sequence of joined-up molecules which are elastic: i.e. they can repeatedly absorb energy when stretched and give it back again when released. One of the characteristics of damaged lungs with COPD is that their elastic recoil function is grossly impaired. Elastin is an unusual molecule since it does not participate in the continual renewal of its chemical constituents, as most protein molecules in living systems do. Unless damaged it lasts indefinitely. Although new elastin can be synthesised during adult life it cannot be laid down appropriately in line with the original structural pattern. Thus loss of someone's original lung elastin cannot be overcome or reversed.

It may be difficult to determine how much of the difficulty that emphysematous people have in breathing out is due to mechanical obstruction of the air passages, e.g. from excessive sticky secretions, and how much is due to loss of elastic recoil of lung tissue. It is easy to measure mechanical obstruction but easy to forget the equally important aspect of COPD – loss of the elasticity of the lungs.

Epidemiology

Chronic airways obstruction is extremely common and becoming commoner in developed countries.[3] It is serious and potentially life-threatening. In the UK, COPD accounts for about 60 deaths annually for every 100,000 men between 55 and 64 and for nearly 900 deaths annually for every 100,000 men over 75. A survey by primary care doctors has estimated that 8% of men in England between 40 and 65 have COPD. Some 6.5% of men and 4% of women will die from it. More than 30 million working days are lost each year in the UK from chronic chest illnesses. In the USA it is estimated that 14 million people have COPD, which accounted for some 41 deaths per 100,000 people in 1997. It has been estimated that it will soon become the third commonest cause of death as people protect themselves with increasing success against arterial diseases of the heart and brain but continue to smoke and pollute city air.

COPD is about four times less common in women than in men at all ages, but we do not know all the reasons for this. Disentangling the relative importance of genetic predisposition, smoking behaviour and atmospheric pollution is exceedingly difficult, though atmospheric pollution is certainly important. In most parts of England the smoke from factories and houses tends to be carried by the prevailing west winds to the east end or east side of English cities. Most wealthy (and consequently healthy) people have lived on the west side of big English cities, and still do despite improvement brought about by the Clean Air Acts. COPD has been repeatedly shown to be closely associated with low household income. But it is difficult to disentangle all the reasons why social and class differences cause profound differences in prevalence of COPD.

Genetics

There has been a great deal of recent work on the circulating blood protein 'alpha-1 antitrypsin'. This protects the lungs from damage by the digestive enzyme 'trypsin' which breaks down proteins. Two observant Swedish scientists (Laurell and Eriksson) had been analysing the soluble proteins of the blood in hospital patients. They noticed that some people with premature emphysema had blood which was deficient in α-1 antitrypsin.

> α-1 antitrypsin is one of a class of naturally-occurring proteins known as 'serpins'. The name derives from 'SERine Protein INhibitors'. It is interesting that this particular serpin is also associated with scarring (cirrhosis) of the liver and also with degenerative changes in the brain. The protein is not actually lacking. Rather it has folded in a fashion technically described as 'loop-sheet polymerisation'.[4] This allows strings of its component molecules to join up together in an abnormal way. The

11

changed structure means that it can no longer neutralise the protein-digesting enzyme 'trypsin', which is normally secreted by the pancreas into the gut but which can severely damage the lungs when it comes into contact with them.

In the last few years increasing numbers of genetic diseases are becoming recognised as due not to *lack* of an important protein enzyme but rather to its misfolding. This might be due to a fault in a single amino-acid of the whole protein chain. Although this may prevent or impair some important enzyme action (as in α1-antitrypsin deficiency) it can also lead to an unwanted gain of function, with abnormal aggregations of proteins, impairing function. Many genetic defects of the nervous system may be of this type: e.g. Alzheimer's (Chapter 19), Parkinson's (Chapter 28) and motor neurone disease (Chapter 42).

Cause

Smoking is of enormous importance in causing chronic airways obstruction and chronic bronchitis. One effect of cigarette smoke is to impair the sweeping function of the 'cilia', the minute hairs lining the airways. These beat regularly and move particles of foreign material and mucus up the airways towards the mouth, where they can be swallowed. Smoking seems also to enormously increase the lung damage associated with several different inherited conditions. Cigarette smoke activates the production of large defensive circulating white blood cells (macrophages). (The Greek name comes from *macros* = large and *phagein* = to eat.) These cells deal with invading bacteria and with various damaging chemicals such as 'tumour necrosis factor α' and interleukins-1 and -8.

Curiously, there is a strong genetic influence on the speed at which smoking damages people's lungs. Some 5–15% of people in various populations are genetically susceptible to lung damage from cigarette smoke, whereas the remainder suffer far less. So far we do not know the cause of the difference, though strenuous efforts are being made to find it.

Only a few per cent of people have α1-antitrypsin deficiency. It accounts only for a small number of victims of COPD. But it must have been the cause of death, at age 53, of Kenneth Tynan, the well-known dramatic critic. Kathleen, his second wife and biographer, has described in detail his last depressing years – suffering from gross emphysema, dependent on supplemental extra oxygen and with the highest blood carbon dioxide tension that his physicians had ever encountered.[5] Ken became aware of his own emphysema at a party when he found himself unable to blow out a candle with his mouth wide open. I have many memories of him as a fellow Magdalen under-graduate at Oxford. One of the strongest is of an inveterate cigarette smoker. Unfortunately smoking can be the last straw for someone with α1-antitrypsin deficiency. It greatly accelerates lung damage.

There is evidence that some substances in tobacco smoke can directly damage lung elastin, thereby causing emphysema. The loss of elastin in the skin coarsens skin folds. It produces the characteristic facial appearance which will be recalled by those who have seen photographs of WH Auden (another inveterate smoker) towards the end of his life.

We do not know all the ways in which various air-borne pollutants may cause disease. I am interested in the possible causal role of minute particles of the intensely inflammatory and ubiquitous material PVC (polyvinyl chloride) being rubbed off household materials. This has not been suggested by anyone else (so far) as a possible cause of longstanding lung damage. PVC is, of course, a solid material. But even at room temperature this material in the form of dust is highly irritant and has already been linked to a specific risk of asthma,[6] which I shall discuss in the next chapter. Inhalation of PVC smoke by fire fighters and fire victims can cause prolonged airways hyperrespon-siveness, asthma and chronic airways obstruction.[7] Factory work involving PVC processing[8] or meat wrapping or checking[9] can all cause respiratory symptoms. PVC is an ubiquitous material in houses. It is used for wrapping food and other goods and for making electrical insulating materials and innumerable other light moulded structures. In the rubbing of coated surfaces which must inevitably accompany normal use, microscopic PVC particles are going to be spread about in the air. Domestic cleaning workers make up one of the occupational groups identified as being specially at risk of asthma.[10] So could PVC plausibly be a culprit in causing COPD? The answer will only be given decisively when carefully controlled epidemiological studies have been done. Might PVC be directly damaging, or indirectly damaging through immune sensitisation? Clearly a short exposure to small amounts is harmless. But we need to know whether long-continued exposure to PVC dust particles could in the end cause lung damage. The rising prevalence of chronic airways obstruction world-wide has not so far been fully explained by the many factors we already know about, such as air pollution from car exhausts.

My speculations about the possible damaging effects of PVC are both wild and difficult to investigate. Science begins with hypotheses, many of which start off wild. It cannot do without them. Thomas Love Peacock, the witty Victorian novelist, made fun of many of his own and Shelley's friends in *Crotchet Castle* (published in 1803). One of Peacock's creations was 'Mr Firedamp' who bores the company by repeating: 'Whenever there is water, there is malaria, and whenever there is malaria there are the elements of death...Get rid of malaria by abolishing duck ponds.'

Many discoveries about the causes of disease begin with amateur observations like these, associating a particular disease with particular living conditions. But then a clinical scientist is needed to sort the wheat from the chaff. It was a century after Mr Firedamp's reflections that Ronald Ross identified the mosquito as the agent of malaria. And it was a century later that removal of 'duck ponds' around the area allowed the Panama Canal to be built.

British susceptibility to COPD

A puzzling feature of the epidemiology of COPD is that one would expect people living in the UK to be relatively protected against COPD. UK residents enjoy a climate that is remarkably temperate compared with that of other northern European or North American countries and states. But the British collectively suffer severely from COPD. I have lived in southern Ontario (Canada) for many winter months, and for a year in Cleveland, Ohio (USA). I have also visited many North American hospitals in that time. During these periods I saw remarkably little end-stage respiratory failure from COPD, even though this is a familiar feature of general medical practice in the UK. I shall hazard a guess which might explain the trans-Atlantic difference.

During my clinical career I recorded the medical history of many people, mostly men, with COPD. It was always my habit to ask my patients whether they slept with their windows open in the winter time. (This is not a feasible practice in much of North America because the cold outside is so intense that it can freeze the bedroom water pipes. I have even seen explicit instructions to British visitors to Canadian hotels not to open the windows in winter!) The invariable indignant answer to my question was that of course he did not close his bedroom windows in the winter. Most of my patients regarded this as a thoroughly unhealthy practice. Yet an important function of the extensive surface of the air passages in the nose (contributed by the turbinate cartilages) is to warm as well as filter the incoming air. Very cold air is a constricting stimulus to the lung airways. In my view it is best avoided.

Doubtless similar observations have been made by many others, though I have not come across a proper epidemiological survey. It might make an interesting study. If correct it would have obvious prophylactic relevance and might perhaps justify some publicity.

Summary

Chronic obstructive pulmonary disease (COPD) is common and becoming commoner as other more preventable causes of disease and death are prevented or deferred. It is usually associated with a chronic productive cough (chronic bronchitis) and with structural changes in the lungs (emphysema) in which the minute terminal air spaces in the lungs are expanded and the residual lung volume is increased. There is notable lack of the normal elastic recoil of the lungs so that even breathing out may require active muscular effort.

Air pollution, most notably from cigarette smoke, is the main causal factor in COPD. One important effect of cigarette smoke is to damage the elasticity of the lungs and to prevent them emptying properly. There are additionally some rare genetic causes of emphysema, particularly that due to deficiency of circulating α1-antitrypsin which normally protects the lungs from damage by the protein-digesting enzyme trypsin.

Undoubtedly there are many significant air pollutants. I have suggested the possibility that minute particles of polyvinyl chloride (PVC) might be particularly irritant. Other possibilities, such as unduly cold bedrooms during wintertime, might also perhaps play a part by damaging the linings of the lung airways.

2

ASTHMA: WHY IS IT INCREASING?

Asthma is very common. It was well known to the Greeks, who gave it its name. Its precise definition has been debated at many international conferences. The diagnosis implies that the asthmatic individual suffers from episodes in which breathing is temporarily obstructed because of narrowing of the airways of the lungs. The obstruction is unlike that described in the last chapter because it is potentially *reversible*, either spontaneously or with treatment.

The background to asthma appears always to be bronchial hyperresponsiveness, i.e. an excessive reaction by the airways to irritants such as cold air or to materials causing 'allergy'.[1] These materials induce muscular spasm of small airways and increased secretion of sticky slime (mucus) by the linings of the larger airways. In the case of the trachea, which is a semi-rigid structure, thick mucus secretion is the cause of narrowing. In the smaller airways there is also active contraction of circular muscle in the airway wall. This makes the internal diameter of the hollow tube concerned (the 'lumen') smaller. A well known relationship in physics (Poiseuille's formula) is that the resistance offered to the flow of gas or fluid through a tube increases as the inverse fourth power of the radius. In the presence of turbulence the resistance is even higher. If, for example, the diameter of a tube through which air is flowing is halved, its resistance to airflow will increase at least sixteen times. This makes for a potential trigger effect. Quite a small reduction in airway calibre can suddenly make someone feel that breathing has become obstructed, a sensation technically referred to as 'dyspnoea' (the Greek word for 'bad breathing'). Lung capacity is reduced in an asthmatic attack. A sufferer finds it very difficult to empty the lungs after taking a deep breath in. Measures of airways obstruction such as the Forced Expiratory Volume in one second (FEV_1) and the peak flow rate are much reduced.

I can testify from my own clinical experience just how suddenly breathing can get obstructed. When I was a junior doctor I had been writing down the medical details of a middle-aged woman admitted to a hospital ward in an attack of asthma. She felt the need to pass urine, excused herself, then walked the length of the open ward. She had not returned after ten minutes or so. I assumed that she must have been constipated. Then a white-faced nurse came out and said that the woman had collapsed in the ward toilets. All efforts at resuscitation were in vain. Post mortem examination (necropsy) showed almost complete obstruction of the trachea and larger bronchi by thick tenacious mucus. It still seems hardly credible to me that someone able to talk freely and walk 40 yards could be so close to fatal asphyxia. The fact that the lavatory and bathroom area was entirely full of flowers may have provided the final trigger.[2] At the time, drug treatment of asthma was primitive. Steroids had not come into use. But this experience made an indelible impression on me which later I always tried to pass on to my students. Someone in a bad asthma attack can be living on a knife edge.

Attacks of asthma may end spontaneously, but they can be so alarming that sufferers usually start treatment by inhaling a dilating drug preparation as soon as they find that breathing has become difficult. Almost all asthmatics (999 out of 1000) improve if they regularly inhale so-called 'steroids'. This treatment is protective – the medical description is 'prophylactic' (Greek: *pro* = before; *phylaxis* = protection). Collectively such steroid drugs are referred to as 'glucocorticoids' because they affect the way glucose is broken down in the body. As I shall discuss later, steroids also suppress inflammation, by inhibiting the release of a gene transcription factor responsible for the local production of inflammation-promoting chemicals ('cytokines', in this context also called 'chemokines'). Obstructed breathing which can be relieved by inhaling steroids is virtually diagnostic of asthma.

Chronic obstructive pulmonary disease (COPD) – discussed in the last chapter – is not much improved by inhalation of steroids, though sensible physicians usually prescribe a full course of steroids at least once to any patient with established COPD, to see whether there is a reversible element in the condition. Some patients with COPD are given inhaled steroids (e.g. fluticasone) to use on a regular basis, even though the improvement obtainable is rather limited.

The term 'asthma' is not nowadays used for diseases of the heart or blood circulation, even though congestion of the lungs in such conditions may produce similar symptoms. Nineteenth-century physicians recognised 'cardiac asthma', which we would now categorise as acute pulmonary oedema (p. 229). The term 'asthma' is also inappropriate to describe the fixed airways obstruction that may be found in chronic bronchitis and which I described in the last chapter. This does not change suddenly and is not much helped by medical treatment. By contrast, an attack of asthma can often be relieved within minutes by the right treatment.

Epidemiology

Asthma is extremely common and getting commoner. Some estimates are of a doubling every decade. This leads to the prediction that almost everyone will have asthma in 100 years' time! At present, in Europe and in the USA, between 1% and 6% of people are affected. Over the last 10 years, incidence has increased by a third in the under-elevens in the UK. Britain is now known as the asthma capital of Europe. The UK has three times the asthma incidence of Germany or Austria and $1\frac{1}{2}$ times that of Ireland. In the UK more than a thousand children with asthma are admitted to hospital on most days of the year. At any one time the prevalence has been about the same in children and adults. Young children with asthma tend to improve with time as their airways grow bigger but some people first develop the disease as adults. About 7% of children in Britain have asthma at some stage of their lives. Many children with episodic wheezing and probable asthma are never given that diagnosis, so the prevalence may be even greater than current estimates. Some infants get a single episode of wheezy bronchitis from a virus infection but never later go on to develop true asthma.

The sexes are affected about equally. There is some evidence that early childhood infections, especially measles, may protect against asthma,[3] though early exposure to 'allergens' (things producing allergy) may be harmful. There is suggestive evidence that miscellaneous endotoxin exposure, e.g. from dirt, or a household pet, may be protective against asthma.[4] It has also been suggested that children who have often been given antibiotics to treat minor bacterial infections may thereby become more liable to asthma. The picture is confusing.

Though asthma is distressing and attacks are disabling, most attacks end spontaneously or after drug treatment. Even in older people – over 55, for example – death rates from asthma in England and Wales are around 8 per year for every 100,000 people. In children the asthma death rates are only about one twentieth of this. Even so, with the disease so common, an appreciable number of children in the UK die in an asthmatic attack each year. The summer months seem to be the worst for children, probably because of increased exposure to pollens and moulds. This contrasts with asthma deaths in the elderly, which are commoner in the winter months. Recently exposure to moulds has been recognised as a factor increasing severity of asthma in adults.

Asthma is manifestly a far from trivial disease. In the USA and some other countries asthma death rates in recent years have been rising despite widespread use of prophylactics, while preventable deaths from most other causes have been steadily falling. In the UK asthma death rates peaked in the 1960s, fell in the 1970s, rose to a peak in the 1980s and are now falling again. We have really no idea why these changes occurred, though the early peak in the 1970s may have been due to over-use of inhalers containing adrenaline-like drugs (see below).

Genetics

Asthma tends to run in families, but its inheritance is complicated. Many different genes are involved. The effects of shared local environments may be difficult to disentangle from genetic factors. Claims have already been made that genes localised on chromosomes 5, 6, 11, 12, 13 and 14 are linked with asthma,[5] but a unique asthma gene has yet to be discovered. The search for it has been described as 'a glorious fishing expedition'. It is unlikely that any one individual gene will prove to be all-important. Everything suggests that the inheritance of asthma involves many different genes.

Recent work in Britain and America has identified a gene called ADAM-33 on chromosome 20 which is strongly associated with bronchial hyperresponsiveness. The protein product of this gene has been identified in lung fibroblasts and bronchial smooth muscle cells. This raises the possibility that this particular genetic defect might operate through modifying reactions of airway muscle rather than modifying immune mechanisms.

Cause

The immediate precipitating cause of an attack of asthma is often exposure to an allergen – that is, to some material, usually inhaled, to which the lungs have become sensitised. Pollens and the excretions (faeces) of house-dust mites are probably the commonest immediate precipitating factors. House-dust mites live off the tiny flakes of skin that humans shed. They like a warm, damp environment to breed. When I was a student I was taught that children with asthma got attacks because of emotional stress at home. This idea seemed to be confirmed because the children quickly got better when they were admitted to hospital. Now we realise that they got better mainly because beds and cots in hospitals have rubber covers and frequently laundered cotton sheets. Both discourage house-dust mites.

Prolonged avoidance of possible allergens by keeping asthmatics for several weeks in a protected hospital environment with filtered air can produce spectacular improvement in symptoms and in excessive airway reactivity.[6] This is rather strong evidence that asthma is provoked, if not actually caused, by something arriving in the air.

Asthma and 'atopy' (Greek: strangeness) are often considered together, but should be considered separately. Between 15 and 50% of people in most parts of the world are atopic. This means that they react strongly and rapidly, with a large skin weal, to pinprick inoculation of many different allergens. Atopic children seem to be specially sensitive to air pollutants. Atopic people have an excess of a particular class of protein antibody in their blood, formerly called 'reagin' but now known as 'immunoglobulin E' (IgE). This reacts with many common allergy-inducing materials. Atopy is partly inherited and partly acquired. It is characterised by the presence of specific proteins ('receptors') which react with cytokines. The occurrence of atopy in an individual may be influenced by the time of birth, being apparently more common in children born in winter months – though this has yet to be confirmed. The difference may reflect the pattern of childhood infections. Some infections (e.g. those due to respiratory syncytial virus) make atopy more likely, but others (e.g. measles, hepatitis A and tuberculosis) make it less likely. Atopy has a definite association with asthma, increasing the risk of asthma about 10-fold, but lots of asthmatics are not atopic.

Do asthma treatments shed light on the cause?

The treatment of asthma is nowadays well established and perhaps sheds some light on its possible cause. Attacks are usually treated by inhaling a 'beta-2 stimulant', a drug related to adrenaline (see below). This switches on chemical receptors in the airways. These tell the muscles in the airways to relax, thus making the air passages larger. The 'beta receptors' also tell the cells lining the airways to stop producing mucus. All this makes it easier to get air in and out. Some people find that strenuous exercise starts off an asthma attack. This may be just because breathing is stepped up, but maybe a rush of cold air constricts the lung air passages. Many people find that inhaling a beta-2 stimulant before exercise prevents an attack. The opposite effect is produced by 'beta-blockers', drugs in common use for treating high blood pressure and angina. These tend to make the air passages in the lungs narrower. Such drugs are not given to asthmatics.

So is asthma caused by the body not having enough natural beta-2 stimulant on board? Probably not – though it is interesting that certain

21

inherited variants of the gene which carries the code for the beta-2 receptor (on chromosome 5q) affect the severity of disease in asthmatic populations. The body's natural beta-2 stimulant is 'adrenaline', which (for historical reasons of American patent rights in its name at the time) is known as 'epinephrine' in the USA. This chemical, a hormone (Greek: *hormao* = to arouse, set in motion) can be released into the bloodstream from the adrenal glands, lying above the kidneys at the back of the abdomen. Similar chemicals are released from specialised nerves supplying the airways. One of the reasons why an attack of asthma may get better without drugs is that the combination of panic and lack of oxygen releases adrenaline into the blood stream. But there is no evidence that lack of adrenaline, or abnormalities in the nerves to the airway muscles, or disorders of the controlling centres in the brain are important causes of asthma.

Immediate treatment of a severe asthma attack always involves giving a steroid drug, though the main use of steroids is prophylactic. Prevention of severe or frequent asthma attacks involves the subject regularly inhaling a fine spray of a glucocorticoid steroid drug (e.g. beclomethasone). Long-acting beta-2 stimulants (e.g. salmeterol) are also used to supplement steroids or to help unusual people who do not respond to steroids. Steroid-resistant asthmatic people can also be helped by 'non-steroidal anti-inflammatory drugs' (NSAIDs), e.g. drugs like indomethacin. This supports the general thesis that asthma is basically an inflammatory condition (see below). Prophylactic drugs, especially steroids, have certainly improved life for asthma sufferers.

So what do steroids do? In the airways they reduce 'inflammation'. This term describes the body's reactions to various insults such as bacterial infections, trauma or burns. The features of bacteria-produced inflammation can be seen on the skin as a boil is starting. There is redness, swelling and pain. Under the microscope specialised non-pigmented 'white' blood cells can be seen to leave the blood stream, accumulate in the inflamed area and destroy invading bacteria. When these cells die and clump together they form the material known as 'pus'. People lacking the appropriate white cells resist bacterial infections very badly. They do not make pus. Steroids are 'immuno-suppressive'. They prevent or diminish allergic inflammatory reactions to inhaled foreign substances.

The action of steroids on glucose metabolism (Greek: *metabole* = change), means that any substantial excess of steroids in the body can raise the blood sugar concentration and cause diabetes. Fortunately the small amounts of inhaled steroids needed to control asthma do not usually cause trouble. In general, all drugs that specifically damp down immune and allergic reactions are helpful to asthmatics. A useful prophylactic against asthma, especially in children, is the inhalation of an anti-allergic and antibody-suppressive drug such as cromoglycate. This also stabilises mast cells and may allow the dose of steroid drugs to be reduced.

Is there inflammation in the lungs in asthma? There always is. Asthmatic individuals don't get pain in the chest from their lung inflammation, because there are very few pain nerves within the lungs. Redness and swelling of the lungs can't be seen on the skin surface. But when sections of lung are examined under the microscope there is evidence of inflammation around the air passages. We now realise that asthmatics, even when not in an attack, have hypersensitive airways which react unduly strongly to irritants or allergens. Such external factors have in common the ability to activate or switch on a large number of genes concerned with inflammation.

The common pathway is an interesting one. Unstimulated cells such as those lining the airways have in their 'cytoplasm' (Greek: *cyt* = cell; *plasm* = something formed: that part of the cell outside the nucleus) a protein complex called nuclear-factor-kappa-B (NFκB). This is technically a 'transcription factor', which is normally held in an inactive form combined with an inhibitor protein (IκB).[7] Many forms of stress release NFκB from its inhibitor, thus allowing it to enter the cell nucleus. That is where the transcription takes place. NFκB binds to the controlling elements of DNA and promotes the synthesis of ribose nucleic acid ('messenger RNA') which is a transcribed copy of the genetic code provided by DNA. This single-stranded nucleic acid molecule then leaves the nucleus and reaches the ribosomes, which manufacture the chemokines involved in lung and airway inflammation. One important effect of steroid drugs – possibly the most important – is to suppress the release of NFκB.

Annexins

Steroids are not the only factors involved in inflammation, or in its suppression. Chemicals collectively known as 'annexins' are proteins which bind to calcium and phospholipids and have many diverse individual actions. Annexin-1 (formerly known as lipocortin 1) is a glucocorticoid-inducible protein which inhibits the synthesis of purines and DNA. By this means it reduces the proliferation of both B- and T-lymphocytes. It also controls the release of hormones from the anterior pituitary and adrenal glands and is an extremely potent anti-inflammatory agent. It inhibits the migration of specialised white cells from the bloodstream into an inflamed area. Transcription of genes is not necessary for the release of annexin-1 by glucocorticoids.

23

Infections and asthma

Is asthma triggered by some low-grade chest infection which releases NFκB and switches on production of damaging inflammation-producing cytokines? Over the years various candidates have been suggested. A widely distributed bacterium, *Chlamydia pneumoniae*, can live inside body cells. When human cells are grown in tissue culture outside the body and then infected with *C. pneumoniae* the infected cells produce a variety of active chemicals. These could be the main cause of lung inflammation in asthma.

Another possibility is that airway inflammation is set off by some non-infective agent polluting inhaled air.[8] There has been some interest in the particles contained in diesel smoke. Diesel engines now power 25% of road vehicles in the UK. Their use is encouraged on the basis of fuel efficiency, low cost and relatively innocuous gaseous emission. Diesel smoke has little immediate constricting effect on airways but it contains about 100 times more particles per unit volume than petrol engine exhaust gases and it undoubtedly has the capacity to produce lung inflammation.[9]

Many different types of specialised blood cells play a part in the inflammatory process in the lungs. These can be recognised under the microscope and have descriptive names such as eosinophils, mast cells, macrophages and T-lymphocytes.

Eosinophils and mast cells seem to cause damage by locally releasing cytokines. Why are normally circulating white blood cells such as eosinophils capable of causing lung damage and inflammatory reactions in asthma? The question has not yet been answered for sure, but a possible explanation for eosinophils is that their normal function is rather specifically to resist an invasion of the body by small creatures like worms. Worm infestation of the lungs brings forth into the blood tremendous quantities of eosinophils, which appear to have a normal defensive role. So perhaps eosinophils appear in some cases of asthma because the allergen or whatever is setting off lung inflammation has some similarity to the chemical substances produced by invading animal parasites.

Cells lining the airways are involved in lung inflammation. Most of these cells can release a mixture of cytokines and other chemicals which cause muscle constriction and mucus secretion. There have been several useful summaries of the complex interacting mechanisms.[10] In asthma some of the cells lining the airways are usually swollen. There is also thickening of muscle in the walls of the larger airways. We do not yet know all the ways in which inflammation narrows airways.

24

There may be active muscle constriction, but excessive secretion of mucus is often a more important cause of airway narrowing. There is also increased exudation of fluid directly from the bloodstream. Usually all the airways in an attack of asthma are narrowed by large amounts of thick sticky mucus. The normal $\frac{3}{4}$ inch (2 cm) internal diameter of the trachea may be reduced to little more than a pinhole. Many of the smaller airways become completely plugged with mucus. This is the image of asthma I have in my mind, from the two necropsies I have attended of people who had died in an asthmatic attack.

Asthma can cause death when not enough air is reaching the alveoli of the lungs. Gases can then no longer be exchanged with the blood. Carbon dioxide, the waste gas produced during the extraction of energy from food, dissolves readily in the fluid part of blood (the plasma). Any difficulty that the body might have in getting rid of carbon dioxide via the lungs can be overcome by the body allowing the concentration (more accurately, the 'partial pressure') of carbon dioxide to increase. This increases the average gradient for outward diffusion. People can still stay alive with twice the normal carbon dioxide concentration in their blood, though they get a bit drowsy. But a bigger problem with reduced ventilation of the lungs is lack of oxygen. In an attack of asthma many parts of the lungs are blocked off though blood still passes through them. In the alveoli there is a mis-match between ventilation (the movement of air in and out) and perfusion (the passage of blood around the air sacs). It may not be possible to get enough oxygen into the blood to keep the body going. People in a really bad asthma attack need to be artificially ventilated and have the mucus in their airways sucked out to survive.

When people die from asthma the lungs are expanded. Air is sucked in with each deep breath, but can't be breathed out fully because the airways are blocked. It is as if the mucus-filled airways act as one-way valves. Failure of lung ventilation may be aggravated by infection (bronchopneumonia) or sometimes even by lung rupture, when air leaks into the space between the lungs and the chest wall – the condition called 'pneumothorax'. I find it difficult to believe that excessive muscular contraction of the airways can by itself ever cause death, without additional mucus blockage, though some people claim that this is possible. I would expect that such a manifestly disadvantageous situation would have been eliminated by natural selection. If severe mucus blockage is not present in an apparently asthmatic death, it is more likely that there has been a catastrophic heart rhythm disorder rather than obstruction to ventilation.

Leukotriene-receptor antagonists

Steroids remain the basic remedies for control and stabilisation of asthma, but other drugs may be useful. The leukotriene receptor antagonists, e.g. montelukast and zafirlukast, help to reduce inflammation in asthma by interfering with the ill effects of 'leukotrienes'.[11] These comprise one of the many groups of chemicals released from inflammatory cells. They play an important role in airway constriction. Leukotrienes increase the production of sticky mucus and reduce the activity of the cilia. However, although leukotriene antagonists have been promoted as being as good as steroid drugs in controlling asthma attacks, trials of antagonists have so far failed to show a very significant reduction of risk compared with the use of steroid drugs, though they may be useful in steroid-resistant patients or as an adjunct to steroid use.

Hyperventilation in asthma

Although in a bad asthma attack lung ventilation becomes severely obstructed, this does not apply in the early stages of an attack. The amount of air going in and out of the lungs each minute (total ventilation) is often actually increased, as is the ventilation of the alveoli. This seems paradoxical, but it can happen because lung inflammation itself and low oxygen both send signals to the brain to increase the rate and depth of breathing. It has even been suggested that overbreathing (hyperventilation) is actually the cause of asthma. This is not correct. Many people habitually overbreathe, usually from anxiety, without getting the pathological changes in the lungs which characterise asthma. But hyperventilation is none the less important. Asthmatics may improve a lot if they are trained to hold their breath and to adopt a slow deliberate breathing pattern. The improvement probably arises because slow breathing gives time for incoming air to warm up. This then reduces the constricting stimulus from cold air. An initial intensive course of steroids to reduce the over-inflation of the lungs will often lead to reduction in hyperventilation and an improvement in symptoms which outlasts the intensive course of steroids. It is always worth making at least one attempt in any severe asthmatic to get rid of every trace of airway narrowing.

Possible environmental factors in the increasing incidence of asthma

Is asthma an allergic reaction to some inhaled material? Or is the stage set by the lungs being chronically inflamed or irritated by some constituent of the air we breathe? The answer is probably 'yes' to both questions. I have mentioned pollens and the faeces of house-dust mites as potential allergens. British farmers are growing increasing amounts of oil seed rape. Could its pollen be a culprit? A large number of different factors and mediators are undoubtedly involved in causing lung inflammation. These include normal body constituents or products: e.g. cytokines, enzymes, transcription factors, prostaglandins, adhesion molecules, endothelins and nitric oxide. I shall not discuss these any further, even though much therapeutic effort is currently directed towards modifying one or more of these systems. This may eventually provide better control of asthma attacks, but it won't solve the main problem of the increasing incidence of asthma. It is unlikely that people are fundamentally changing. There must be external factors involved.

Some individuals are allergic to certain foods or chemicals which may trigger off an attack of asthma, e.g. peanuts and aspirin. Other environmental contacts, e.g. cats, may also provide allergens. Asthma is getting more common even though the environment in many respects is getting cleaner. Although car exhaust fumes are increasing as the number of cars goes up, no damaging material has yet been clearly identified in car exhaust emissions, though diesel exhaust fumes are definitely not good for you. Dust particles, crop sprays, refrigeration chemicals and a vast number of other air contaminants are under suspicion. It would be wonderful if we could find the main culprit, if there is a single main one. Then we would have some idea of how to stop asthma getting progressively worse, as it is becoming at present in most developed countries. A huge collaborative epidemiological investigation is under way: the International Study of Asthma and Allergies in Childhood (ISAAC). Self-administered questionnaire data have been collected on children aged 13–14 in 155 centres in 56 countries.[12]

Do animals get asthma? Not often; but domestic cats can get spontaneous asthma attacks. Asthma can be precipitated in cats by exposing them to allergens. This can make their airways narrower, secrete excess amounts of sticky mucus, and produce a great increase in white (eosinophil) blood cells. Similar reactions to allergens have been produced in human volunteers. But so far no single allergen has been firmly identified as the main culprit for human asthma, though pollens and house-dust mites certainly make a contribution. Perhaps there is something in the construction or equipment of modern houses which can trigger asthma in humans and sometimes in cats. Is it that we keep the temperature of modern houses much higher than we used to do, so that some unusual bacterium or virus can flourish? Severe virus infections of the lungs have been observed to predispose to the later development of asthma. Some airborne infections were not identified for many years, e.g. so-called 'legionnaires' disease', which is caused by a bacterium that can grow and multiply in the hot water tanks of large hotels and establishments. (Incidentally, this is why all big hotels now keep their hot water supplies extremely hot, to kill these bacteria.)

Is asthma anything to do with television sets? Television tubes need very high positive voltages (10–20 kv) to attract negatively charged electrons to the screen. There is likely to be a cloud of positively charged particles (ions) around the very high voltage transformer, capacitor and screen. Such components electrostatically attract dust, as anyone who has looked at these components inside an old television set knows. Is it possible that clouds of ions around television sets could conceivably accrete and electrically charge dust particles which might then act as lung irritants?

There is a tantalisingly large number of other possibilities. It is unlikely that the current increase in asthma incidence can be accounted for by better diagnosis or reporting. Perhaps the reduction of childhood infections, because of better living conditions and increased antibiotic use, increases all allergic responses.[13] This has been suggested as one of the causes for increased asthma incidence. A similar situation has been recognised in other diseases. There is a fascinating animal example. Mice of the inbred strain known as 'NOD' spontaneously develop diabetes, probably because of auto-immune destruction[14] of the insulin-secreting cells of their pancreas; but the disease can be completely prevented by deliberately infecting young animals with a gut parasite. Many other agents or organisms have a similarly protective effect. So it is a plausible hypothesis that asthma may actually be made worse or even precipitated by preventing certain childhood infections.

This line of reasoning does not explain why domestic cats get asthma. A provocative report came from Ethiopia a few years ago. In that country asthma is almost unknown in the country districts, but is common in the towns. The particular interest of this report is that diet is hardly different in the two places. There are very few motor vehicles in either place. Atopy in Ethiopia appears to be protective rather than damaging. The authors suggested that the increase in asthma was 'consistent with an effect of new environmental exposures' in towns.[15] A further report from the same group has confirmed this, pointing a finger at urban kerosene, and tobacco use.[16]

Whatever the mysterious environmental factor causing the current nearly-worldwide increase in asthma may be, it probably arrives in the air. Some factor (or factors) peculiar to living in towns seems to be its immediate provocative cause. Apart from my previous suggestion of electrically charged dust particles from television sets, I also considered, in the last chapter, whether fine particles of polyvinyl chloride (PVC) rubbed off coated surfaces might trigger airway inflammation and hence predispose to asthma. The problem with investigating this or any other possible damaging material lies in determining whether long-lasting exposure over months or years can set up inflammatory processes in the lungs. In the first instance, long-range animal studies are needed. It will then be necessary to study matched human population pairs, if enough can be found in which there is a difference in long-continued exposure to some environmental factor such as PVC, or to one of its plasticisers. This is easier said than done. But so are all really challenging and important problems.

Summary

'Asthma' describes attacks of difficult breathing due to reversible narrowing of lung airways caused by muscle constriction, swelling of lining cells and secretion of sticky mucus. Force is needed to expel air from the lungs, which become expanded. Gas exchange is impaired. In severe cases lack of oxygen can be fatal.

The disease arises on a background of excessive reaction of lung airways to a variety of external allergic or inflammation-producing agents. Although the immediate precipitating factors are often not known, the final common pathway may involve the release of so-called transcription factors which produce and release inflammation-producing chemicals.

Asthma tends to run in families, but many genes are involved and no simple pattern of inheritance can be found. External factors are probably more important than heredity. The condition is getting commoner, especially in towns, but traffic fumes are probably not its main cause, which has not been identified. Diesel smoke may have slowly-developing injurious effects. My own guesses are that charged dust particles around television sets, or minute amounts of polyvinyl chloride (PVC) (in increasing use in innumerable domestic contexts) might be responsible agents; but hundreds of other possible contenders are under suspicion.

3

MULTIPLE SCLEROSIS

In many parts of the world multiple sclerosis (MS) is the commonest serious disease of the brain and nervous system. The proportion of the population newly diagnosed with the disease each year (the incidence) is extraordinarily variable. In one part of the world it is very rare, e.g. only one new case per year for every million people in the population. In other places it is much commoner, e.g. 30 cases per year per million population. The proportion of the whole population suffering from the disease at any particular time (the prevalence) is also variable. At the present time about 80,000 people in the UK have the disease. In the USA the estimate is about 300,000.

MS characteristically gives rise to episodic and often sudden appearances of neurological symptoms and signs. Some of these get better after a few days. Others leave permanent nerve defects. Increasing disability often results over the next 30 or 40 years, though the speed of deterioration is extremely variable. Women are two to three times more often affected than men.

Many different neurological functions may be damaged. The commonest damaged parts (lesions) are in the motor neurone pathways which control the leg muscles. The word 'neurone'[1] is used to refer both to the body of a nerve cell and to all the nerve fibres which branch from it. 'Motor' means that the neurone controls muscle movements. 'Upper' motor neurones in the outer layers of the brain (the cortex) are linked through nerve fibres with the brain stem and spinal cord (Fig. 3). A second set of large nerve cells (the 'lower' motor neurones) gives rise to nerve fibres which directly supply muscles. The junctions (synapses) between the two sets of nerves allow other neurones to influence the pathways. For example, this makes it possible for someone's conscious intention to make a muscle move – by sending nerve impulses down the motor nerves – to be coordinated by the unconscious automatic harmonised relaxation of opposing muscles and by the contraction of other muscles needed to stabilise joints.

In MS the disease mainly damages upper motor neurones in the brain and spinal cord. Lesions seem to be randomly distributed in

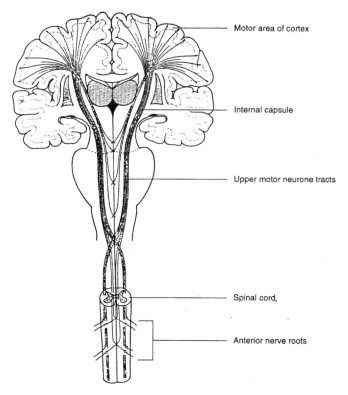

Motor area of cortex

Internal capsule

Upper motor neurone tracts

Spinal cord,

Anterior nerve roots

Figure 3 Diagram of the main nerve tracts in the brain and spinal cord which convey electrical impulses to muscles. Multiple sclerosis mainly affects the upper motor neurone tracts. The nerve fibres come from cell bodies in the motor area of the brain cortex and pass down to the brain stem and spinal cord, where they make connection with the lower motor neurones which supply muscles through the anterior nerve roots.

nerve tracts, especially in those running close to the central fluid-filled brain cavities (the ventricles). Individual lesions are usually only the size of a pinhead, but can be larger. Nerve tracts controlling the leg muscles are usually interrupted first, probably because they run longer paths. This leads to a stiff (spastic) weakness of the legs which is the commonest first symptom of the disease. Coordination of muscle movement is impaired, often with shaking, because of involvement of the cerebellum (part of the brain responsible for coordination and balance). Sometimes an episode of double vision lasting a few weeks is the first symptom of the disease. This may precede other symptoms by many years. Weakness and stiffness of muscles rather than pain is the cardinal symptom of established MS, but pain may follow from

32

prolonged immobility, bad posture and difficulties in walking. Pain in the face (trigeminal neuralgia) is an occasional symptom.

Different types of MS have been recognised. The commonest, accounting for about 80% of cases, occurs in young adults. It is described as 'relapsing remitting'. The affected individual runs a stable course between relapses. This form of the disease in about half the cases passes into the 'secondary progressive' form, in which gradual neurological deterioration occurs without sudden relapses. In later life, from the ages of about 40 to 60, the 'primary progressive' form comprises about 10% of all cases. In this there is a gradual neurological deterioration without any well-marked sudden relapses. Some patients with this form of disease suffer later episodic relapses, in which case the condition is described as 'progressive relapsing'. It is not clear whether these apparently different manifestations are really different. It may just be a matter of the size of new lesions and the frequency with which they appear.

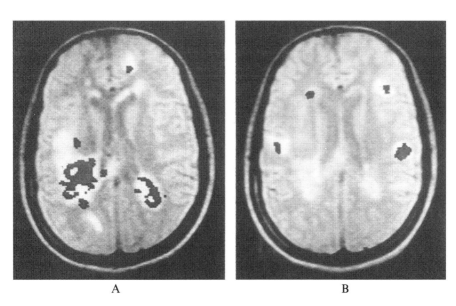

A   B

Figure 4 Successive brain MRI scans in a woman of 26 with relapsing/remitting multiple sclerosis which was beginning to enter the secondary progressive phase. The scan on the right (B) was made 3 months after that on the left (A). The dark blobs (with white surround) on both scans show the sites of inflammatory lesions disrupting the blood/brain barrier (identified by a technique involving the injection of a gadolinium compound). Note that all evidence of acute inflammatory foci in the earlier scan (A) has disappeared in scan (B), but 4 new small inflammatory lesions have appeared. (Adapted from an original illustration, from McDonald WI and Barnes D, Trends in Neuroscience 1989; 12: 376–379, by permission of Elsevier Science Inc.).

Sequential studies of the living brain by magnetic resonance imaging (MRI)[2] show new MS lesions regularly appearing and disappearing, though at greatly different rates (Figs. 4A & 4B). Those lesions which do not disappear presumably account for persisting neurological defects, although it has proved surprisingly difficult to correlate new MRI-visible lesions with new neurological symptoms. One reason is that the brain opens up new nerve pathways to bypass damaged neurones. This accounts for the (usually) near-complete recovery of sight in an eye affected by 'retrobulbar neuritis' – a common occurrence in MS. In normal people the main nerve tracts pass from the retina of the eye to an area at the back of the brain, the occipital cortex. After recovery from retrobulbar neuritis due to MS, dynamic brain imaging reveals that many new and changed connections have been established between the retina and other parts of the brain. So even though visual acuity may return to normal after an attack of retrobulbar neuritis, reflex paths involving muscle movement may be longer than normal and fixation of objects by the eyes may consequently be unduly sluggish. Patients often find reading difficult because coordination of eye movement is not as rapid and accurate as it was before the attack.

The primary progressive variety of multiple sclerosis is probably the form taken when each successive lesion is so small that the functional defect is difficult for either patient or doctor to recognise when it occurs. Under the microscope, all MS lesions in brain or spinal cord have in common 'demyelination' of the larger nerve fibres. In brain and spinal cord these nerve fibres ('axons') are sheathed by an electrical-insulating layer containing fat and protein – 'myelin'. This allows faster transmission of nerve impulses and insulates each nerve fibre from other adjacent fibres. In MS, in areas which may be only a millimetre or two across, the larger nerve fibres lose their normal myelin sheaths. Individual lesions of MS seem to arise close to blood vessels, in which there are signs of inflammation and accumulation of white blood cells. Loss of myelin sheaths slows down and impairs nerve impulse transmission. There may also be actual axon breaks, which make impulse transmission impossible. Figure 4 shows two successive MRI scans of the brain in the same patient on two different occasions, three months apart. They illustrate the dynamic nature of multiple sclerosis, with discrete lesions coming and going.

Epidemiology

Multiple sclerosis is commoner in cold northern climates than in hot countries. It is commoner in cool southern parts in the southern hemisphere than in the warm northern parts (e.g. of Australia). This is not a universally applicable rule: for example, it does not apply within Japan. In Europe the distribution of cases does not bear any clear relation to geographical latitude, but the enormous differences in incidence in different places in the world point towards important environmental influences. Ultraviolet light appears to suppress immune reactions. It has been suggested that sunlight may protect against MS because of this, and account for some of the geographical differences in incidence of the disease.

There are some well recognised influences on relapse rate in people already diagnosed with MS. In the period from two weeks before until five weeks after the onset of one of the common virus infections of childhood (such as measles, mumps and chicken pox) the relapse rate of MS increases nearly three-fold. Although pregnancy does not alter the natural history of the disease, relapse frequency is much reduced during the last three months of pregnancy, but much increased in the three months after delivery.

The other main influences on relapses of MS are other specific virus infections. These appear to activate the body's immune defence system. Specific changes take place in anti-inflammatory white blood cells (specialised T-lymphocytes: see below) towards the end of pregnancy, and reverse after delivery. Sudden deterioration, usually coinciding with the appearance of a new MRI-identifiable lesion in the brain, can usually be reversed or cut short by giving large doses of steroids (immunosuppressive glucocorticoid drugs such as prednisone and methylprednisone).

Genetics

The lifetime risk of developing multiple sclerosis is about 0.2% for members of the general population in developed countries. There is undoubtedly a genetic element in MS, though an unidentified environmental factor in the home could account for some apparently inherited cases within families. Relatives of patients with MS have a 10- to 50-fold higher risk of developing the disease than do people without affected relatives. The risk of a brother or sister of an MS patient developing MS is several times increased if the affected individual got the disease early in life. The absolute risk to a first-degree relative (brother, sister, son or daughter of someone with MS) is only between 2% and 6%. The concordance rate of the disease between twins (the percentage of cases in which a twin is affected when its sibling has the disease) is about 30% for identical 'monozygotic' twins, but only 2%

for non-identical 'dizygotic' twins. Clearly this points to some genetic influence, but an external environmental factor (or factors) is much more important than heredity in causing MS.

Cause

Studies of people migrating to different parts of the world at different periods of their lives suggest that whatever the environmental factor may be, it is acquired before puberty.[3] Adolescence seems to be a critical time for later developing MS. The different rates of attack in different geographical areas may give us clues about the possible cause of the disease. A virus[4] infection seems much the most probable environmental trigger. But no one has yet clearly identified either viruses or portions of viruses in those parts of the nervous system damaged by the disease.

Many viruses selectively attack specific parts of the brain and spinal cord. 'Polio' is a good example. The poliomyelitis virus has been firmly established as the cause of that disease (formerly called infantile paralysis). The virus almost exclusively attacks the lower motor nerves which supply muscles, but it usually leaves other parts of the nervous system alone. The damaged parts of the brain can be identified under the microscope. Virtually complete protection can be provided by immunisation with a preparation derived from inactivated virus.

Although there have been reports of clusters of cases of MS in some restricted locations, e.g. in the Hebrides, it is exceedingly difficult to establish whether these are outside the bounds of statistical chance. In defined regions in which the disease has been well studied, the annual incidence of newly diagnosed cases is very variable over time. This is characteristic of most epidemics of infectious disease. There has been some evidence suggesting that bird viruses might be involved.[5]

A promising lead suggests that a retrovirus[6] is strongly associated with MS and is only rarely found in normal individuals.[7] It has also been suggested that infection with the Epstein-Barr (E-B) virus (technically a ubiquitous 'B-lymphotropic' herpes virus which causes glandular fever when acquired in adult life) may pave the way for a retrovirus infection which triggers MS in susceptible individuals. People with very high levels of antibodies against the E-B virus have been observed to have an increased risk of later developing MS. Furthermore, there is astonishing molecular structural similarity between a peptide of the E-B virus and that of a basic protein peptide from myelin, despite their dissimilarity in respect of protein sequences.

Another virus which can attack the nervous system is Japanese

36

encephalitis virus (JEV), which can be acquired from pigs and spread by mosquitoes. In parts of south-east Asia many children are infected, with little morbidity, but infection acquired later in life can give rise to nerve damage resembling poliomyelitis. This scenario resembles infection with the E-B virus: i.e. childhood infection is often harmless but infection acquired as an adult may be potentially damaging.

Progressive multifocal encephalopathy (PML) is an interesting virus infection which produces ill effects more or less exclusively in so-called immunocompromised patients whose immune defences are seriously impaired. This commonly happens with 'Human Immunodeficiency Virus' (HIV) infection, which causes 'acquired immune deficiency syndrome' (commonly abbreviated to 'AIDS'). PML is almost unknown in normal individuals, but has occurred in as many as 5% of AIDS patients, whose specialised protective T-lymphocytes[8] in the blood are severely reduced in numbers. PML is due to infection with a usually harmless papova virus, known as the 'JC' virus (so named from the first patient in whom it was recognised). Since antibodies to JC virus can be detected in more than 70% of normal adults, infection is obviously harmless to most people. The situation is similar to that with E-B virus, mentioned above. Since PML can produce clinical symptoms and brain image changes looking very much like multiple sclerosis on X-rays and MRI scans, investigators into the cause of MS remain interested in the JC virus.

But no virus has yet been convincingly identified or confirmed in the brain cells of MS patients, or incriminated as the immediate cause of the disease. Though the evidence is not strong enough to point the finger at any specific virus at present, a virus trigger still seems the most likely primary cause of MS.

Immunological aspects

There are many reasons to suppose that the body's immune defence system is in some way involved in causing or perpetuating the disease. Conditions closely similar to MS can be produced in animals by repeated exposure to certain provocative agents, including components of myelin, the material which ensheaths large nerve fibres. The suggestion has often been made that there is a vicious circle in MS: destruction of myelin might lead to exposure of the body's immune system to myelin components which might then act as antigens.[9] These might then produce further immune reactions directed towards myelin, whose destruction might then complete a vicious circle. It seems possible that a vicious circle of this sort could be started by a virus infection and later be kept going by the body's own immunological defence system, without the original virus necessarily being involved.

But if so why should the disease affect different parts of the nervous system at different times?

Another clue suggesting that immune reactions are involved in causing MS is the recent report that the 'statin' drugs (used to lower cholesterol and protect against arterial disease) may have some mild immuno-suppressive effects and reduce symptoms in MS. Another recently introduced drug which suppresses inflammation (mitoxantrone) may also be able to reduce the rate of progression of the disease and reduce the severity of relapses. Most trials in multiple sclerosis suggest that beta-interferons also reduce the rate and severity of relapses. The anti-inflammatory agents interferon beta-1b, interferon beta-1a and glatiramer acetate may also favourably modify the course of the disease, though many questions remain.

Cells carrying the strongly anti-inflammatory material annexin-1 have been identified in high concentration at the site of nerve lesions in MS, suggesting that the body's defences have been mobilised against the inflammatory effect of some harmful material.

Following on from previous work in mice, Romagnani and colleagues recognised two main categories of T-lymphocytes concerned with immune reactions in man. These so-called 'helper' cells have been roughly categorised as those promoting inflammation (Th1) and those inhibiting it (Th2).[10] Th1 cells secrete inflammation-producing 'cytokines' such as tumour-necrosis factor alpha (TNFα), interleukin-2 (IL-2) and gamma-interferon. Th2 cells secrete many anti-inflammatory cytokines such as IL-4 and IL-13. But it would be naive to regard Th1 cells as damaging and Th2 as protective. The actions of these two types of T-cells complement each other in most immune defence reactions. Th2 cells seem to be the main agents involved in various organ-specific immune diseases such as Crohn's disease. They also accelerate the progression of 'human immunodeficiency virus' (HIV) infection into full-blown 'acquired-immune deficiency syndrome' (AIDS).

Lymphocytes circulating in the blood get into the nervous system by sticking to the 'endothelium' of small brain blood vessels in regions of inflammation, using chemicals known as 'integrins'. Chemicals known collectively as 'selective adhesion molecule inhibitors' have recently been reported to reduce the rate and severity of relapses in MS (e.g. an antibody against the a_4 integrin – natalizumab.[11]

Demyelination and axon breaks

Hitherto a lot of research has concentrated on looking for the cause of demyelination of nerve fibres in MS. People have tried to control the disease by supplying extra dietary amounts of some of the chemical constituents of myelin. The oil of the evening primrose is a popular though unproven remedy. Unfortunately, careful microscopic examination of axons (the central thread-like structures conducting nerve impulses) in MS lesions has revealed that there are actual breaks in many axons, with egg-shaped swellings at the breaks. Such observations were made more than a century ago by the French neurologist Jean Charcot. They have been recently intensively studied[12] and rather convincingly explain why permanent nerve damage can follow a sudden worsening of neurological symptoms. The possibility has also to be considered that loss of myelin sheaths could come first and make axons unduly fragile.

Therapeutic efforts need to be directed towards prevention rather than cure because reversal of the established lesions of MS seems hopelessly optimistic. Some protection against attacks of brain inflammation (easily identified by MRI of the brain) has been achieved by the selective removal of specialised T-lymphocytes by injecting an appropriate antibody. The idea is that such lymphocytes are immunologically active cells which are destroying myelin. The long-term merit of this treatment is uncertain, especially as it may cause auto-immune disease of the thyroid gland.

Summary

Multiple sclerosis is a common disabling neurological disease. It may start in early adult life, with an episode of double vision or difficulty in walking. Progression is usually by brief attacks in which symptoms increase and disabilities develop. Some attacks clear up completely, but others result in permanent loss of function.

The condition is probably initiated by infection with a virus in late childhood or in early adult life. This might be with an (as yet) unknown retrovirus. It is commoner in colder parts of the world than hotter. This might mean that transmission of the virus from person to person is commoner where people live closely together in poorly ventilated rooms with the windows shut, and is rarer in hotter places where there is less overcrowding and windows stay open. Such ideas suggest that infection may be acquired by breathing in the exhalations of infected people. The initial infection may lead to a state in which neurological damage progresses because of damaging auto-immune mechanisms.

Other routes of infection are possible. I do not know the figures, but would suspect that infestation of houses by rodents is commoner in temperate than in hotter climates, so that chance contact of humans with rodents is greater. Rats, particularly, are known to carry many diseases which infect man. There is no convincing epidemiological evidence incriminating domestic animals of any sort in triggering MS. Perhaps we need some 'lateral thinking' to identify other possible routes for a virus infection. For example, hepatitis A (p. 252) is an infection of the liver usually acquired through eating or drinking material contaminated with the virus.

Complete solution of the mystery of multiple sclerosis will not necessarily lead to an immediate cure or substantial prevention. AIDS is an example of a virus infection where understanding of the cause of the disease has come long before a cure has been found. But seeing the rapid progress now being made in slowing down or arresting progression of HIV infection – the cause of AIDS – I am hopeful that once the causative agent or agents of MS has been identified, control or suppression of the disease will soon follow. I expect that this will come about within the next decade.

4

SLEEP AND SLEEP DISORDERS

Physiological changes during sleep

Sleep is not a uniform state. Everyone recognises that sleep can be 'deep' or 'light', or 'disturbed' by frequent episodic wakings. A more subtle analysis of sleep was made some 50 years ago by Nathaniel Kleitman. He had been recording fluttering eye movements in somnolent animals and recognised similar eye movements in man, sometimes accompanied by twitching of hands and feet. When human subjects were woken up while their eyelids were fluttering they reported: (1) that they had definitely been asleep, and (2) that they had been dreaming and could often recall their dreams. It is now generally accepted that paradoxical or 'rapid eye movement' (REM) sleep (as Kleitman named it and as it is now usually known) is strongly associated with dreaming. Many mammals, including dogs and cats, have comparable episodes of rapid eye movements when apparently asleep. It seems likely that such animals have been dreaming. Birds also have episodes of apparent REM sleep.

When rapid eye movements are correlated with electrical activity from nerve cells in the brain, recorded through the intact skull by electrodes on the skin – the technique known as 'electroencephalography' (EEG) – REM sleep is regularly observed to be accompanied by a specific pattern of brain waves. These can identify REM sleep episodes without the need to record eye movements. The EEG record in quiet wakefulness comprises low amplitude waves and a characteristic ('alpha') rhythm. Ordinary sleep not accompanied by rapid eye movements is usually classified as quiet or 'non-rapid eye movement' (NREM) sleep. The EEG in NREM sleep has been described as 'slow, synchronised idling activity'. Four different patterns of EEG activity have been recognised. Stage I is the lightest and stage IV the heaviest. Stages III and IV are often lumped together.

Human adults vary a lot, but after going to bed usually begin with a period of NREM sleep. Later on average about one quarter or one fifth of their sleeping time is spent in two to six short episodes of REM sleep, interposed with a similar number of longer episodes of

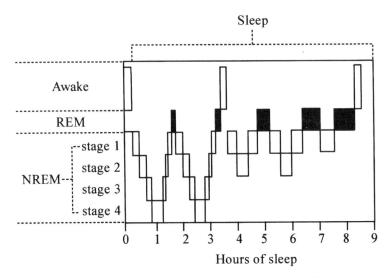

Figure 5 Diagram of a typical sleep pattern of a young adult. The time scale at the bottom of the graph covers 9 hours of the night, running from left to right. The 5 stages of normal sleep, described in the text, merge into each other. Each stage is recognised by characteristic patterns of electrical brain activity.

NREM sleep. Infants spend much of their sleeping time (more than half) in REM sleep, the episodes often lasting 50–60 minutes. As they grow up their periods of REM sleep become shorter and less frequent.[1] They dream less. Figure 5 shows a typical record of the sleep patterns of a young adult.

Once NREM sleep is established, slow coordinated waves appear in the EEG record. Blood pressure usually falls to a stable low level. The same applies to heart rate. The total blood flow to the brain falls as the depth of sleep increases. Breathing gets slower and the body temperature falls slightly. Thereafter the EEG pattern changes progressively to the lighter stages of sleep until the next night, in which the same sequence of events occurs:

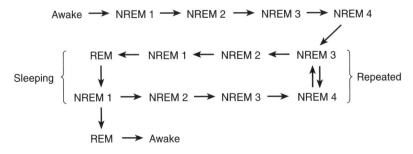

42

The cycle typically repeats two or three times at about 90–100 minute intervals. NREM predominates in the early hours of sleep, whereas episodes of REM sleep typically occur more often in the early morning hours. Figure 5 shows the typical successive sleep stages which might be seen in a young man. Sleep is deepest at first. Later, episodes of REM sleep become longer.

REM sleep has been described as one of the great biological mysteries of the last century. It is accompanied by several interesting physiological changes. The most striking is relaxation of stiffness (tone) in most of the body muscles. All the limbs become floppy (atonic). Spinal reflexes such as the 'knee jerk' cannot be obtained. Blood flow to most muscles is reduced. The brain, especially its outer layers (cortex), is active during REM sleep with nerve messages passing to and fro. Most investigators, though finding that brain blood flow is greater in REM than in NREM sleep, report that it is about the same as in quiet wakefulness.[2] There is general agreement that: (1) the total blood flow and oxygen consumption of the brain both fall as the depth of sleep increases, and (2) both rise again, either to normal waking values or slightly above them, during REM sleep.

The brain structures involved in sleep initiation and in the bodily

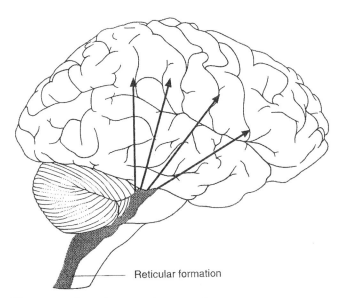

Reticular formation

Figure 6 Diagram to show the general course of nerve tracts comprising the reticular activating system, arising at the sides of the brain stem, extending over a considerable part of its length, and spreading forwards and upwards to make contact with the cerebral cortex.

changes which accompany sleep depend on the brain stem, as Bremer worked out many years ago by his observations in cats. All the changes known to occur in sleep can still take place in animals lacking a cerebral cortex. During wakefulness, the reticular formation of the brain stem (Fig. 6) is continually sending activating ('keep awake') nerve messages to the cerebral cortex.[3] If these messages are interfered with by damage to the nerve tracts concerned, the electrical activity of the cortex diminishes, its blood flow decreases and the cortex in effect goes off to sleep. Selective damage to various parts of the nerve circuits can induce the whole gamut of sleep stages and the electroencephalographic changes which normally accompany them. Electrical stimulation of the reticular formation in the brain stem reverses these changes. I shall summarise in Chapter 38 my hypothesis that chronic fatigue syndrome (so-called 'ME') could be due to previous damage, perhaps from a virus infection, to the reticular formation of the brain stem or to some of its nerve connections – thus causing sleepiness, decreased energy and weakness of muscles.[4] More severe damage to the brain stem, e.g. from trauma or a large tumour, can cause coma and persistent slow waves in the electroencephalographic record. Sleep disturbances are almost invariable after a severe stroke.[5]

Vegetative changes during sleep

After a spell of what can be called 'quiet wakefulness' someone goes off to sleep. Consciousness is suspended. Body temperature normally goes down one degree centigrade (from about 37.2 to 36.1 degrees C on average). Heart rate, blood pressure and metabolic rate (judged by the rate of oxygen consumption) all descend to base-line values during the first hour of sleep. The rate of nerve impulses coming from the brain and travelling out in sympathetic nerves (p. 481) decreases during sleep. The activity of parasympathetic nerves increases. Both these effects reduce both blood pressure and heart rate. The effects reverse shortly before a subject wakes. Blood pressure rises slightly and may fluctuate during episodes of REM sleep. Heart rate follows the same general pattern.

There is recent evidence that the chemical adenosine, involved in energy storage through its phosphate derivative ATP (p. 464), is a sleep promoter. Growth hormone released from the pituitary gland is closely associated with the initiation of sleep. Many substances have been identified in the cerebrospinal fluid surrounding the brain of sleep-deprived dogs and goats which, when injected into another animal, induce sleep. Human sleep is probably initiated and regulated by the integrated action of many chemicals which act on

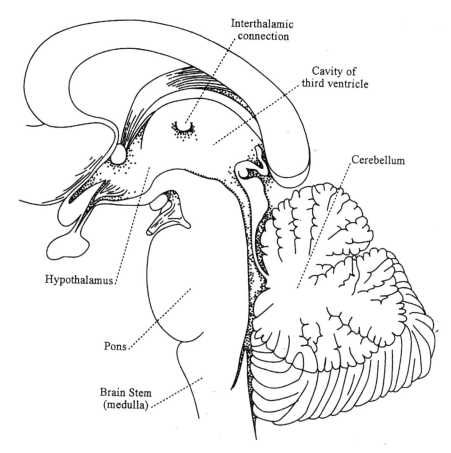

Interthalamic connection

Cavity of third ventricle

Cerebellum

Hypothalamus

Pons

Brain Stem (medulla)

Figure 7 Diagram of the mid-brain, brain stem and cerebellum showing their relative positions in a vertical (sagittal) section through the cavity of the third ventricle. The groups of nerve nuclei which comprise the hypothalamus occupy the floor of the 3rd ventricle. The hypothalamus has chemical connections with the pituitary gland lying below it and nerve connections to higher and lower brain centres.

the sleep-generating nerve cells in the brain stem and hypothalamus (Fig. 7).[6]

During sleep the well-known cardiovascular reflexes remain in action. If blood pressure is gently but artificially raised or lowered during sleep (e.g. by intravenous infusion of drugs) appropriate reflex changes in heart rate ensue. This is the so-called 'baroreflex'. It is brought about by interconnecting nerve centres in the brain stem which get information about blood pressure changes from the arterial baroreceptors (described in Chapter 31). Spontaneous and induced

45

baroreflex changes may be greater during sleep than when subjects are awake.

Physiological mechanisms and structures which cause or influence sleep

Many body organs and tissues – not just the brain – contain intrinsic free-running chemical oscillators which have an approximately 24-hour rhythm. 'Free running' means that the intermittent rhythmic production of chemicals by the structure under consideration does not depend on external stimulation of any sort. Chemical oscillation can continue indefinitely as long as the tissue has access to basic materials and an energy supply.

The rhythm is described as 'circadian' (Latin: *circa* = around; *die* = day). These other potential oscillators are normally subservient to a master rhythm controller which is located in the brain about an inch behind the eyes, just above the 'chiasma' (Greek: crossing) where the optic nerves from the two eyes cross. This master rhythm controller is a small paired structure, the size of a pinhead. It comprises a group of only about 20,000 nerve cells, known as the 'suprachiasmatic nucleus' (SCN) of the hypothalamus (Fig. 7). If this tiny structure is removed from a mammal's brain and put into a test tube containing appropriately nutritious fluid it will continue to secrete chemicals in an approximately circadian oscillating fashion. The retina of the eye also contains a similar chemical clock, located in its deeper layers. This also repeatedly secretes active chemicals into the blood flowing through it, again with a circadian rhythm. Electrical impulses from the SCN and adjacent forebrain structures pass to lower structures in the brain stem which control body temperature, blood pressure, heart rate and lung ventilation. Although most of these observations have been made in mice, most mammals possess similar structures which probably have similar functions.

In human beings synchronisation of the SCN to the normal day/night, light/dark cycle – the phenomenon described as 'entrainment' – is possible because the SCN is supplied by nerves which connect it to the retina of the eye. But people who have lost their sight still retain most of the same normal circadian oscillatory production of chemicals by their brains as do sighted people. Presumably they get their day/night clues from sounds, temperature, touch and smell.

The SCN is connected to the pineal gland, another small structure in the mid-brain. Early in the course of evolution – many million years ago – the pineal gland contained cells which were light-sensitive. Now its main function seems to be to secrete a chemical called melatonin,

46

mainly at night. The human pineal gland usually contains between 50 and 100 mg of melatonin. Ingestion of synthetic melatonin promotes sleep. There is much interest in its use to correct sleep disturbances caused by long-distance flights and rapid transition of time zones. In birds, removal of the pineal gland destroys the sleep/wake cycle. Transplantation of the pineal gland restores the cycle.

Curiously, in human beings the sleep-promoting effects of melatonin are most effective when it is given during daylight hours rather than at night-time. Although it has been tried as a sleep-promoting drug the normal function of melatonin is not entirely clear. It has many actions, not only on the brain. It can act as an anti-oxidant in defensive white blood cells, limiting the potentially damaging effects of oxygen. It may have a part to play in resistance to infections and to other harmful external agents. Unfortunately, synthetic melatonin has been somewhat prematurely released for public use in the USA and elsewhere. Many people are taking it regularly to induce sleep. This may prove to be unwise. The long-term effects are unknown.

Insomnia

Difficulty in sleeping has to take into account the normal duration of sleep at different ages. Children of 6 on average sleep $10\frac{1}{2}$ to $13\frac{1}{2}$ hours per night, 15-year-olds 9 to 10, adults $7\frac{1}{2}$ to $8\frac{1}{2}$. Women sleep slightly longer than men, on average. Insomnia can be defined as 'difficulty in initiating and/or maintaining sleep'. It is a common complaint. About 12% of members of the general adult population complain that they can't sleep as well as they feel they should. Complaints of insomnia are commonest in the dark periods of the year and in countries where the sun is low on the horizon. A distinction is usually made between difficulty in falling asleep (a particular problem in the young) and difficulty in remaining asleep (a problem for the elderly). A particularly common complaint in the elderly is early morning wakening, often brought about by a wake-up call from the elderly bladder.

Sleep disorders are extremely common after a serious or stressful traumatic event. They may require treatment if the problem is severe enough for the victim to seek medical help. People regularly exposed to stressful events (bus drivers, for example) are often troubled by insomnia.

Several drugs can cause insomnia. Although alcohol promotes stages III and IV deep sleep it is one of the drugs which can interfere with refreshing sleep, possibly by reducing REM sleep. Others are the methylxanthines (in tea and coffee), non-sedating antidepressants, and drugs used to treat people with Parkinson's disease (Chapter 28). Medical conditions, especially chronic airways obstruction, asthma, indigestion, and musculoskeletal pains can all keep people awake. Lack of sunlight can be a problem. Comprehensive surveys in Scandinavia have reported that insomnia is common there. Only half of adults felt that they regularly enjoyed a good night's sleep. In Sweden 14% of men and 22% of women use hypnotics regularly.

Insomnia is a major complaint of many elderly people but sometimes it has a simple explanation. They go to bed too early. The older you get, the less sleep you need. By the age of 80 few normal people not on drugs can expect to sleep much more than 6 hours. Consequently those who retire to bed at 10 p.m. – which may have been a lifetime's habit – are likely to wake spontaneously at 4 a.m. and complain that they don't sleep properly. Television and radio are boons here. Simple devices such as making a cup of tea and reading a book can dissipate the boredom of early wakening. My personal recommendation to elderly patients complaining of insomnia is that they should get into the habit of always staying up at least till midnight or 1 a.m. by reading or watching television.

Genetics of sleep disturbances

So far some 8 genes have been identified which influence the biological clocks in the body and determine the sleep/waking cycle. In animals (notably in the fruit fly and the mouse) it has proved possible to delete or inactivate individual genes and produce effects on the circadian cycle. Undoubtedly many minor genetic abnormalities will be identified in future years. Some may be difficult to recognise. But in man there is a dominant[7] familial inherited abnormality known as the 'advanced sleep syndrome'. People with this 'defect' (hardly an appropriate name for it!) go to sleep earlier in the night than most people do, and get up earlier in the morning. I imagine that inheriting the advanced sleep syndrome is a positive advantage for postmen and dairy farmers. It has probably influenced their choice of job.

Snoring

Snoring is produced while a sleeping individual with partial obstruction of his upper airway is breathing in. It is caused by vibrations of the soft palate and the sides of the mouth at the back. Most questionnaires confirm that between 6% and 30% of adults habitually snore and that up to 7% of children do so. The condition is almost invariably found in people who suffer from the 'obstructive sleep apnoea syndrome' in which (as its name suggests) breathing intermittently

48

stops (Greek: *apnoia* = lack of breath) in people whose breathing is partially obstructed. Such people are commonly obese, their parents or spouses are often smokers and their blood pressure is above average. Snoring and intermittent apnoea usually disappear when someone loses weight and clears his airways. People with the sleep apnoea syndrome often have raised blood pressure which comes down to normal values when the respiratory obstruction is relieved.

Narcolepsy and cataplexy

Narcolepsy describes an 'organic' (i.e. structural) brain disease – as opposed to one which is functional, without any identifiable specific features. It has an estimated prevalence of about 2 in every 10,000 adults. It results in the victim getting irresistible episodes of (usually) short spells of sleep, lasting a few minutes and recurring at short intervals of time. Attacks may also, rarely, last longer, e.g. for an hour or two. Individual attacks can sometimes be precipitated by emotion, especially laughter. People with narcolepsy often report feeling sleepy much of the time. Patients have often been confused with sufferers from chronic fatigue syndrome – so-called 'ME' (Chapter 38) – because being given a firm diagnosis of the disease 'narcolepsy' can prevent sufferers obtaining and retaining paid employment. Narcolepsy has been reported in most ethnic groups in the world and in a variety of cultural backgrounds. It presents itself in a similar way at about the same time in life – typically in the early twenties.

Narcolepsy has a strong genetic basis and most sufferers have a characteristic HLA (p. 474) inheritance of Class II genes. This suggests that the condition may have been initiated by some factor from the environment, most probably a virus infection. There is suggestive evidence that people born in March are slightly more liable to narcolepsy than those born in other months. If so, perhaps a virus infection common in springtime might be a precipitating cause – but the evidence at present is no more than suggestive. When the attacks are also accompanied by sudden episodes of muscle weakness (causing falls) the condition is described as cataplexy. In this situation, the episodes of sleep appear to be of the REM type. Animal experiments and a few human observations suggest that narcolepsy is triggered from the brain stem, more specifically from the reticular formation of the lower pons.

An interesting link has recently been established between narcolepsy and the secretion of 'hypocretins' (otherwise known as orexins), which are appetite stimulants[8] (see Chapter 16). Loss of hypocretin-producing

49

nerve cells in the hypothalamus is associated with narcolepsy and cataplexy.[9] Some dogs (Dobermann pinschers) and mice, with signs and symptoms resembling human narcolepsy, have been found to have mutations in a hypocretin receptor gene. Canine narcolepsy can be improved by administration of hypocretin-1.

Why do we sleep?

I have been absurdly presumptuous to have devoted a short chapter to sleep and its disorders, when in most other conditions and diseases I have reviewed in this book I have been able at least to approach the subjects with some general physiological understanding. But I feel entitled to discuss the subject briefly because of a lifetime's experience as a general physician (internist) and physiologist. I have watched people go to sleep and wake from sleep. I have watched people in various stages of sleep, in various depths of coma, and in light and deep anaesthesia. I have also made many observations of respiratory and cardiovascular function in man, in cats, dogs, rabbits and rats, both when conscious and anaesthetised. Some of these observations I have described at length in published work.[10]

All mammals sleep but no one knows why. It is obvious that sleep must have some restorative function, but we don't know what is being restored. We know that sleep deprivation is bad for human adults and that various functions are disturbed. For example, sleep deprivation tends to raise blood pressure. Francis Crick (the co-discoverer of the structure of DNA) at one time suggested that REM sleep might be regarded as a device to clear the brain of unwanted memories. He noted that animals without the REM sleep phase had particularly large brains.[11] The main trouble about this theory is that the well-developed fetus still in the womb spends about half its time in REM sleep. It is difficult to imagine that a fetus in the womb has acquired any large number of memories needing removal.

There have been many other suggestions and theories not only about the function of REM sleep, but also about the function of sleep itself. For example, the opossum sleeps for about 18 hours each day, whereas the elephant sleeps only 3 hours. Why? Dolphins spend little or no time in REM sleep, but have excellent learning and reasoning ability. Many fascinating mysteries about sleep remain to be solved.

Summary

Stages of sleep can be recognised by their characteristic pattern of electrical waves, which can be recorded through the intact skull – the electroencephalogram (EEG). There are four well-recognised stages of sleep: rapid-eye-movement sleep (REM), and three or four successive phases of increasing depth of non-rapid-eye-movement (NREM) sleep. Sleep grades III and IV are the deepest, when body temperature and blood pressure are at their lowest and lung ventilation is least. Episodes of REM sleep are frequent in the fetus (in the womb) and get gradually shorter and less frequent with increasing age. Total sleep duration also gets less with age.

There is a circadian clock in the suprachiasmatic nucleus in the hypothalamus. It has overriding control of the sleep/wake cycle. Its nervous connections pass to the brain stem from which control of many functions is exercised by activating nerve impulses that in effect keep the cerebral cortex awake. Many chemicals which influence sleep are secreted at the various neuro-chemical pathways involved. One such chemical is melatonin, produced by the pineal gland.

Difficulty in initiating or maintaining sleep (insomnia) has many causes, most of which are psychological rather than physiological, e.g. recent emotional or stressful events. Many drugs can either stimulate or inhibit sleep, according to which nerve pathway is activated or inhibited.

Narcolepsy and cataplexy are syndromes usually due to previous brain damage which leaves affected individuals with electrically unstable brains that can unduly readily and very rapidly enter and leave REM sleep. This is often accompanied by bizarre features.

5

PSORIASIS

Psoriasis is a common inflammatory skin condition which at some time of their lives affects between 1% and 3% of the world's population, more than 2% of Europeans, and about 8 million people in the USA. It typically produces sharply demarcated scaly raised red plaques or patches. The lesions are usually roughly symmetrical. The elbows, knees, back of the forearm and back of the upper arm are commonly involved, as well as the scalp, penis and vulva (Fig. 8). These are all places where there is pressure or rubbing. Both seem to be provocative factors. But in severe cases almost the whole skin surface can be involved. The nails are often pitted and deformed, especially if the disease has also involved the joints (a situation described as psoriatic arthropathy). This joint disease produces deformities, especially of the hands, which resemble those seen in rheumatoid arthritis (Chapter 9). However, the rheumatoid factor (p. 95) in psoriatic arthropathy is negative.

In Dennis Potter's BBC television play *The Singing Detective* the chief character spent a long period in hospital being treated for extensive psoriasis with joint involvement. The realistic depiction of his sufferings came from the author's own experiences. He was able to dramatise his illness in this unusual vicarious manner. The American novelist John Updike has also dramatised the sufferings of a severely affected psoriatic patient from his personal knowledge. For most people psoriasis is fortunately a mild, though tiresome, disease. It affects general health very little unless large areas of skin are involved, or if there is much inflammation, as there can be in generalised pustular psoriasis.

Psoriasis can appear at any age but it typically appears for the first time between 20 and 25, though there is another smaller peak at around age 50. It does not shorten life. Although there is excessive growth and proliferation of certain skin layers, psoriasis does not itself predispose to cancer. Certain treatments which make use of controlled exposure to ultraviolet light can increase the risk of skin cancer but it has also been suggested that spontaneous skin cancer may be less common in people with psoriasis than in those without

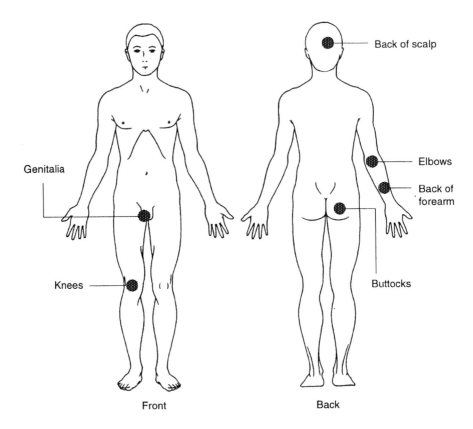

Figure 8 Diagrams showing the common sites of psoriatic lesions.

the condition. Long-term controlled epidemiological studies may resolve the matter.

There seems to be a relative excess of factors encouraging growth of blood vessels in the outer layer of the skin (the epidermis) and also in its deeper layers. There is also a relative deficiency of factors normally suppressing growth of blood vessels. (Blood vessel growth and restriction of blood vessel growth will be discussed further in Chapter 7.) The epidermis is abnormally thickened, even in areas where the skin appears normal to the naked eye. The rich network of blood vessels in psoriatic lesions can be shown by gently scraping their scaly surface. This (painless) procedure produces minute drops of blood on the surface of the lesions.

A number of other skin conditions look like psoriasis in their early stages, but the outstanding characteristic is the absence or relative mildness of itching, compared with conditions such as seborrhoeic dermatitis, chronic eczema and drug-induced eruptions, in which itching is usually more severe. (It is ironic that the word 'psoriasis' derives from Greek: *psora* = the itch.) The other diagnostic clue is that family members may also suffer or have suffered from the disease. A 'positive' family history is often reported by people with psoriasis, especially by those whose disease started early in life. In case of doubt, a biopsy (Greek: *bios* = life; *opsis* = vision) of a skin lesion can be examined under the microscope. On the surface of affected skin there is a thick layer of scale, a hard insoluble protein-containing crust, with loss of the layer of cells just beneath it. The word 'keratin' (Greek: *keras* = horn) has a less specific meaning. 'Scale' is a better term.

Genetics

Identical twins are 35–45% 'concordant' for the disease, i.e. one twin has a 35–45% chance of getting the disease if his or her identical twin has it. This is a striking observation. It emphasises the importance of someone's genetic inheritance, but also points to the almost equal importance of some external environmental factor such as chance exposure to some noxious or infective agent. Non-identical twins are only 10–15% concordant. The inheritance is evidently polygenic. What is inherited seems to be a predisposition which needs an environmental stimulus for its expression, as in so many of the medical mysteries described in this book.

Since the initial report of a gene locus on chromosome 17, which is now recognised as specially linked to psoriatic arthropathy, other genes on chromosomes 2, 8 and 20 have been weakly linked with psoriasis. A gene or genes on chromosome 6 is the strongest genetic link so far identified.[1] This chromosome contains the 'HLA' determinants, which suggests a possible link between infections and psoriasis.

Cause

In the affected parts of the skin there appears to be a great (ten fold) increase in the rate of growth of the cells which form the epidermal layer. Apparently normal skin also shows an increase in cell growth rate, though the turnover rate of cells is not as rapid as in the lesions themselves. It is difficult to grow scale-forming cells in tissue culture and thereby to measure the rate of cell turnover. Approximate estimates suggest that replication rate can probably vary from one cell division per day to one every month. Scale presumably forms when the rate of growth of the epidermal cells exceeds the rate of their destruction. An underlying defect in psoriasis seems to be in the processes concerned with wound healing.

When fibre-forming cells in skin from people with psoriasis are grown in tissue culture, completely outside the body, it has been reported that they synthesise at a faster rate than normal the fibre protein 'collagen', which is important in skin structure. If this is confirmed, we may still need to find out whether the problem is excessive stimulation of the cell division cycle, or whether there is reduced activity of inhibitors of cell growth. Curiously, despite the increased growth rate, skin thickness is not increased in uninvolved skin in psoriasis.

Many possible factors have been studied, but no single one has been incriminated as the main functional defect in psoriasis. Increased production of inflammation-promoting factors such as cytokines IL-1β, TNFα, and IL-8 is particularly notable, but the reason for the excessive production of these chemicals is not known. Recent discoveries in asthma have revealed the key role of NFκB in switching on the transcription of genes coding for inflammation-mediating cytokines. It is likely that NFκB in scale-forming skin cells plays a key role in the inflammation which characterises psoriasis. There has already been a hint of this possibility. Other cytokines suppress rather than stimulate inflammation. Recent reports suggest that the cytokine IL-4, produced by specialised 'helper' T-lymphocytes (Th2 cells), may be able to reduce the extent and severity of the skin lesions of psoriasis.

Immunological factors

The fact that steroid drugs (glucocorticoids) can reduce inflammation in psoriasis suggests that the disease might have an auto-immune cause (p. 472). The association is not proved, because steroids suppress the production of many inflammation-producing cytokines. Stopping steroids can exacerbate the disease. On the other hand, complete disappearance of psoriatic lesions can only rarely be obtained by the use of steroids, which in any case sometimes seem to destabilise scaly skin and make it pustular.

Psoriasis is reported to have been transmitted to a previously normal individual by a bone marrow transplant from a patient with psoriasis. This probably means that T-lymphocytes (p. 473) can themselves initiate the disease. The immunosuppressive drug cyclosporin specifically inhibits T-cell activation. It is notably effective in treating psoriasis. The involvement of T-cells in causing psoriatic lesions is also supported by ingenious animal experiments in which mice were made immuno-deficient so that they could tolerate a graft of human skin. Then it was found that lymphocytes from patients with psoriasis, even when taken from apparently normal skin, could induce the changes of psoriasis in human skin grafts in the mice.[2]

There is an association of psoriasis with certain specific inherited human leucocyte antigens (HLA), especially Cw6 and DR7. The association with Cw6 is specially close in young people. None the less, only 10% of people with this antigen develop the disease. The type of disease described as generalised pustular psoriasis has a different genetic HLA association, with A1, B37 and DRw10. Although particular HLA antigens may confer susceptibility to psoriasis, they are not of great causal significance. The inheritance of psoriasis, like most conditions of variable severity, certainly involves many genes. Probably a genetic predisposition from the HLA system needs to coincide with one, or a few, additional common genetic variations. Much collateral evidence suggests that a predisposition to develop auto-immunity is an inherited dominant trait and that HLA genes determine the type of auto-immunity.

The effectiveness of immunosuppressive drugs such as cyclosporin and azathioprine in psoriasis is a further pointer towards the disease involving a T-cell auto-immune response.

Although experiments in animals have not yet brought a breakthrough to solve the enigma of the disease, the creation of genetically modified ('transgenic') mice has opened up an enormous field of research in which human genes that determine the severity, type and location of psoriatic lesions will be gradually identified. Psoriasis is not unique to man and has been observed in primates. Typical lesions have not been identified in lower animals, though mice can develop a large variety of scaly skin conditions.

Environmental triggers

Environmental factors may be nearly as important as heredity. Obesity, smoking and certain drugs aggravate psoriasis. Lithium (a treatment for serious depressive illness) has been recorded as making psoriatic lesions worse. The importance of psychological factors is disputed, though physical or emotional stress sometimes appear to be trigger factors. I remember a striking case. On the first day that a senior colleague was to start a particularly responsible and demanding medical job he had to be admitted to hospital for a bad attack of psoriasis affecting his entire body. But it is unwise to make deductions from anecdotes surrounding such a common disease.

57

Physical trauma (the Koebner effect) is probably an aggravating factor, accounting for the localisation of psoriatic plaques on areas such as the elbows which are often pressed and rubbed. Mechanical strain can release a powerful stimulant of inflammation (the cytokine IL-1).

Infection and psoriasis

The appearance of new lesions has often seemed to follow a streptococcal sore throat, suggesting that the *Streptococcus haemolyticus* bacterium is a cause of psoriasis. Antistreptococcal antibiotics may improve the disease. Streptococci have been found in the skin lesions of a few patients who have responded well to antibiotics. There are close chemical similarities between some of the proteins from streptococcal bacteria and keratin protein in normal human skin. So perhaps the body starts treating its own skin scale as if it was an invading bacterium. There is also an association between psoriasis and infections with the bacterium *Staphylococcus aureus* which causes boils and other skin infections.

> Streptococcal and staphylococcal bacteria can both embody 'superantigens', a group of proteins which can activate many different T-cells.[3] Some people have suggested that psoriasis is a T-cell mediated autoimmune reaction triggered by bacterial superantigens, releasing damaging cytokines. So far the jury is out. Pus-producing ('pyogenic') infections may not be needed to maintain psoriasis, but they may be exacerbating or triggering factors in some patients.

Despite these observations there is very little to suggest that bacterial infection is normally a cause of psoriasis. It just seems sometimes to start the disease off. Yeasts of the genus *Pityrosporum* have often been found in psoriatic skin lesions and skin scales. They are so often found in normal individuals that it is difficult to believe that these yeasts can have a unique causal role; but since man and yeasts share many genes in common it remains possible that a yeast could yet be a trigger for psoriasis.

> Recently successful trials have been made in psoriasis using drugs which block the action of two of the damaging cytokines which contribute to the inflammation underlying the disease. One is that against TNFα (etanercept), the other is against material produced by white blood cells which helps them stick to their targets (efalizumab). Although these observations do not immediately shed light on the cause or causes of

psoriasis, it is certain that many similar drugs will be introduced over the next few years and perhaps will lead to a better understanding of a most mysterious disease.

Summary

Psoriasis is a common skin disease which in its mildest form produces scaly non-itchy patches on elbows and knees, but in its most violent form may involve large skin surfaces with raised and sometimes pustular lesions. It may also cause joint pains and deformities resembling those of rheumatoid arthritis.

Sufferers are not born with psoriasis, but are genetically predisposed to develop the condition when they encounter one of a number of possible environmental factors, especially infections. These act as triggers to set the disease off, but no consistently responsible trigger has yet been identified. Psychological factors may be important, but this is unproven. Many different genes seem able to confer susceptibility, but so far none has been recognised as invariably associated with psoriasis. The disease is probably maintained by T-lymphocytes, which can by themselves carry or transmit the disease.

6

THYROID DISORDERS

The thyroid gland was first identified by the Greek physician Galen nearly two thousand years ago. Its name describes its shape: Greek: *thyreos* = oblong shield; *eidos* = shape. It comprises two soft pear-shaped lobes, each about 2 inches long and an inch thick, lying on either side of the windpipe (trachea) in the lower part of the neck. The two lobes are joined across the midline, in front of the trachea, by an isthmus (Fig. 9).

The thyroid is the largest of the 'ductless glands'. A 'gland' can be defined as an organ which produces a fluid secretion, e.g. sweat glands in the skin, tear glands in the eyes, glands producing saliva in the cheeks, and acid-secreting glands in the lining of the stomach. In each case the secretion acts at or close to where it is produced. But ductless glands secrete soluble chemicals directly into the bloodstream (hormones: p. 22). They can therefore exert their effects anywhere in the body.

The main secretion of the thyroid gland is an iodine-containing protein called thyroglobulin. This is produced by and stored in thousands of minute 'follicles' – fluid-filled cysts which have been likened to microscopic clusters of berries. Thyroglobulin breaks down into the hormones 'T3' and 'T4' which can be released into the blood-stream when required.[1] When T4 reaches body tissues, T4 is converted into T3 (the active hormone) by losing one of its four iodine atoms. T3 can bind on to specific T3 receptors in many tissues, thus bringing about its various physiological actions. Some 90% of circulating T3 is formed directly from T4. This explains why thyroxine (T4) is so effective a treatment for thyroid deficiency.

T3 and T4 both circulate combined with specific carrier proteins, but T3 is less strongly protein-bound than T4. The effect of protein binding is that the biological activity of both hormones is much less than would be expected from the total quantities in the blood, because only the unbound 'free' hormones are active.

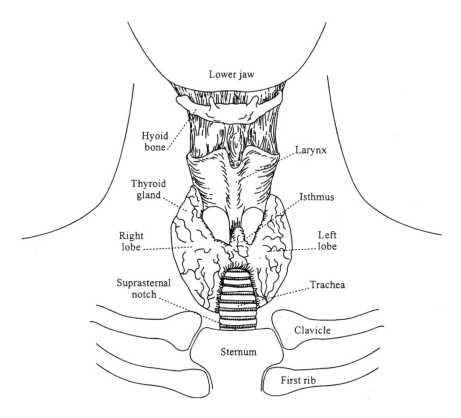

Figure 9 Diagrammatic view of the front of the neck showing the position and size of the two lobes of the thyroid gland. These are joined by an 'isthmus' which lies in front of the trachea. The 4 small parathyroid glands cannot be seen from the front because they lie behind the thyroid gland itself, commonly at its lower and middle parts.

Effects of thyroid hormones

In fetal and early life thyroid hormones promote growth and are especially important for brain growth. The fetus usually gets enough thyroid hormones from its mother to grow normally in the womb. But there are some conditions arising after birth when the infant thyroid gland is absent or fails to develop. Lack of enough thyroid hormones in infancy causes cretinism – mental deficiency associated with a characteristic facial appearance. This is preventable if thyroid hormones are given in good time.

When growth has ceased, in adult life, thyroid hormones have other important actions, the most important of which is the regulation of body heat. T3 increases body heat, by mechanisms which are not entirely understood.

I was taught as a student that thyroid hormones increased body heat by 'uncoupling oxidative phosphorylation'. Oxidative phosphorylation describes the chemical reactions by means of which the oxidation of foodstuffs provides energy. This makes it possible for a phosphate group to be added to each molecule of adenosine diphosphate (ADP), thus converting it into adenosine triphosphate (ATP). ATP is a bottled-up flexible energy source. It can power muscle contraction, gland secretion, protein synthesis and many chemical reactions when it loses a phosphate group and turns back into ADP.

Until recently, it was thought that thyroid hormones disturbed the link between the oxidation of food and the generation of ATP, thus dissipating energy in the form of heat. This interpretation is now disputed, because the main receptors for thyroid hormones appear to be in cell nuclei. In general terms, current thinking is that heat is generated in the body by thyroid hormones breaking up complex molecules like proteins then using ATP to build them up again. However, the discovery that thyroid hormone receptors are also present on mitochondria (minute structures inside cells in which oxidative phosphorylation takes place) has renewed interest in the old ideas about how thyroid hormones act. There are still mysteries to be solved here. Historians of science can delight that not all old ideas are necessarily wrong. Scientists don't recognise 'facts' but only hypotheses, which represent the best current explanations for phenomena and which account for the greatest number of observations.

One consequence of overactivity of the thyroid gland is that some food eaten is not converted into body tissues nor immediately used to power muscles or make glands secrete. The energy which the food could have provided is simply dissipated as heat. Specific thyroid hormone receptors are located in many organs of the body, including the cells of the liver, the kidneys and the heart. There are also specific receptors in some circulating white blood cells (lymphocytes). All these sites can generate heat when acted on by thyroid hormones.

Body temperature is regulated by a temperature-sensing organ in the centre of the brain (the hypothalamus: Fig. 7, p. 45). Any potentially damaging rise of temperature is prevented because the brain sends out messages to sweat glands in the skin, chiefly via specialised nerves connected to the glands. The evaporation of sweat cools the skin and hence the body. Excessive sweating is a cardinal symptom of thyroid hormone excess, which is also known as 'thyrotoxicosis' or hyperthyroidism. Unless food intake goes up appropriately, people with thyrotoxicosis lose weight. T3 and T4 are well absorbed by mouth and have often been prescribed by unscrupulous doctors and taken (unwisely) by people desperate to lose weight.

I have seen the full-blown picture of congestive heart failure (Chapter 21) precipitated by severe thyrotoxicosis in a young woman without any previous heart disease. Fortunately the condition quickly got better when appropriate anti-thyroid drug treatment was cautiously given. I have also seen two deaths in middle-aged women during inadvisably energetic treatment of thyrotoxicosis: in one case the patient was in atrial flutter which suddenly converted to fatal ventricular fibrillation. In the other an unduly large therapeutic dose of radioactive iodine temporarily increased thyroid hormone release, again with a fatal disorder of cardiac rhythm. With doctors' greater knowledge and experience such catastrophes are now fortunately rare.

The general effects of excess thyroid hormones resemble excess activity of the sympathetic nervous system (p. 481). I have seen an adrenaline-secreting adrenal gland tumour in a woman producing symptoms which so closely resembled thyrotoxicosis that the unfortunate patient was subjected to an unnecessary operation to cut out part of her thyroid gland, before the correct diagnosis was made. Minor degrees of hyperthyroidism can be difficult to diagnose. The condition may show itself by otherwise inexplicable fatigue and by heart rhythm disorders, especially atrial fibrillation – but with no other notable symptoms. It has often masqueraded as chronic fatigue syndrome, so-called 'ME', as described in Chapter 38.

Thyroid hormone deficiency

I have already mentioned that thyroid hormone deficiency in the infant impairs growth, notably of the brain. In the adult, thyroid deficiency (hypothyroidism) produces many effects which are the opposite of thyroid excess. The body tends to become cold. Curiously I have not noticed such patients shivering, even though they feel very cold to touch. All body movements slow down, notably the beating heart and regular breathing, as also does mental activity. The skin becomes dry because of reduction in sweating. The reduction in metabolism of food tends towards obesity (Chapter 16). This is often aggravated by excess fluid retention, which is also a symptom of hypothyroidism. There is often 'myxoedema'. This rather unsuitable term means 'mucus swelling'. It was chosen to describe the rather firm enlargement, mainly of the legs, which does not deform easily on pressure as does swelling due to simple fluid excess. Similar swelling of the vocal cords often makes the voice characteristically hoarse. The face looks puffy, though its texture is firm. Longstanding hypothyroidism is usually accompanied by increased arterial blockages, notably in the coronary arteries. Death from heart attacks is common.

Very occasionally – I have not seen it myself – a patient with myxoedema develops psychotic behaviour described as 'myxoedema madness' – the diagnosis of which made the young hero's clinical reputation in AJ Cronin's novel *The Citadel*.

Control of thyroid function

The rate of release of T3 and T4 from the thyroid gland into the bloodstream is controlled by 'thyroid-stimulating hormone' (TSH for short – also called 'thyrotropin'). TSH is a secretion of the anterior pituitary gland, lying below and in front of the hypothalamus in the centre of the skull. There is a classical negative feedback system. TSH stimulates release of thyroid hormones and tends to make the gland bigger, but thyroid hormones inhibit the release of TSH from the pituitary gland and make the gland smaller. TSH secretion is itself stimulated by 'thyrotrophin-releasing hormone' (TRH: a simple tripeptide[2]) synthesised in and released from the hypothalamus. But the main feedback control is mediated by thyroid hormones inhibiting TSH release.

A thyroid gland of normal size is quite soft and difficult to feel clearly. It has much the same consistency as the strap muscles in the neck. But an enlarged gland, called a 'goitre', may be both visible and easy to feel. When in doubt a doctor will ask the patient to swallow. This makes the whole gland move upwards.

The commonest cause of goitre in the world is lack of enough dietary iodine. This inevitably reduces the body's production of thyroid hormones, which in turn increases TSH secretion. This is the usual cause of goitre. Many years ago, in the English midlands, gross enlargement of the thyroid gland was common. It gave rise to what became known as 'Derbyshire neck' – due to TSH overproduction in a low iodine region. This is no longer seen today because of changes in the habitual UK diet.

In urban communities throughout the world, without endemic goitre, the average daily intake of iodine is 1/10 milligram (100 micrograms: μg). The absolute minimum intake for health is not known but may be less than this. The World Health Organisation, to be on the safe side, currently recommends that adolescents and adults should take 150 μg daily, that pregnant and lactating women should take 200 μg, children aged 1–2 should take 90–120 μg, and younger children should take 50 μg daily. However, the average dietary intake of iodine by adults in the UK is now so high (200–300 μg daily) that taking substantial amounts of extra iodine could be positively harmful.

Epidemiology of medical thyroid disorders

Overproduction of thyroid hormones (thyrotoxicosis) is a common condition. It has been seen at some stage of their lives in nearly 3% of all adult women in the UK, most commonly between the ages of 30 and 50. The condition is usually associated with a soft goitre which is very 'vascular': i.e. it has an exuberant blood supply. This may create a rushing noise, in time with each heart beat, which can be heard when the diaphragm of a stethoscope is placed over the gland. The combination of a soft vascular goitre and thyrotoxicosis is often called 'Graves' Disease', after one of the physicians who first described it. (Pedants put an 'apostrophe' after the name to mean 'described by Graves'.) Graves' disease is often accompanied by characteristic signs in the eyes – lid retraction and sometimes actual bulging of the eyes (exophthalmos). A connection between emotional stress and the occurrence of Graves' disease has been quite firmly established. The association is thought to be related to overproduction of glucocorticoids by stress, but the connection is not completely understood.

Many people with a 'nodular' goitre, i.e. one with discrete palpable lumps of firm tissue in its substance, also develop thyrotoxicosis but do not, as a rule, get exophthalmos. Nor do people who get cancer of the thyroid gland, even though such cancers sometimes cause thyrotoxicosis by making excessive amounts of T3 and T4.

Spontaneous decrease of thyroid hormone secretion (hypothyroidism) is also common. The gland is usually smaller than normal and atrophic, but it can also become larger and harder than normal (so-called 'Hashimoto's thyroiditis') even though it is producing less than normal amounts of T3 and T4. Hypothyroidism has a prevalence of nearly 2% in women. I have seen several patients who first complained of symptoms of thyrotoxicosis (which was confirmed by blood tests[3]) but who later went in the opposite direction and developed hypothyroidism.

It is obvious that in the control system I have described hypothyroidism could also result from failure of production of TSH by the anterior pituitary gland. Indeed, lack of thyroid hormones produces many of the symptoms and signs of pituitary gland failure, though in that condition there are additional effects due to lack of adrenal and sex gland function. I vividly recall an occasion when I was a medical officer in the British Army and had admitted under my care an ex-soldier from the Royal Hospital in Chelsea. When I first saw him he was lying immobile under a pile of blankets, though the ward was warm. He complained of weakness, tiredness and feeling the cold. His skin was pale and cold and he had little body hair. He presented the typical picture of 'panhypopituitarism' (Greek: *pan* = all; *hypo* = under: i.e. lacking all the pituitary hormones). X-ray of his skull showed a curious round shadow in the pituitary gland area. X-rays of his thighs showed numerous small opaque linear shadows, evidently containing calcium. These were typical of cysticercosis, a manifestation of previous pork tapeworm infection. It seemed almost certain that the round shadow in the position of the pituitary gland was a calcified cysticercus larva which had replaced the gland. Research in the library revealed that cysticercosis was specially common in soldiers who had served in India and who were either cooks or bandsmen. My patient had served in the Indian Army as a cook. I have described his clinical presentation elsewhere.[4]

At the time I saw him, reliable blood tests for thyroid function were not available. We measured thyroid function by the 'basal metabolic rate' (BMR), i.e. the rate of oxygen consumption by an individual at rest. The BMR is increased by thyroid hormone excess and diminished by hormone deficiency. I measured the BMR in my patient by filling with oxygen a closed gas circuit connected to a breathing recorder (spirometer). The patient rebreathed his own expired air through a tubular glass column filled with soda lime, to absorb carbon dioxide. Under these circumstances the rate of fall of gas volume in the system should correspond to the rate of oxygen consumption. This is determined by the slope of the spirometer trace. Imagine my astonishment to find that this man with evident gross deficiency of thyroid and other hormones was using oxygen at three times the normal rate for subjects at rest. The problem was solved by examination of his ear drums, one of which had a large hole in it, caused by a previous middle ear infection. Oxygen was steadily leaking out of the system through the eustachian tube which connected his nasal passages to his damaged middle ear. I later found that this old soldier capitalised on his condition by making successful bets in local Chelsea pubs that he could hold his breath for five minutes with his face under water, breathing in and out through his perforated ear drum.

To measure thyroid function nowadays physicians just sign a form and send a specimen of blood off to the lab to measure thyroid function, but they miss a lot of fun.

Cause

The common occurrence of both thyroid excess and thyroid deficiency, sometimes manifesting successively at different times in the same individual, has always been something of a mystery. Understanding has advanced a great deal in the last half century. I remember being intrigued in 1953 by finding that patients with hypothyroidism (some six of whom I looked after as a junior doctor) all had a raised 'erythrocyte sedimentation rate' (ESR) – a blood test which suggests the presence of some inflammatory process. I also recall being rebuked by one of my chiefs (the late John Nabarro) for having been slow to draw this phenomenon to his special attention.

There are other curious aspects of these medical thyroid diseases. In the Middlesex Hospital in London, where I was working in 1957, I often had lunch with Deborah Doniach, a scientist who was working in the Department of Immunology with Ivan Roitt. 'Immunology' is the study of the various protective mechanisms which help the body attack and neutralise foreign substances or organisms. One way in which the body does this is by generating 'antibodies' – protein molecules which circulate in the blood and combine with and render harmless various toxins and parts of infecting organisms. Antibodies are synthesised by specialised cells ('B-lymphocytes') in lymph glands. Antibodies combine with and neutralise any foreign chemicals which have not been identified as belonging to 'self', i.e. to the individual concerned.

Deborah told me about her work on circulating thyroid antibodies in patients with medical thyroid diseases. She had measured the concentration (titre) of the circulating proteins (antibodies) which combined with extracts of normal thyroid gland in patients with several thyroid diseases. She had found them often increased in both hypo- and hyperthyroidism. Their occurrence in hypothyroidism suggested that circulating anti-thyroid antibodies could be the reason for impaired thyroid function and atrophy of the gland. But anti-thyroid antibodies were also present in many patients with thyrotoxicosis. This seemed totally anomalous. Here were antibodies which in some patients were damaging the thyroid gland and making patients hypothyroid but which in other patients were associated with overactivity of the gland and 'thyrotoxic' symptoms.

The first steps in solution of the puzzle came with the discovery that some antibodies were themselves stimulators of thyroid hormone production. The first to be recognised was called 'long-acting thyroid stimulator' (LATS), because in animal assays it had a long time course of action. Its chemical structure was that of an 'immunoglobulin' a typical protein antibody generated by B-lymphocytes (see above). One generally thinks of antibodies as substances which combine with and neutralise or inactivate damaging or toxic chemicals and which are produced after repeated exposure to such damaging or toxic chemicals. But LATS does not neutralise either T3 or T4 and may even increase their blood concentrations. Thyroid-stimulating activity is present in virtually all people with Graves' disease. The question obviously arises: how can an antibody act as a stimulant to an organ's function when antibodies, as their name suggests, impair organ function? The problem remains, to challenge the next generation of clinical scientists.

Many, perhaps half, of all patients with primary Graves' disease have classic eye signs, including lid retraction and eye muscle weakness. These can make the eye look larger than normal. In severe cases there may be actual protuberance of the globe because of enlarged lymphatic tissue in the orbit. Occasionally these eye signs can develop without any evidence of thyroid gland overactivity. They may even get worse while hyperthyroidism is being successfully treated. At present there is no generally agreed cause of the eye signs in typical Graves' disease, but they are thought to have an auto-immune basis and to be produced by the local liberation of cytokines (p. 474) acting on connective tissues in the eye socket. Many thyroid antigens are expressed in the orbit. Curiously, exophthalmos is strongly and positively associated with smoking.

Diseases associated with and caused by so-called 'organ-specific' antibodies (e.g. pernicious anaemia, adrenal gland atrophy, Type 1 diabetes, rheumatoid arthritis and the medical thyroid diseases I have been describing) often occur together in the same patient. They may also run in families. Liability to these auto-immune diseases is clearly an inheritable trait but the exact nature of the genetic predisposition is not known. It is probably related to the HLA DR3 haplotype. Hypothyroidism itself has been found associated with several different antibodies. Some are directed against thyroglobulin, some against the enzyme which makes thyroid hormone (thyroid peroxidase) and some against the TSH receptor.

Damage to the thyroid gland can also result from auto-immune attack by T-cells which have been primed to destroy thyroid structures. A wide variety of thyroid cell antigens are likely to be targets. It is this type of cell-mediated damage which is also thought to underlie hypothyroidism due to so-called 'Hashimoto's thyroiditis' in which the gland itself is enlarged and firm, though producing very small amounts of thyroid hormones.

The interested reader should refer to a useful review.[5]

What is the trigger for auto-immune diseases?

Why should the body produce damaging antibodies against parts of itself such as the TSH receptors? There is no generally agreed answer.

But some clues suggest that the trigger may be an infection, most probably by a virus, which either itself contains an antigen or which releases or creates from body tissues an antigen which the body's immune system has not previously encountered. We know from the work of Peter Medawar and others that the adult body is normally tolerant of organs, tissues and chemicals which are present before birth. Shortly after birth this tolerance switches off. Many foreign materials can then potentially act as antigens, exciting an immune response.

If this interpretation for auto-immune thyroid diseases is correct, we need to identify possible agents which can trigger immune attack either by B-cells or T-cells. This may be difficult since there are so many known infectious agents. Or could some common article of food be responsible? Twin studies comparing the occurrence of Graves' disease in identical and non-identical twins show a moderately strong genetic component of the disease – identical twins having a 22% concordance for the disease – but environmental factors clearly have at least the same order of importance. Today almost all research into auto-immune thyroid diseases has been directed into identifying the various immunological steps by which thyroid damage occurs. But some imaginative epidemiology is urgently needed to provide clues about possible environmental trigger factors. Paradoxically the very commonness of these medical thyroid diseases makes epidemiology more rather than less difficult.

Aspects of treatment

The treatment of thyroid deficiency is obvious and straightforward: i.e. to supply the missing hormone. Fortunately thyroid hormones are well absorbed by mouth and do not have to be injected. Many different treatment protocols have been tried because there have been so many deaths during treatment – usually from a heart attack (myocardial infarction). The two deaths I mentioned earlier both occurred while the patients appeared to be getting better during treatment. T3 has been used in the past to initiate treatment but is now thought to be unduly abrupt in its effect. Some physicians use very gradual treatment with slowly increasing doses of thyroxine (T4). However, I remember the late Donald Hunter, a very experienced physician, saying that it had never been proved conclusively that gradual treatment was better than giving full replacement doses from the start and that the gradual approach wasted time. I am unsure whether this problem has ever been unequivocally solved. A reasonable compromise (now recommended by the British National Formulary) is to give most people full replacement doses of T4 from the start except for elderly people and those with known heart disease, who should start with lower doses, gradually increasing at 4–6 week intervals.

The treatment of thyroid excess is also controversial. In my early clinical life I assisted at many operations called 'partial thyroidectomy' in which some three-quarters of the whole gland tissue was simply cut away. It was a bloody operation, because of the numerous blood vessels in the overactive gland. But I never saw any catastrophies. All my patients seemed to do well, achieving normal thyroid function with no late disasters. Surgery is still recommended today by some surgeons who claim that it 'continues to offer the highest cure rate in the shortest period of time'.[6] Temporary suppression of thyroid hormone oversecretion can be achieved by many drugs, notably propylthiouracil or methimazole. These can often damp down damaging immunological reactions. But medical treatment only leads to permanent, or at least long-lasting, thyroid suppression in about 50% of cases. In about the same number of cases the condition recurs when treatment stops. Giving a dose of radioactive iodine (^{131}I) by mouth is today probably the most commonly used treatment, but it is difficult to judge the dose correctly because the damage inflicted on the gland continues for a long time. In my observation all thyrotoxic patients adequately controlled by radioactive iodine therapy finish up needing thyroid replacement therapy in the end. So if tomorrow I developed thyrotoxicosis myself, I would ask to be given a full suppressive dose of radioactive iodine. (This has not yet been incriminated in causing thyroid cancer.) I would, of course, have to resign myself to taking thyroxine tablets daily for the rest of my life. But perhaps a younger physician might disagree!

Summary

The main secretions of the twin-lobed thyroid gland in the lower part of the neck comprise the iodine-containing hormones tri-iodotyrosine (T3) and tetra-iodotyrosine (T4: also known as thyroxine). T4 is converted into T3 (the active hormone) in body tissues. Hormone secretion rate and thyroid growth are controlled by a pituitary hormone known as 'thyroid stimulating hormone' (TSH). This is in turn controlled by the secretion of a simple tripeptide hormone called 'thyrotropin-releasing hormone' (TRH) by the pituitary gland, in the skull base.

Excess thyroid hormones increase the generation of heat in the body, with increased sweating and many other associated symptoms including weight loss and tremor. Lack of thyroid hormones cause the opposite symptoms, i.e. lack of body heat and tiredness. It also predisposes to arterial disease.

In both situations the causes are usually 'auto-immune' resulting from antibodies which may either stimulate the gland or block its normal function. Some antibodies may be able to do both at different times.

7

THE BLOOD SUPPLY OF TUMOURS

Thirty years ago I wrote in *The Encyclopaedia of Medical Ignorance* that the way in which tumours got themselves a blood supply was a notable area of ignorance.[1] It still is, but vast strides have been made in our understanding. The subject is at the forefront of current cancer research. It has implications for many other normal and disease processes, such as fetal growth, wound healing and scarring.

Cancer starts when a cell in the body has suffered a sequence of 'somatic mutations' (see below), sometimes augmented by damage to genes involved in DNA repair or by a mutation in the tumour-suppressor protein (p53) which controls the programmed self-destruction of abnormal cells. Inherited abnormalities of DNA often predispose to cancer in later life. This means that a cell in a newborn child may start off already part way towards cancer. For example, the BrCa genes make breast cancer more likely in women who inherit them. (Two are known already, but clues from family breast cancer pedigrees suggest that several more await identification.)

A mutation can be defined as a change in some part of the DNA contained in a chromosome in the cell nucleus. A 'somatic' mutation means one pertaining to the body (Latin: *soma* = body), i.e. one which develops after fertilisation of the egg. A skin papilloma is the consequence of a somatic mutation. Such a lesion tends very slowly to get bigger, but almost never disappears spontaneously. If one of its cells develops one or more further somatic mutations the tumour might become a so-called 'rodent ulcer', which is a localised form of skin cancer. This can get progressively bigger and destroy local tissues, but it does not spread from the skin into internal organs. To become an epithelioma (a 'malignant' skin tumour, i.e. one capable of causing death) it needs to produces enzymes which can digest proteins and fibrous tissue. This can then let cancer cells into the blood flowing through a local vein and thus allow such cells to spread throughout the body – a process known as metastasis. Cancer cells may also spread indirectly by stimulating normal blood macrophages to produce the necessary enzymes to clear a path for cancer cells to spread. In either case a certain minimum bulk of tumour tissue is needed.

The number of divisions of most body cells is limited because a portion of the end of each chromosome – the 'telomere' (Greek: *telos* = end) – is lost with each successive cell division. Each chromosome gets progressively shorter at each division until the cell which contains it has lost too many of the vital genes it needs to survive. Between 50 and 100 units of DNA (technically 'base pairs') are lost from the ends of each chromosome at each cell division. Since there are several thousand redundant non-functional 6-unit DNA sequences (the telomeres) at the end of each chromosome, no harm ensues when a cell divides, providing that the important coding sequences of DNA are not lost. The presence of a string of telomeres at the end of each chromosome also may prevent chromosomes from joining up in tangles. It allows many replications to take place before cell function is compromised. But eventually, after perhaps 50 cell divisions, a cell loses vital genes and dies.

We have known for many years that most cancer cell lines grown in culture, away from the body, are immortal. They can continue to divide indefinitely without losing genetic material. The reason is that in about 90% of cancer cells an enzyme (telomerase) is active: technically, 'upregulated'. This is a DNA polymerase, composed of ribose nucleic acid (RNA) and protein sub-units. Telomerase reconstructs the truncated or damaged ends of each chromosome each time the cell divides. The process may not be necessary to start cancer off because some two extra cancer genes ('oncogenes') are usually also needed, but it is highly relevant for the later disastrous growth and spread of cancer around the body. Cancer cells can also become immortal by recruiting yet another mechanism for repairing chromosome ends, the 'alternative lengthening telomeres' (ALT) system.

How do tumours get a blood supply?

The mystery I want to discuss in this chapter is not why a cell escapes from its normal controls and starts dividing, but rather how it manages to build up a mass of tumour tissue. How does it get itself a blood supply? All cells require a supply of food and oxygen to provide energy to remain alive. If the main artery supplying a tumour is tied off the tumour shrivels up and dies. A malignant tumour – one which has lost all control over its cells dividing – cannot grow to more than about one tenth of an inch (2 mm) in diameter unless it gets new blood vessels to supply its component cells with nutrients. The reason is the time it takes for materials to diffuse through the jelly-like material between cells. Dissolved particles or genetic materials have to get through the walls of blood vessels and then eventually diffuse into recipient cells before they can make normal cells behave like cancer.

Although diffusion is extremely rapid across short distances it is extremely slow across large distances. This is, of course, why all except the tiniest of animals and plants have developed some form of fluid circulation to allow nutrients to be brought to tissues, and waste products to be removed. Table 1 shows the calculated rates of diffusion of a small molecule (glucose) and a larger one (a small protein) across various distances.

Table 1 Typical rates of diffusion in water of molecules of two different sizes

Time for 50% of molecular particles (molecules) to move by diffusion alone distance of	Glucose	Small protein
1 micron (1/1000 mm)	1/1000 second	1/100 second
10 microns (1/100 mm)	1/10 second	1 second
1 mm	16 minutes	4 hours
1 cm	26 hours	17 days
10 cm	4 months	5 years

Before new blood vessels can grow into a tumour, to nourish the malignant cells, a path must be cleared through the surrounding tissue. This is performed by the synthesis by many cancer cells of zinc-containing 'matrix-degrading metalloproteinases' (MMPs), especially one known as stromelysin (MMP-3). Once the way is cleared, new blood vessels have room to grow.

Angiogenesis (Greek: *angio* = vessel; *genesis* = creation) has been described as driven by a cocktail of growth factors and pro-angiogenic cytokines, tempered by an equally diverse group of inhibitors of new blood vessel formation. Some 20 blood vessel growth stimulators and inhibitors are known, including 'epidermal growth factor' (EGF), 'platelet-derived growth factor' (PDGF), 'fibroblast growth factor-1' (FGF) and 'transforming growth factor-beta' (TGFβ). Most of these chemicals, possibly all of them, work by facilitating the production of one of the 'vascular endothelial growth factor' (VEGF) family of cytokines. These vary in their permeability and chemical properties. The basic molecule of VEGF closely resembles that of PDGF. Both are technically 'dimers', i.e. paired molecules. They combine with those parts of receptors which stimulate cell synthetic functions. Nitric oxide seems also to be needed. The main receptors are known as VEGFR1 (Flt-1) and VEGFR2 (Flk-1 or KDR) for VEGF, and the beta receptor for PDGF. There are natural stimuli which switch on or increase production of all these substances. Increased metabolic rate, which increases oxygen consumption and lowers its availability, is much the most important stimulus for blood vessel growth. Increased metabolic rate also increases the activity of another growth factor distinct from VEGF (angiopoietin-1) which promotes growth when it combines with a receptor called Tie-2, also known as TEK. The latter is located particularly in the thin inner lining membrane of blood vessels (the endothelium). This combination has recently been shown to stimulate smooth muscle proliferation in blood vessels of the lung, thereby causing pulmonary hypertension. This will be discussed further in Chapter 36. Figure 10 illustrates the relation between some of the main angiogenic factors. All this sounds complicated enough, but any idea that the story is nearing completion should

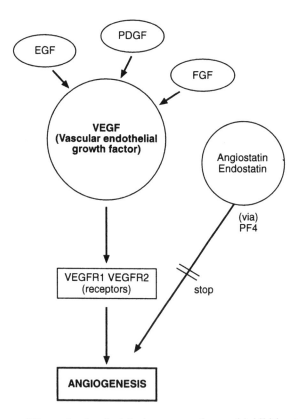

Figure 10 Some of the main chemical factors promoting and inhibiting the growth of blood vessels: EGF = epithelial growth factor; PDGF = platelet-derived growth factor; FGF = fibroblast growth factor; VEGFRI&2 = vascular endothelial growth factor receptors; PF4 = an angiogenesis inhibitor.

be dispelled by current estimates that there are about 50,000 discretely different proteins and protein sub-units in each cell of the body.

The normal rate of division of the endothelial cells lining blood vessels is about one division every 6 months, but under appropriate stimulation in rapidly growing tumours the replication rate can be at least 50, possibly 500 times faster. The relevance of endothelial growth stimulators to tumour growth is attested by observations that a high rate of VEGF production in breast cancers is associated with a shorter than average survival of the patient, presumably because the tumour can grow without being held back by shortage of nutrients.

Current interest in angiogenesis is growing because it opens up the possibility of inhibiting growth or spread of tumours by interfering with their blood supply. This can be done in many ways. The most obvious is to make an antibody to VEGF and inject it into the bloodstream. Alternatively, VEGF might be linked to a toxin (e.g. diphtheria toxin,)[2] thus producing damage to any cells which have receptors for VEGF. It might also be possible to prepare a chemical similar to VEGF but which would block its receptor. There are many possibilities. The main problem is that angiogenesis is also involved in wound healing, so that damaging side-effects might limit this form of therapy. But despite the potential problems, inhibition of angiogenesis has already been envisaged for the treatment of tumours which are known to have a large blood supply.

New blood vessels can also be inhibited by naturally occurring anti-angiogenic, usually called 'angiostatic' factors (e.g. angiopoietin-2, a naturally occurring antagonist for the Tie-2 receptor: see above). There is a particular family of related cytokines, the 'CXC chemokines', which can be either stimulators (e.g. IL-8) or inhibitors (e.g. PF4) of angiogenesis, depending whether or not one end of the molecule contains a specific sequence of three amino-acids, the 'ELR' group. Two further potent inhibitory factors have been identified by Judah Folkman's research group in Boston. (Folkman has been a leader since 1970 in the search for inhibitors of cancer angiogenesis.) 'Angiostatin' is a powerful inhibitor of the growth of endothelial cells. It has been observed to slow down the body-wide spread of some types of cancer in animals. It has turned out to be a fragment of plasminogen, a naturally occurring protein present in blood plasma and which is part of the system of interacting chemicals in the blood that dissolves clots.

The action of angiostatin was noted in a most interesting way. A single large cancerous tumour growing in a mouse seemed to inhibit the growth of smaller tumours round about the main tumour mass. The responsible chemical was purified and then identified, after immensely painstaking work extending over many years.[3] The same group of investigators have since discovered an even more powerful inhibitor of blood vessel growth, 'endostatin'. This is part of the structural protein 'collagen XVIII' which is found exclusively in blood vessels. It is present in detectable amounts in human circulating blood. A particularly exciting feature of endostatin function is that not only is it effective in shrinking malignant tumours in mice, it does not seem to induce resistance to its anti-tumour effects, as all standard anti-tumour drugs do. A report of the combined use of angiostatin and endostatin produced banner headlines in national newspapers because of the spectacular inhibition of malignant tumours in mice, even after they had spread widely. There has been recent difficulty in confirming all claims, but the subject remains a potentially exciting one. Several other fragments of normal body proteins, not themselves anti-angiogenic, have also been found to have anti-angiogenic activity (e.g. part of the hormone prolactin).[4]

Another interesting recent discovery is that the notorious drug thalidomide (which when taken by pregnant mothers sometimes causes maldevelopment of childrens' limbs) is an immunosuppressive drug which also has anti-angiogenic properties. It has already been used successfully to treat multiple myeloma, a highly vascular malignant condition.

Angiogenesis and anti-angiogenesis are part of a normally nicely balanced system in all tissues (Fig. 11). Given an appropriate local oxygen concentration, blood vessels will grow until the needs of a tissue or organ are fully met, after which the angiogenic stimulus is shut off and angiostatic factors turned on.

There is currently a fast rate of discovery of new stimulating and inhibiting factors. The large numbers of names and abbreviations is very confusing to entrants to this field. But to an onlooker like myself

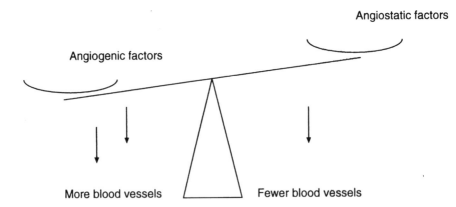

Figure 11 Cartoon emphasising that the density of blood vessels in any tissue is a balance between factors encouraging and factors inhibiting blood vessel growth.

it appears that cancer research may be in the process of changing its direction or at least its emphasis, in an extraordinarily interesting way.

Other requirements for the successful spread of tumours include increased extracellular matrix degradation by tumour- and host-secreted proteases (enzymes which can destroy protein), actual movement or migration of cells into host tissues, and reduction of cell-to-cell adhesion. In addition, programmed cell destruction (apoptosis: p. 97) has to be switched off or inhibited before unrestrained cell growth becomes possible.

In years to come many of the mysteries of cancer will be solved, though others will doubtless appear. The sort of mystery which studies of angiogenesis may help to solve is exemplified by a patient of mine who had a 'radical mastectomy' to remove a cancer of the breast, leaving a long scar over the site of her breast. (This unpleasant and mutilating operation has now been mostly abandoned, because careful controlled trials have shown that as good results can in most cases be achieved with much less radical surgery.) My patient remained well for 5 years, with no signs of recurrence of the tumour, until she had an attack of pneumonia, whereupon multiple individual nodules of cancerous tissue started growing all along the scar. In retrospect, it seems likely that a lot of individual cancer cells had been scattered in the wound during the initial operation, but that they had insufficient blood supply to multiply and grow. Then along came an infection which produced a lot of stimulatory circulating cytokines which switched on angiogenesis and got all the tiny lumps of residual tumour growing again.

Another patient, a man of 50, was sent to me with multiple circular shadows, about $\frac{3}{4}$ inch diameter, visible all over the lung fields in a chest X-ray. Other evidence suggested that he had an underlying cancer of the bowel which had spread (metastasised) to the lungs. He felt well: so well, indeed, that he refused to give permission for one of the presumed tumour nodules to be removed and examined under the microscope, though there could be no reasonable doubt that he had multiple lumps of a malignant tumour of some sort. I watched him at increasingly long intervals with chest X-rays for about 10 years until I left my clinical service at St. Bartholomew's Hospital in London. The tumour nodules never got any bigger, but never went away. In retrospect it seems likely that some powerful angiostatic factor had stopped the tumours spreading. Unhappily such phenomena are extremely rare. This is the only example I have ever seen myself of the spontaneous arrest of already widely spread tumours. But however rare such occurrences may be, they give us hope that at least some cancers may eventually prove to be controllable by anti-angiogenic therapy. The first human trials of this type of therapy are getting under way. A recent report suggested that the administration of an antibody against vascular endothelial growth factor may have (slightly) slowed down the progression of nodules of already disseminated cancer of the kidney.[5]

Other aspects of angiogenesis

All that I have done in this short chapter is to introduce some of the many remaining mysteries about cancer. There is an interesting shift in research away from exclusive concentration on identifying the genetic make-up of malignant cells towards understanding how such cells can invade normal tissues and secure themselves a blood supply when they do. Such studies overlap with many aspects of physiology. For example, each month an egg (ovum) is shed from a fertile woman's ovary and is conveyed to the womb. New tissue starts growing in the bed of the egg in the ovary, forming the 'corpus luteum' (Latin: 'yellow body'). This shrivels up if the egg is not fertilised; but if it is, the corpus luteum continues to grow. It then secretes hormones which support the first three months or so of the pregnancy.

There is much current interest in the interplay of angiogenic and angiostatic factors in the growth and shrivelling up of each corpus luteum. VEGF and its receptors have been identified as playing a major role, as also have insulin-like growth factor (IGF) and its receptors. Sex steroids play some part both in angiogenesis of new lining tissue (endometrium) of the womb at the beginning of the menstrual cycle and in shutting down endometrial blood vessels if pregnancy does not occur, so that the endometrium is shed. This latter action is made use of in 'hormone replacement therapy' (HRT). For example, the 17-αhydroxyprogesterone derivatives incorporated in HRT preparations prevent undue endometrial growth by shutting down the blood vessels of the womb.

New blood vessel formation is also an important factor in the healing of all but the smallest wounds. The excessive formation of new blood vessels in the retina of the eye in people with diabetes is nowadays the commonest cause of acquired blindness. I shall explain in Chapter 22 why I suggested that PDGF might be the immediate cause of clubbing of the fingers. New blood vessel formation (angiogenesis) is a necessary part of the formation of pannus (p. 94) in rheumatoid joints. There is current interest in the possibility of limiting joint damage by preventing pannus formation, by angiostatic treatment.

Angiogenesis is also relevant to the formation of plaques of atheroma (Greek: *athere* = gruel, porridge), the cholesterol-rich deposits which narrow and obstruct large arteries and which are the main cause of heart attacks and strokes (Chapter 20). Angiogenesis is necessary for new small blood vessels to grow in blood vessel walls and also to nourish damaging lumps of atheroma and allow them to grow. Drug or dietary treatment of arterial disease can directly lessen atheroma plaques and at the same time reduce the number of new blood vessels in the plaques.

Anti-angiogenic drugs may act directly, or perhaps by the subtle but so far rather disappointing 'anti-sense' approach[6] in which synthetic DNA fragments are designed to combine with and inactivate a damaging gene. Anti-angiogenesis treatment may also interfere with normal wound healing, and with the processes of recovery from blocked arteries in the heart and elsewhere.

Summary

The study of new blood vessel formation is a very fast-moving field at present. Angiogenesis is involved in many processes: e.g. in wound healing, in the growth and decay of the ovarian corpus luteum in women's reproductive life and in the formation of destructive pannus in rheumatoid joints. Recently there has been great interest in the possibilities of inhibition of growth of new blood vessels in cancer. Since no tumour can get to a damaging size unless it has an adequate blood supply, there is enormous current excitement in the possibilities of anti-angiogenic treatments. At present this approach looks (to me) as if it might even match or overtake drugs which directly attack and kill cancer cells.

An anti-cancer treatment designed to prevent tumours getting an adequate blood supply has to be very selective to interfere with the damaging formation of new blood vessels supplying tumours without interfering with important normal functions, but results in animals using this approach look promising. Watch this space!

8

OSTEOARTHRITIS

The word itself is misleading. The combination of the two Greek words, *osteon* = bone and *arthron* = joint, is fine as far as it goes. But the suffix '-itis' denotes 'inflammation of'. A current textbook defines osteoarthritis (OA) as 'an inherently *non*-inflammatory disorder of movable joints characterised by deterioration of articular cartilage and by the formation of new bone at the joint surfaces and margins'. The word 'inflammation' suggests 'flaming within'. Inflamed joints certainly feel hot to the touch. Under the microscope such joints as are seen in acute rheumatoid arthritis (described in the next chapter) are full of white cells from the blood. These appear to be attacking invading organisms or damaged tissues. In osteoarthritis, on the other hand, affected joints are typically cool. The joint tissues are not packed with attacking or defending white blood cells. So the name is misleading. Perhaps we do best to call osteoarthritis simply 'degenerative joint disease'. Continental Europeans sometimes call OA 'osteoarthrosis', but this is also misleading because the suffix '-osis' in ordinary medical use in the UK signifies 'too much of'.

Bone is hard; but the surfaces of bones which come together in a joint are normally prevented from damaging each other's hard surfaces because these are covered by a 2–4 mm thick layer of cartilage (Latin: *cartilago* = gristle). Lubrication is supplied by 'hyaluronan', a matrix material which enables joint surfaces to slide over one another without causing damage. Hyaluronan is produced by the 'synovium', a thin layer of cells lining the joints. The word was invented by Paracelsus to mean 'joint oil'. In complex joints which involve movement in several planes further support is provided by an intervening articular disc of cartilage. Figure 12 illustrates diagrammatically the main structures of a simple synovial joint. Any or all these structures can be involved in an osteoarthritic joint.

Pain can arise from all parts of a joint except from cartilage, which is not usually supplied with pain nerves. Although the inside of bone is not pain sensitive either, the membrane covering bone (the periosteum) is, and so also is the synovium. The pathological changes of OA involve thinning and destruction of cartilage and remodelling of the

83

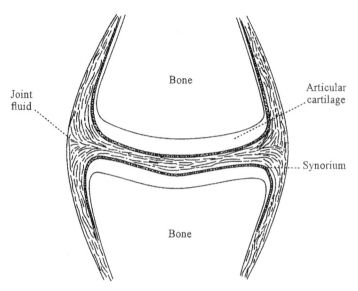

Figure 12 Diagrammatic section through a joint showing its various constituents. The hard end surface of each bone is covered by a thin layer of cartilage, itself covered by a thinner layer of cells (the synovium), which secretes joint fluid.

bone underneath it. In OA the articular cartilage becomes very thin or may even be absent, with consequent accelerated wear and tear of the bone surface underneath. The early changes in OA cartilage are increased water content – from the normal 70% by weight, to about 80%. Fine splits in cartilage can be seen under the microscope. The volume of fluid in affected joints may be increased, but there is no great increase in the number of its contained cells, such as are seen in inflamed joints. In severely osteoarthritic joints actual crystals of pyrophosphate are sometimes seen and deposited in joint cavities. They probably contribute to the wear and tear of joint surfaces.

There are various ways in which OA presents itself to a patient, and thence to the doctor. The main one is pain. This is usually aggravated by moving the joint. In most cases pain coming from an osteoarthritic joint stops quickly once the joint is at rest. This obviously suggests that pain has a protective function by making the sufferer avoid further injury. Experimentally, OA of a joint gets worse if the joint has been rendered pain free by cutting the posterior nerve roots carrying pain nerves from the joint up to the brain. At first sight this seems to prove the important protective function of pain nerves. But like many plausible interpretations and explanations of body functions, it is wrong. Alongside pain nerves from joints run nerves which convey to the brain the spatial position of each joint (the 'proprioceptive' nerves). It is the cutting off of information passing to the brain from these nerves that is mainly responsible for damaging joints.

Chemicals called 'prostaglandins', released from damaged joints, can cause inflammation and consequent pain. Aspirin, and so-called 'non-steroidal anti-inflammatory drugs' (NSAIDs) suppress prostaglandin release. There is continuing argument whether treatment of OA with NSAIDs like ibuprofen or diclofenac protects joints as well as reducing pain. In the UK at any time 85,000 people are regularly taking NSAIDs. These are really dangerous drugs, especially in the elderly. Each year about 12,000 hospital admissions are due to bleeding from the stomach, provoked by taking NSAIDs. About 1200 people, mostly elderly women, die each year from this complication. There are comparable figures from the USA: 100,000 hospital admissions, with 16,500 deaths. NSAIDs are not strictly pain-relieving (analgesic). They do not, like morphine, take pain away by acting directly on the brain. But they can unquestionably reduce pain, in most situations, by interfering with the local release of pain-producing chemicals. I do not know whether NSAIDs have any long-term effect on the progression or slowing down of OA. Long-term trial results are awaited.

Good pain relief with less danger of gut bleeding has been observed with selective inhibitors of inflammation-producing prostaglandins ('type-2 coxibs').[1] Unfortunately, one of these drugs (rofecoxib) was found to cause blood clotting and has been withdrawn. As far as I am aware, oral glucosamine (a normal nutritional supplement and a constituent of cartilage matrix and of synovial fluid) is the only material which has so far been shown in randomised double-blind placebo-controlled trials actually to slow down progression of OA (in the knee joint)[2] – even though it is largely metabolised in the gut.

OA of the hip is the most crippling manifestation of the disease. The hip joint comprises a 'ball' at the upper end of the thigh bone (the femur) and a 'socket' in the pelvis into which the ball fits snugly. The typical male former athlete, now much heavier than he was in his twenties, finds that weight-bearing and movements of one of his hips have become gradually more and more painful. Even the range of passive hip movement (i.e. manipulation of the leg by someone else) becomes gradually restricted. A good way to quantify the extent of hip disease is for a subject to lie supine on a flat surface with the knee of the affected leg bent to a right angle. Then the examiner can gently try to move the knee outwards (technically the process of abduction – from the Latin word *abductio* = movement away from the midline).

This process stretches the pain-sensitive fibrous capsule surrounding the hip joint and reveals any restriction of joint movement.

Many other large weight-bearing joints, notably the knee, are also affected by OA. Wear and tear can be surprisingly focal: i.e. only one portion of the articular surfaces of a joint may be affected by OA. The lower joints between the bones of the spine (the vertebral column) are commonly involved, as indeed can be almost any joint which is exposed to heavy compression and (still worse) sharp impacts across the joint plane. By contrast, frequent and repeated non-compressing movements of joints does not cause OA and need not wear out joints prematurely. Repair processes such as the renewal of cartilage by active cells (chondrocytes) can easily keep pace with minimal wear from repeated but lightly loaded joint movements.

As a lifelong clavier player myself I have marvelled at the pianistic prowess of 80-year-old concert pianists like Vladislav Richter, whose finger joints remained virtually as mobile as they were when he was in his teens. And this despite practising at the piano for many hours a day throughout his life and moving all the joints of all his fingers through their ranges, without any notable deterioration in function.

Epidemiology

OA is not present in the newborn, but its prevalence steadily increases with age. In most series and at most ages OA has been reported to be about twice as common in women as in men. Changes of osteoarthritis accompanied by pain or restriction of joint movement are present in about 10% of the general population. Above age 65 more than 50% of people in the UK have OA in one or more joints. Above age 75, 80% have the disease. Weight-bearing joints typically suffer from OA, but so also do joints through which extreme pressures and impacts have been applied. According to one evolutionary hypothesis, OA of the thumb base, which is common in man, is rare in Rhesus monkeys because monkeys do not grip objects between thumb and fingers.

Malformed joints often become prematurely osteoarthritic, presumably because they are subject to new forces which were not present in the course of evolution of the species. Surgical correction of joint deformities can reduce later development of OA.

A distinction is often made between 'primary' and 'secondary' osteoarthritis. 'Primary' is used to describe OA when there is no obvious precipitating factor and where the gross anatomy of the joint appears normal. There is controversy whether sufferers from hip OA already have structural differences from normal people before they experience joint pain. Most investigators have not been able to find any significant differences. The arthritis of Dachshund dogs is well known and usually ascribed to arthritis secondary to their tiny legs having to carry too big a weight burden. But I dislike a 'primary/ secondary' classification of osteoarthritis being applied in man. How can the stresses and wear on joint surfaces over many years be classified as primary when perhaps some trauma to a joint many years before has been forgotten? Unfortunate individuals can undoubtedly inherit a considerable genetic predisposition to OA. This most probably lies in cartilage metabolism and in different inherited rates of cartilage repair. Genetic OA would clearly have to be classed as primary.

Genetics

In the last few years we have heard a lot about 'Dolly', the first mammal successfully cloned from a single body cell – not an egg or sperm – taken from an adult sheep. As I write (in 2005) there has been great interest, and in some quarters, alarm, that Dolly apparently developed premature arthritis in a back leg joint. She needed methotrexate to control the inflammation, and had eventually to be killed. Although Dolly's body cells would have had the same basic genetic make-up (i.e. DNA) as that of the sheep which provided the original cell, Dolly was reported to have 20% shorter telomeres (p. 74) in the chromosomes of her body cells than normal sheep have in their chromosomes. One theory of ageing is that as each body cell divides during growth and development a small length of telomere is lost from each chromosome, and that when this exceeds a certain length, after perhaps about 50 divisions, future cell divisions do not work properly. Nuclear material is then lost, causing most of the symptoms and signs that we recognise as 'ageing'. Loss of skin elasticity is an obvious example. A recent report has suggested that rats successfully cloned from a single body cell do not live as long as rats conceived and born naturally. This again suggests that cloned individuals may not behave exactly as did their progenitors.

This concept of ageing, if correct, is fascinating on several counts. Clearly during the creation of each single strand of DNA, before it becomes part of a sperm or egg cell, there must be some mechanism for generating extra redundant telomeres on each chromosome in the new embryo. If this mechanism fails, the embryo would start life already partly aged. We do not know when this process begins or ends.

The rate at which cartilage cells (chondrocytes) become incapable of dividing further in single-layered cell cultures outside the body depends on the animal from which they have been taken. Chondrocytes from old rabbits age rapidly and often turn into fibrous tissue prematurely, whereas cells from young rabbits last longer. Human chondrocytes have not yet been observed to become incapable of dividing in culture,[3] but I suspect that they would become so eventually. These observations are fascinating because human OA is so strongly age-related. Maybe the human race has only been provided with a fixed life span for all its cartilage cells.

If the current accounts of Dolly in the popular press are correct, there may be a rather poor prospect for the successful cloning of human beings. Few people created through cloning will relish the prospect of finding themselves already prematurely aged when they become old enough to understand how they had been created! But Dolly also reminds us of the potential genetic component of osteoarthritis. This is being revealed by twin studies. Identical twins each tend to develop OA at about the same time in life, in the same joints, whereas non-identical twins usually do not behave in this way. But there is also an inherited predisposition to OA in general – shown, for example, by frequent 'Heberden's nodes' (small bony lumps on the back of the joints at the last segment of the fingers). People with many Heberden's nodes on their fingers have been shown to have more hip OA than those without them. Siblings of people who have undergone hip surgery, and who presumably have had hip OA, have a five-fold higher than expected risk of having hip OA themselves. The same applies to OA of the knee joints. Siblings have a 30% higher risk of developing knee OA if their sibling already has the condition.

Family clusters are commonly seen in many joint diseases as well as in OA. Most joint diseases, certainly OA, are influenced by many genes. We have not as yet been able to identify one or two specially important major genes, the inheritance of which leads to someone developing OA. The inheritance of osteoarthritis is evidently polygenic. What is inherited seems to be a predisposition which needs an environmental stimulus for its expression, as in so many of the medical mysteries described in this book.

Genetic studies in identical twins suggest that OA susceptibility may be particularly due to differences in cartilage composition and rates of cartilage repair. This is suggested by the observation that certain single gene defects can cause premature OA, e.g. collagen type II mutations. Apparent site specificity (e.g. the tendency of some families to have, say, OA of one particular joint) is most likely to be due to individual differences in body build inheritance and in muscle and joint ligament strength. It is also possible that there can be at least some additional element of site-specificity of cartilage metabolism as well.

Cause

Most research suggest that osteoarthritis probably involves 'interaction between intrinsic cartilage metabolism and extrinsic mechanical factors'. Cartilage metabolism (e.g. the rate of oxygen consumption) is increased in OA, possibly due to an action of hyaluronan.[4] Bone and probably cartilage growth can be stimulated by a single traumatic event, but in most situations a series of cumulative insults are usually needed to produce disease. There are lots of well known examples of bone outgrowth and OA being stimulated by undue repeated pressures: examples are 'wicket keepers' hand', 'ticket collectors' thumb', 'Zulu dancers' hip', 'coal miners' back', 'foundry workers' elbow' and 'whipkickers' knee': this last in competitive breast stroke swimmers. Approximate estimates suggest that regularly lifting weights of at least 22 pounds (10 kg) more than ten times a week, kneeling or squatting more than 1 hour a day, or getting up from kneeling or squatting more than 30 times daily carry high risks of knee OA. Excessive pressure is probably needed. It is well known that runners, for example, do not often suffer from OA of their hip and leg joints. But we have also to consider that successful runners may have been born with predisposing good features in their body structure of bones and joints which minimise traumatic pressures.

A search has been made for local factors which may cause damage to cartilage. Various cartilage-degrading and protein-degrading enzymes, especially the metalloproteinases, have been examined in OA to explore the possibility that OA might be prevented or alleviated by giving enzyme inhibitors. Another possibility is that abnormalities in the structure or function of bone immediately under cartilage in joints might cause OA. It has been reported that bone thickening sometimes precedes fine splits appearing in cartilage.[5]

Pressures in joints

There have been many investigations of the fluid pressures in joints, in case abnormal joint fluid pressures might be directly damaging, e.g. by restricting blood supply. Pressures can be measured by inserting a fluid-filled needle connected to a pressure-measuring device into the joint cavity. This has been done in man and in many animals, and in many joints. When normal joints are at rest and not under stress the pressures are usually sub-atmospheric. These negative pressures are generated by the osmotic pressure of the plasma proteins which in effect are sucking fluid from the joint cavities and returning it to the blood stream. This gives the shoulder, notably, some protection against dislocation additional to that provided by ligaments around the joint. In inflamed joints (e.g. in rheumatoid arthritis), the pressure in joints is invariably above atmospheric. This is a marker for joint inflammation.[6]

Any increase of pressure in a large joint is detected by sensory nerve endings in the joint capsule. Curiously, distension of an uninflamed joint does not cause pain, but has a profound direct inhibitory effect on the spinal cord neurones which supply the muscles working on the joint concerned. The magnitude of the inhibition is directly related to the pressure in the joint capsule. The consequent reduction in the force of contraction of all the muscles acting on the joint immediately reduces the pressure distending the joint.[7] I imagine that in the course of human evolution this inhibiting reflex has evolved to protect inflamed joints against undue mechanical damage, but it must be a major factor causing leg weakness in people with osteoarthritic joints.

Few investigations have been made of pressures inside osteoarthritic joints, but even slight distension of a joint capsule reduces muscle power. One recent investigation reported positive pressures of 7–21 mmHg in OA knee joints at rest, increasing to 20–116 mmHg during forceful isometric contraction of the knee muscles.[8] (Pressures between 7 and 116 mmHg correspond roughly in SI units to a range of 1–15 kPa). High pressures, maintained for any significant time, could reduce local blood flow to the joint tissues and risk metabolic damage. Pressures inside the hip joint in osteoarthritic hip fractures may rise to 60 mmHg or more even with the limb at rest. Consequentially impaired blood supply might be a main cause of so-called 'avascular' necrosis of the head of the main bone of the thigh (the femur).

Throughout life cartilage is being continually synthesised, but loss of cartilage thickness may occur in OA when the rate of cartilage synthesis is overwhelmed by increased rate of destruction of its collagen matrix. In an OA joint there may be islands of cartilage proliferation interspersed with areas of new bone formation.

The earliest change in OA joints is the appearance of microscopic splits (fibrillation) in the cartilage and reduction in its thickness. Is this due to increased stiffness of the underlying bone? Are the cells which make cartilage matrix (chondrocytes) abnormal, or is there an unduly fast breakdown rate of the collagen matrix? There have been many studies suggesting abnormal metabolism and enzyme function in OA cartilage, including increased breakdown of cartilage protein by enzymes (proteases). This may be stimulated by the generation of cytokines such as IL-1, IL-6 and TNFα which increase the rate at which destructive enzymes are synthesised.

A possible cause of abnormal cartilage and hence of undue propensity to OA is the presence of abnormal pigment in cartilage. One example is the common disease haemochromatosis, in which there is deposition of excessive amounts of inorganic iron (see Chapter 26). Another example is the rare disease ochronosis.

Excessive bone growth in joints

Bony overgrowth surrounding or in joints is a major cause of disability. One cause of excess bone growth is a single episode of localised bone trauma. I had the opportunity a few years ago to watch a Heberden's node develop on one of my fingers. My squash partner had accidentally hit me a hard blow with the wood frame of his squash racquet on the upper and outside surface of the end bone (the terminal phalanx) of my left index finger. (It was probably my fault for getting in his way.) The point of impact was tender for only a few days, but during the ensuing month there was growth of new bone at the site. I finished with a typical hard round bony Heberden's node of about 4 mm diameter at the original impact site. The bones and joints of my other fingers were unaffected. But an observation such as this suggests that a sudden blow or pressure on one of the bones of a joint can stimulate local bone growth and cause restriction of mobility – one of the features of an osteoarthritic joint.

To generalise, it appears that pressure on bone stimulates it to grow thicker. Sometimes this can get in the way of free movement of a joint. I have also had personal experience of this process. As a lifetime's squash player, I must have unduly stressed one of the joints above my right shoulder (technically, my acromio-clavicular joint). This caused the growth of extra bone around the joint. To relieve pain and restore full shoulder movements the bony excrescence had to be removed. After a minor surgical operation and a course of appropriate physiotherapy this restored a pain-free full range of shoulder movements.

Lack of the normal pressure and stress on any bone leads to reduction in bone density (osteoporosis: see Chapter 30). Astronauts living long periods in zero gravity spaceships need to stress all their bones regularly to prevent the rapid development of osteoporosis.

Environmental factors

Moose in Michigan's National Park have suffered a great recent increase in OA, suggesting the possibility that some infective agent may have been introduced into the Park. Around the same time there was also an epidemic of severe undernutrition. This suggests an alternative explanation: that the nutritional health of cartilage and its repair systems in the moose might have been irreparably damaged.[9] I am not aware of any reliable human observations suggesting either infection or specific undernutrition as a major cause of human OA, though the observation that concentrations of 'C-reactive protein' (a marker for inflammation) are often increased in human OA suggests the possibility of underlying infection.[10] Experimental transmission of OA to man by blood or joint fluids has not been reported, as far as I can discover.

Summary

Osteoarthritis (OA) is a longstanding (chronic) disorder of movable joints characterised by deterioration of the articular cartilage and by the formation of new bone at the joint surfaces and margins. It causes pain on movement. The new bone formation often limits full joint movement.

Muscle weakness and instability of a joint from any cause are strong predictors of the later development of osteoarthritis. In addition trauma, especially repetitive sharp trauma with heavy loading of joints, damages cartilage and may also lead to OA. Pre-existing structural abnormalities of bones and muscles may also favour its development. Cartilage defects can be solely responsible for OA, and a few inherited abnormalities of cartilage metabolism have been recognised. Cartilage implants are being increasingly used to repair osteoarthritic joints. But in most cases osteoarthritis involves a combination of muscle weakness, mechanical factors and impaired cartilage function.

9

RHEUMATOID ARTHRITIS

Rheumatoid arthritis (RA) is one of the commonest disabling diseases. A strict definition is impossible because its symptoms, signs and findings on investigation overlap with many other conditions. Because of this, the incidence of the disease (the number of new cases per year) has to be inferred by comparisons of prevalence estimates (the numbers of the population affected by the disease) made at different points in time. Such comparisons suggest that at least two in every 10,000 people will develop definite rheumatoid arthritis each year. At any time at least one in every 100 of the population will be suffering from the condition. This estimate of prevalence has been made using strict criteria for diagnosis. Everyday observation suggests that the real prevalence is much higher than this. Many mild cases are undoubtedly overlooked or not recorded. Although RA is not thought of as a fatal disease, about 1000 deaths per year in the United Kingdom are attributed to it, though many of these are misadventures with anti-rheumatoid therapy. The disease causes a lot of disability. About 75% of sufferers become significantly disabled within 3 years. Early diagnosis and consequently the early use of disease-modifying anti-rheumatic drugs have been shown to reduce eventual disability.

RA cannot be diagnosed by a single laboratory test or X-ray, but accepted criteria are (1) the presence of morning stiffness, (2) pain in three or more joint areas, (3) arthritis of the hand joints, (4) symmetrical joint involvement, (5) the presence of rheumatoid nodules, (6) raised levels of rheumatoid factor in blood, and (7) X-ray changes of bony erosions at joint surfaces. The first four of these must have been present for at least 6 weeks before the diagnosis can be established. The reason for the delay is that doctors cannot tell at the time whether an illness presenting in this way will clear up on its own or whether it will pass into the chronic stage we recognise as established rheumatoid arthritis. Smoking is associated with rheumatoid arthritis in men and may make the symptoms worse, but it seems to have no effect on RA in women.

Bone is hard; but bone surfaces in joints are covered with cartilage, which is smooth and relatively soft. As I described in the last chapter,

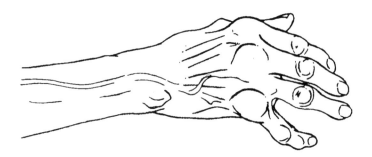

Figure 13 Drawing of a hand seriously affected by rheumatoid arthritis. The knuckles (the metacarpo-phalangeal joints) are severly swollen and the fingers are deviated in the opposite direction to the thumb (so-called 'ulnar deviation'). There is also considerable wasting of the small (intrinsic) hand and finger muscles.

lubrication is supplied by the matrix material (hyaluronan) secreted by the synovium. Several features are common to most cases of rheumatoid arthritis. One is that the synovium is mainly involved. In RA there is widespread inflammation of many synovial membranes, especially in the hands. The knuckles of the fingers (the metacarpo-phalangeal (MCP) joints), the first finger joints (the proximal inter-phalangeal (PIP) joints) are particularly affected and swell up (Fig. 13). The wrists, the knees and sometimes other joints may also be involved. The disease is roughly symmetrical in its manifestations: i.e. if a particular joint on one side is affected, the same joint on the other side is almost always involved, to a similar extent. There is also the formation of 'pannus' (Latin: cloth), a destructive tumour-like growth within joints caused by synovium invading cartilage and acquiring a blood supply of its own. This restricts joint movement and further damages joint surfaces. Another rather constant feature is the appearance of hard, usually painless, nodules under the skin of the elbows and forearms.

The bone around affected joints is often weakened or destroyed. One possible reason for this is the behaviour of certain white blood cells which accumulate in the synovial cavities of affected joints. When they are cultured outside the body they can aggregate and turn into single large cells with several nuclei. These have all the characteristics of 'osteoclasts', which are specialised cells able to remove bone. The same thing happening in rheumatoid arthritis probably accounts for the bone destruction which is always found around severely affected joints. This is also aggravated, and perhaps caused, by the secretion of many chemical growth factors, especially vascular endothelial growth factor (VEGF), which stimulate the development of blood vessels. I have already discussed VEGF in Chapter 7, in the context of blood vessels in tumours.

Growth factors are activated, i.e. their secretion is switched on, by the release of nuclear factor kappa B (NFκB). I have already mentioned this powerful activating factor in Chapter 2, in relation to asthma. It is notable that steroids antagonise the actions of NFκB, which probably explains why steroids are such effective treatment both for rheumatoid arthritis and asthma.

Rheumatoid factors and complement

'Rheumatoid factors' are specialised antibodies known as auto-antibodies.[1] These chemicals react with some of the body's own normal constituents – hence the term 'auto' (self). Rheumatoid factors are usually present in the blood in RA, though RA can occur without rheumatoid factors being present and rheumatoid factors can be found without RA. In general, rheumatoid factors are found associated with severe rather than mild disease. These circulating antibodies are produced by specialised cells in lymph glands and tissues, the B-lymphocytes. These comprise some of the non-pigmented white cells of the blood and seem to be particularly involved in RA. B-lymphocytes produce specialised Y-shaped protein molecules. The variable parts of these molecules can take on many shapes, allowing them to combine with and in effect wrap up many different foreign chemical molecules, making them harmless. In RA, unfortunately, there seems to be an abnormal survival and excess of B-lymphocytes, which attack synovial membranes and seem to treat them as foreign material.

An antigen-antibody complex or an antibody can set in motion (activate) a complicated sequence of linked chemical changes in certain constituents of the blood plasma (the fluid part not containing any cells). The chemicals concerned are all proteins or large polypeptides, predominantly made in the liver and present in the form of inactive enzyme precursors. Collectively they are referred to as 'complement'. More than 25 separate complement proteins have been identified. These can make an amplifying cascade of enzyme reactions reminiscent of the amplifying cascade of reactions involved in blood clotting. The so-called 'classical' complement pathway is activated by antibody-antigen complexes. A slower 'alternative' pathway can be activated by antibody alone or directly by invading microbes. A third activation pathway is associated with 'mannose-binding protein'.

Complement damages the membranes of cells perceived as foreign or coats the cells with a combination of complement proteins, forming the

95

so-called membrane attack complex (MAC). The body's defensive white blood cells then swallow up the coated cells. At different stages of the cascade of chemical reactions, cytokines are released. Complement activation and cytokine release play an important part in causing tissue damage in conditions such as rheumatoid arthritis. The complement system is also involved in causing hypersensitivity and in most immune reactions.[2] It makes potential targets for the suppression of damaging reactions. Despite this, complement effects are overall beneficial. Deficiencies of complement factors can have serious consequences. For example, a genetic defect in mannose-binding protein predisposes to particularly severe bacterial infections (e.g. those causing meningitis). The serious human disease, systemic lupus erythematosus, is strongly associated with (inherited) deficiencies of complement proteins (especially C1).

T-lymphocytes, mast cells and cytokines

The T-lymphocytes are involved in RA.[3] These cells are concerned with immune defences against direct attacks on body cells, rather than with resisting indirect attacks by the circulating defensive antibodies produced by B-lymphocytes. T-lymphocytes have been identified in rheumatoid-affected joint tissues. Arthritis can readily be induced in rats which have been first primed to respond to a foreign chemical antigen and then given injections of the same material into a joint. Although this sounds unlikely to occur naturally, defensive macrophage cells can carry foreign antigens into joint cavities.

At present the precise role of T-lymphocytes in RA is uncertain, though they are probably involved in the release of damaging cytokines. Treatment of patients with an antibody to the cytokine TNFα has been spectacularly successful in relieving RA patients of pain and disability, although there is some concern that this treatment may damage long nerve tracts. Unfortunately the improvement does not last long because the anti-TNFα-antibodies are themselves soon recognised by the body as foreign chemicals. The body then produces antibodies which inactivate them. This is unfortunately the story in many of the treatments for RA which have been tried over the years. Some patients initially improve, but problems appear with longer term therapy. Fortunately, newer synthetic and less immunogenic materials are coming along. In addition, prolonged relief of symptoms in rheumatoid arthritis can be obtained by giving anti-TNFα-antibodies combined with the anti-cell-dividing drug methotrexate, which decreases the production of antibodies. The ill effects of TNFα can also be blocked by etanercept, a synthetic protein which binds to receptors for TNFα and inactivates them. Its combination with metho-trexate is particularly effective in RA[4] though the combination can seriously lower the body's resistance to bacterial infection. Metho-trexate alone is already well established as a main treatment for rheumatoid arthritis, despite its potential ill effects.

Attempts have been made to treat severe rheumatoid arthritis by irradiating all lymphocyte-containing tissues with X-rays, thus destroying the T-cells which are (presumably) doing the damage. Unfortunately improvement was only short lived.

Certain specialised cells play an accessory role in the inflammation which characterises RA. One type is the 'mast' cell which is activated when an antigen becomes bound to a circulating IgE antibody. Mast cells derive from the bone marrow and contain granules which are released when the cells are activated. The granules notably contain the intensely destructive enzyme tumour necrosis factor alpha (TNFα) as well as histamine and other cytokines.

Other similar conditions: systemic lupus erythematosus

The best known rheumatoid arthritis lookalike is 'systemic lupus erythematosus' (SLE). The name describes the full-blown skin condi-tion with complications ('systemic' = involving organs and systems apart from, or in addition to, the skin; Latin: *lupus* = wolf – signifying destruction of flesh; Greek: *erythema* = redness of the skin). SLE is a more severe and aggressive inflammatory condition than RA. Vital organs such as heart, lungs and kidneys may be involved and damaged. In SLE there is deranged function of the B-lymphocytes as in many similar conditions, but the characteristic antibodies are unusual, being directed against the double-stranded DNA of cell nuclei: these are 'anti-nuclear antibodies'. Inherited deficiencies of certain complement proteins can strongly predispose someone to develop SLE.

During growth and indeed throughout life many body cells have to die at the end of their life span so that they can be replaced by new cells, during the remodelling of tissues and organs. Programmed death of cells is rapid and can take place without inflammation or the production of sensitising factors. The process has been named apoptosis (Greek: *apo* = from; *ptosis* = falling) – the word having been used originally to describe the normal shedding of leaves from trees in the autumn. Apop-tosis is brought about by a set of complex proteins called *caspases*.[5] These cause a rapid (20–30 minutes) controlled dissolution of the cell, without the production of inflammation.

But cells that are traumatised or infected can die in a different and potentially damaging way ('necrosis'), accompanied by inflammation. In RA and particularly in SLE it seems that apoptosis goes wrong and doesn't lead to a quiet and harmless programmed death of cells.[6] Certain chemicals (possibly phosphatidylserine) are left on the surfaces of dying cells. Such cells may then be treated as foreign material by the rest of the body. The consequence seems to be the start of a much more extensive process which damages many tissues other than simply joints, even though in its early stages SLE can produce similar symptoms and signs as RA.

Cause

Proper scientists disdain anecdotes. They are so often misleading. Despite this I shall start with a true story. Its message is difficult to ignore. I had been a regular visiting professor in a Canadian university medical school. My wife and I had used the occasion to take two splendid holidays in a small fishing lodge in Ontario. The owner was a highly athletic man in his early forties who was an expert water skier. When we first met him he took pride in his skill and seemed to have inexhaustible energy. But when we stayed at the lodge in the following year he was a changed man. He had been struck down quite suddenly, within a week or two, with severe pain in wrists, knees and ankles, which swelled up. He told us that tests had shown that he had developed severe rheumatoid arthritis. His athletic activities were greatly curtailed.

This example convinced me that whatever other causes of rheumatoid arthritis may sometimes operate, some external environmental factor must have set the disease in motion in this man. It is true, of course, that there are inherited diseases of middle age which can arise in people who had previously appeared entirely normal. Huntington's disease is an example. This causes incoordination, progressive dementia and death in middle age. But neither it nor any other disease determined by a single gene defect starts in a middle-aged adult as suddenly as rheumatoid arthritis did in the case I described. There is some genetic influence on rheumatoid arthritis, as indeed there is in virtually all diseases and conditions – even on liability to road traffic accidents! But Danish studies looking at concordance rates in nearly 40,000 twin pairs showed surprisingly little influence of heredity. Identical twins had only slightly greater mutual resemblance in respect of RA than did non-identical (dizygotic) twin pairs.[7]

More is known about the cause of a less serious and usually self-limiting disease known as 'reactive arthritis' (previously known as

'Reiter's disease'). This is usually triggered either by a bacterial sexually-transmitted infection, usually with *Chlamydia trachomatis* (which causes discharge from the penis in men) or by a gut infection causing diarrhoea. After a few weeks one or more large joints swell up and become painful. The reaction occurs because a small portion of the protein constituents of an infecting organism, perhaps only a sequence of 10 or 12 amino-acids, acts as an antigen and brings about a damaging T-cell defence reaction. Certain genetic variants of the HLA system (see note 9, p. 474), especially HLA B27, when triggered by an appropriate infecting organism, may cause 'ankylosing spondylitis', a serious and disabling disease.

Although some environmental factor such as an infection may well be the 'seed' of RA as well as of reactive arthritis, an appropriate genetic inheritance (the 'soil') is usually also needed. As in reactive arthritis, certain inherited human leucocyte antigens (HLA) seem to predispose to the disease, though an external trigger is needed to start the disease off. There is a lot of evidence incriminating infections in many varieties of infective-immune disease, but so far no single infectious agent has been identified as the trigger for rheumatoid arthritis.

Atopy describes a common partly inherited allergic constitution, discussed in Chapter 2. It seems to confer some protection against rheumatoid arthritis, but is associated with asthma. Since atopy describes an individual's strong allergic reaction to external agents, its lack of association with RA provides some further evidence in favour of RA being initiated by an infection. Retroviruses (p. 473) and gut bacteria have been the most intensively studied candidates so far.[8] *Parvovirus B19*, which causes 'erythema infectiosum' (also known as 'fifth disease'), is common and found worldwide. In children the disease is usually mild and self-limiting, though it is sometimes associated with transient joint pains. Most children acquire the infection between the ages of 4 and 10. It appears to be specially associated with juvenile rheumatoid arthritis. The connection with adult rheumatoid arthritis is less certain, since antibodies to the virus are found in the majority of adults, but evidence incriminating *parvovirus B19* seems to be getting stronger.[9]

Many other infections have been suspected of triggering rheumatoid arthritis, e.g. Lyme disease and flavivirus. Both these infections can be carried by ticks. Sufferers from RA seem to have been more often exposed to cats in the home than those not so exposed, though more data are needed for this association to be convincing.

If an external infecting agent is involved in causing rheumatoid arthritis, there should often be time and space clustering of cases: i.e. there should be many cases in a particular district, or many cases should occur at around the same time. Such evidence of external infection has been looked for, but not convincingly shown.[10] As far as it goes, this is evidence against an ubiquitous virus infection spread by the air, or by water supplies. However, there is some fascinating historical evidence suggesting the existence of an extrinsic triggering infection. Severe rheumatoid arthritis produces characteristic bone changes. Old skeletons in North America show that rheumatoid arthritis has occurred there for thousands of years, whereas there is no such evidence from buried bones in Europe until the end of the fifteenth century. Columbus's sailors returned to Europe in 1493 and are often blamed for the epidemic of syphilis which spread across Europe at that time. It is tempting to suggest that they might have also brought another infection, perhaps *parvovirus B19*, which might have played some part in rheumatoid arthritis taking hold in Europe. But this can only be regarded at present as just an intriguing speculation.

There may be a parallel with the Epstein-Barr (E-B) virus, which has sometimes been thought to be involved in causing rheumatoid arthritis. As I have already mentioned in Chapter 3, the E-B virus is an ubiquitous herpes virus which infects most children in Europe and North America. Such children may show no evidence of infection at all, or at worst have a mild respiratory illness or sore throat and think nothing of it. Thereafter they become immune to further infections with the same virus. Those who are unlucky enough not to get infected in childhood, but who acquire infection as adults, may suffer from 'glandular fever' (also known as 'infectious mononucleosis'). In my observation of many cases of this common illness, the symptoms are more severe the older you are when you get it. This is not due to any change in the virus itself, so it must be due to older people having less active or effective immune protection. Glandular fever usually clears up in a few weeks: but it can also occasionally lead to more serious conditions such as Hodgkin's lymphoma.

An analogous scenario could be envisaged for human *parvovirus B19*. This infects the majority of young children. Is it possible that those unlucky enough to escape childhood infections but who encounter the virus as adults might react adversely and develop rheumatoid arthritis? If the great majority of adults are already immune to *parvovirus B19*, time and space clustering of new cases of rheumatoid arthritis might not necessarily be expected even if the parvovirus was its immediate cause. A large prospective study would be needed to investigate the possibility. It would involve screening young adults for evidence of previous *parvovirus B19* infection, to find whether those previously uninfected were those who later developed rheumatoid arthritis and at the same time developed antibody evidence of parvovirus infection. The possibility is an exciting one, because of the possibilities not only of opening up more specific therapy than exists at present but also of developing some kind of protective vaccination against RA.

Summary

Rheumatoid arthritis is a common disabling disease which may affect many joints, but particularly the smaller joints of the hands. Joints are usually affected symmetrically. The joint lining (synovium) is inflamed. Both sections of the body's immune system (both 'B' and 'T' lymphocytes) are involved. Damage occurs by release of cytokines such as tumour necrosis factor alpha (TNFα). The blood often contains auto-antibodies known as 'rheumatoid factors'.

Probably the best general statement about the cause of rheumatoid arthritis is that it is an 'infective-immune' disease. That is, the disease is a response by the body's immune system to a variety of common infective agents, especially viruses. There is probably no inescapable need to regard it as an 'auto-immune' disease, i.e. one set in motion by the body's immune defences treating one of the parts or organs of the body as if it was foreign. It might rather be that the body's immune defences against an infecting organism may not be specific or targeted accurately enough to attack the invader without harming the individual.

Many viruses and bacteria have at times been linked with rheumatoid arthritis, though no apparent link has been entirely consistent or stood the test of time. An attractive possibility, not yet disproved, is that an infection of an adult by Epstein-Barr virus, or (more plausibly) *parvovirus B19*, might initiate rheumatoid changes when someone previously unexposed in childhood first encounters the infection.

10

DUODENAL AND STOMACH ULCERS

An ulcer in the stomach or duodenum normally implies a 'chronic' (i.e. non-sudden) hole or break in any lining surface of the body. People can get ulcers anywhere on their skin surface. They can also get them in any part of the gut, which in the human embryo is formed by infolding of the skin. The designation 'peptic' (from the Greek: *pepsis* = digestion), when applied to an ulcer, refers to ulcers in the stomach or duodenum. It appears that the lining wall of the organ concerned has been digested by the powerful stomach juices. At this site the gut has presumably lost its protective coat. Its raw surface is the ulcer.

The gullet (oesophagus) leads from the mouth cavity (pharynx) to the upper part of the stomach (the fundus). The lower part of the stomach leads to its exit portal, the pylorus (Greek: *pyloros* = gatekeeper) which joins it to the duodenum (Fig. 14). The duodenum was so called because it was reckoned to be as long as twelve times the thickness of a finger (Latin: *duodeni* = twelve). The stomach lining produces hydrochloric acid and also protein-degrading chemicals (enzymes) collectively described as 'pepsin'. Although the duodenal contents are normally alkaline, acid juice is squirted into the duodenum by active contractions of the lower part of the stomach every time the muscle of the pylorus relaxes. The typical site for a duodenal ulcer is that part of the duodenum which first receives the squirt of stomach acid. The lining membrane of both organs is described as 'mucous', i.e. covered by 'mucus' – a translucent viscid fluid secretion which lines the inner walls of the organs and which is a powerful protection against self-digestion.

Most of our body, except for the skin and gut, comprises what the great nineteenth-century French physiologist Claude Bernard described as the *milieu intérieur*, in which physical changes such as temperature and acidity are controlled within narrow limits and from which potentially damaging infectious material is excluded. But the upper part of the gut is quite different. This is where the outside world, in the shape of food and drink, comes suddenly into massive, uncontrolled and potentially threatening intimate contact with the *milieu intérieur*.

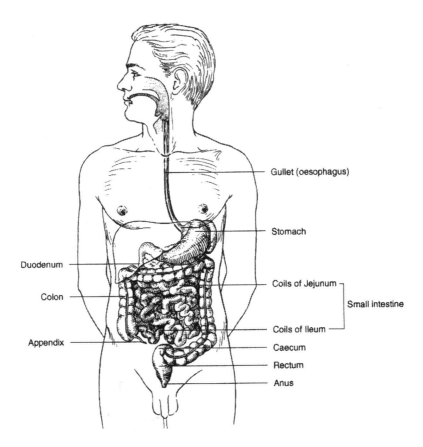

Figure 14 Diagram of the main structures of the gut. The gullet (oesophagus) takes food from the back of the mouth (the pharynx) to the stomach. The stomach leads into the duodenum, which itself leads into coils of jejunum and ileum – all comprising the 'small intestine'. The ileum leads into the 'large intestine' which comprises the colon, the appendix, the caecum and the rectum, before terminating at the anus.

The normal processes of food digestion and absorption

Some digestion starts even before food reaches the stomach. Saliva contains amylase (an enzyme which breaks down starch and sugars) as well as other chemicals which help to destroy harmful bacteria. But stomach acid is a more important first line of defence. Human beings and many animals secrete hydrochloric acid into the stomach from the gland cells which line its walls.

Hydrochloric is, to a chemist, a 'strong'[1] acid. In concentrated form it can be bought from ironmongers' shops, where (in the UK) it is known as 'spirits of salt'. The bottle gives off acrid fumes. Hydrochloric acid can dissolve many metals and break down many potentially harmful organic compounds. It is remarkable that the human stomach makes use of such a dangerous material. The stomach secretes hydrochloric acid at about 5% strength (150 mmoles/litre), at a rate which varies a lot between different people. Its rate when maximally stimulated is between 10 and 80 mmoles per hour.

The acid/base status of the body as a whole is very close to neutrality (pH = 7.0). Blood and most body fluids other than stomach secretions are slightly alkaline (pH greater than 7.0) and would turn litmus paper blue. On the other hand, fluids inside most body cells are slightly on the acid side of neutrality (pH less than 7.0) and would turn litmus paper red. The production of a strongly acid secretion like stomach juice is performed by specialised (parietal) cells which line the main body of the stomach – the upper part. This process requires a considerable supply of energy, which is derived from 'ATP' (adenosine triphosphate: p. 464). Between meals these cells are kept at rest (inhibited) by a circulating chemical (a hormone), a peptide called 'somatostatin'. This is produced by so-called 'S' cells which are widely distributed in every part of the stomach but particularly concentrated in its lower part.

When food gets to the lower part of the stomach (the 'antrum': Latin = cave) it triggers the release into the bloodstream of two other hormones collectively called 'gastrin',[2] secreted by other cells which line the stomach (known as 'G' cells: Fig. 15). Secretion reaches a peak about an hour after a meal. Gastrin circulates throughout the body but comes back to the stomach and acts on it to increase the rate of synthesis and release of hydrochloric acid. Gastrin not only directly stimulates the parietal cells of the stomach, it also releases another chemical (histamine), which is concerned elsewhere in the body with allergic reactions. Histamine is secreted by specialised cells which lie close to the acid-secreting cells in the stomach wall. In the stomach histamine acts in concert with gastrin to increase acid secretion. Simply distending the stomach also directly stimulates its lining cells to produce acid.

There is a useful short review available of the normal physiology of the processes of digestion and the disturbances which underlie peptic ulcers.[3]

Stomach secretions not only contain hydrochloric acid, they also start off the digestive processes with protein-degrading enzymes collectively described as 'pepsin'. These work in the acid medium which the stomach provides. The secretion of slimy mucus is also important and gives some

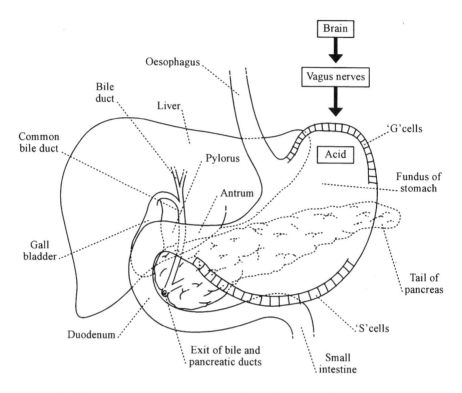

Figure 15   The main structures concerned with acid secretion by the stomach.

protection against self-digestion of the stomach lining, as does its contained bicarbonate (a weak alkali).

In addition to the control of acid secretion by gastrin, acid secretion
can also be switched on by the vagus nerves which arise in the lower
part of the brain (the medulla) and travel down the neck. The vagus
nerve endings release the chemical neurotransmitter acetylcholine. This
is the main mechanism involved in the secretion of stomach acid in
response to the sight, smell and taste of food, even before any food has
entered the stomach. Other branches of the vagus nerves can directly
activate the G cells to release gastrin.

These complex pathways have been investigated by observing the
effects of various blocking drugs: e.g. atropine to block acetylcholine
release from the endings of the vagus nerves, and a specific class of anti-
histamine drugs to block histamine released from stomach-lining cells.
For many years such drugs provided the best available treatment for
peptic ulcers. They greatly reduced hydrochloric acid secretion and
helped to heal peptic ulcers. In many countries of the world they were at
one time the single class of drugs most commonly prescribed by doctors.

When acid gastric juices pass out of the stomach into the duodenum they stimulate the release of another hormone (secretin) which, like gastrin, circulates in the blood.[4] When it comes back to the pancreas it triggers the release of alkaline pancreatic juices. These contain powerful digestive enzymes which break down food to enable it to be absorbed further down the gut.

Yet another hormone is released from cells in the wall of the duodenum when food and acid reach them – cholecystokinin/pancreozymin (CCK/PZ). This single hormone acquired a double name because of its double properties. It circulates in the blood and stimulates the gall bladder to contract, thus releasing bile – hence the name 'cholecystokinin'. CCK/PZ also travels round to the pancreas in the blood circulation and stimulates that organ to release its digestive juices – hence the name 'pancreozymin'. It was only after the two chemical compounds were elucidated that CCK and PZ were found to be identical. CCK/PZ is closely related chemically to gastrin and shares some degree of cross-reactivity with gastrin.

When all goes well a coordinated set of chemical reactions are set off as food passes through the stomach and on through the duodenum to the rest of the gut. The initially sterilising strong acid in the stomach is neutralised in the duodenum by alkali in the pancreatic secretions and in bile. This allows the powerful enzyme trypsin from the pancreas to break down proteins. Trypsin also activates several other digestive enzymes secreted into the duodenum. This indirect action normally helps to protect the pancreas from digesting itself. But when it fails to do this the consequences can be catastrophic and fatal (Chapter 12). Pancreatic secretions also contain many other enzymes which break down fats, starches and sugars.

Bile, like pancreatic juice, is alkaline. Bile also contains 'bile salts'. These act like detergents. They help to emulsify fats and make them soluble, so that they can be acted on by other pancreatic enzymes (lipases).

Peptic ulcers

The walls of both stomach and duodenum are supplied with nerves which control their movements and their secretions. They also contain sensory nerves which signal pain sensations to the brain when local damage releases pain-producing chemicals. Ulcers may be of any size from $\frac{1}{4}$ inch to an inch or more across (5-25 mm). They can occur in either the stomach or duodenum. Duodenal ulcers (DUs) are commoner than simple gastric ulcers (GUs). Usually there is loss only of the superficial lining layers of the walls of the duodenum or stomach, but ulcers in either site can 'perforate' – i.e. produce a hole right through the wall into the peritoneal cavity, or sometimes into an adjacent organ. A leak of strong acid into the peritoneal cavity can produce severe and agonising pain. It is a well-recognised and often fatal surgical emergency. But at University College Hospital one morning I examined a local flower-seller from Warren Street Underground station who insisted on returning to his stall after I had made a firm clinical diagnosis of stomach perforation and confirmed this by an X-ray which showed the presence of gas below his diaphragm. He told me that his future livelihood absolutely depended on selling all his flower stock that day. Happily, he survived that agonising day after a surgeon had closed up the stomach perforation in the evening.

Pain from a stomach ulcer is typically felt centrally in the upper abdomen (the epigastrium). A doctor will strongly suspect that abdominal pain is coming from the stomach if the pain comes on soon after eating. The suspicion will increase if the pain can be relieved by neutralising stomach acid with an alkali like baking soda (sodium bicarbonate). Conversely, if sodium bicarbonate provides no relief from pain, there may be some other explanation. The chemical equation

$$HCl \text{ (hydrochloric acid)} + NaHCO_3 \text{ (sodium bicarbonate)} \rightarrow \text{turns into } NaCl \text{ (salt)} + H_2O \text{ (water)} + CO_2 \text{ (carbon dioxide)}$$

reminds us that stomach acid acting on baking soda produces carbon dioxide gas – hence the 'burping' which accompanies this treatment.

Ulcers in the wall lining the duodenum can produce pain of similar intensity and location to that from a stomach ulcer. It is very variable from day to day. Traditionally medical students are taught that stomach ulcer pain comes on within a few minutes after eating a meal, whereas duodenal ulcer pain comes on later, half and hour to 2 hours after a meal, when food has had time to reach the duodenum. It is also commonly felt in association with hunger. Excess acid may be secreted in anticipation of a meal, even before food has entered the stomach.

Food can relieve the pain of a DU, at least temporarily, by providing a chemical buffer which reduces the acidity of stomach contents. Pain from a DU may occur at night and wake its victim. But my experience is that the clinical distinction between DU and GU symptoms is often difficult. Furthermore, peptic ulcer pain can be confused with pain from the pancreas gland or from the gall bladder. Both organs lie in a similar region of the abdomen and are supplied with nerves which can convey rather similar pain sensations when inflamed or stretched.

There are also other sources of central upper abdominal (epigastric) pain. One of the most notorious is myocardial infarction – a 'heart attack' due to a blocked coronary artery (p. 214). Both the patient and his doctor may think that the pain is some form of 'indigestion' – an imprecise and often misleading term – when it is in fact coming from a damaged heart. I have also several times been confused by pain from an abdominal aneurysm leaking blood into the back or (less commonly) into the abdominal cavity. An aneurysm is an abnormally overstretched main artery (the aorta). A leak of blood from an aneurysm can produce pain in the front of the abdomen as well as in the back. Ulcer-mimicking pain can also derive from the spine, or from a partly obstructed main gut artery. Fortunately nowadays it is almost always possible to make a precise diagnosis of peptic ulcer by directly inspecting the stomach and the upper part of the duodenum after passing down the throat a flexible gastroscope with a light at its end. An X-ray of the stomach (a barium meal) can also sometimes reveal and locate an ulcer, but has the serious disadvantage that it does not allow the removal of a small bit of the ulcer tissue, so that it can be examined under the microscope and checked for cancer.

A tissue (histological) diagnosis is absolutely necessary in middle-aged or elderly people whose pain may be caused by stomach cancer rather than by a simple ulcer. Gastric ulcers at any age need to be properly investigated because cancer of the stomach has a bad outlook anyway and an even worse one if diagnosis and proper treatment are delayed.

There is ongoing argument about the cost/benefit ratio of different levels and frequencies of investigation of possible duodenal ulcers at different ages, taking account of the serious consequences of overlooking stomach cancer. Although in the past I have several times refused – on grounds of national economy – to arrange further investigations of young men who gave entirely typical stories of duodenal ulcer, I would now prefer to make the certain diagnosis which gastroscopy provides. I have sometimes been slow to appreciate that patients may need to have an exact diagnosis for all sorts of strange and unlikely reasons – e.g. life insurance – and that it is not my job to prevent them getting accurate information. The modern appreciation that duodenal ulcers are often caused by infection (see below) suggests a better strategy: i.e. to treat with appropriate antibiotics for a week or two and reserve further investigation for people whose symptoms are not relieved. This line of management is becoming increasingly used.

Clinical decisions can be difficult. In my general medical NHS clinic at Barts I was once consulted by an enormously obese world-famous musician in his eighties who had recently suffered emotional stress and who described entirely typical symptoms of a duodenal ulcer. When I examined him there were no sinister features except that at his age stomach cancer was very likely. But because of his extreme obesity I could envisage little realistic prospect of successful cancer surgery. I therefore arranged no investigations whatsoever, reassured him, and gave him H2-blockers and antacids. These relieved his symptoms. I did not see him again until we met on a social occasion some years later. Fortunately he (and, I suppose, I) were lucky. We both 'got away with it'. He died later of an entirely different condition. Medical practice sometimes involves judging possible risk against probable benefit, not only for choice of treatment but even for medical investigation.

Bleeding

I have mentioned perforation as a complication of peptic ulcers. The other important complication is bleeding. Any inflammation or loss of the stomach lining can obviously produce acute bleeding. I remember seeing in the emergency department of University College Hospital a young woman complaining of abdominal pain and vomiting blood with a lot of mucus in it. She said that the pain started soon after eating a coconut ice sweet, given to her by a man working in the same chemist's establishment where she worked. The symptoms seemed so odd that I suspected poisoning and called in the police, who later arrested the man involved. It turned out that he had sprinkled cantharidic acid powder over the sweets which he had given to my patient and to her girlfriend. He had been trying to excite the girls sexually. My patient was admitted to our medical wards, her friend to another hospital.

Cantharidic acid is the active principle extracted from so-called 'Spanish Fly'. It causes an intense inflammatory reaction in any human tissue with which it comes into contact. Both unfortunate girls died 2 days later from extensive damage to their gut. The man was convicted of manslaughter.

Sometimes bleeding from the stomach lining can be very slight and intermittent, but so persistent that it causes iron deficiency anaemia. In my experience this is very uncommon with simple peptic ulcers. A sudden massive haemorrhage, resulting in the vomiting of large amounts of blood (a 'haematemesis') is much more characteristic. It may be followed by the passage of a loose, tarry, black stool (faeces) comprising partly digested blood. It is in this situation that endoscopic investigation – looking directly into the stomach and duodenum with an instrument – really comes into its own. It enables a precise diagnosis to be made and may allow the source of bleeding to be dealt with directly.

Stomach bleeding is often provoked and is especially common in elderly women who have been treating their painful joints with non-steroidal anti-inflammatory drugs (NSAIDs) like ibuprofen and diclo-fenac. A recent survey suggested that about 15% of retired people in the UK are regularly taking NSAIDs. Infection of the stomach with a bacterium called *Helicobacter pylori* (see below) seems to act in combination with NSAIDs to precipitate bleeding from the stomach.[5]

Many years ago I asked a surgeon to operate on a middle-aged man with an X-ray-confirmed duodenal ulcer which had apparently been insidiously bleeding, causing an iron-deficiency type of anaemia. The surgeon and I agreed that the patient needed removal of the acid-secreting parts of the stomach (a so-called partial gastrectomy). At the time this was considered to be the best treatment for DU. At operation my patient certainly had a duodenal ulcer, but the surgeon had a look around inside the abdomen before proceeding further. He found an obvious cancer of the transverse colon and dealt with this rather than with the duodenal ulcer which had been thought to have been the source of the bleeding. This experience reinforced my clinical impression that peptic ulcers often cause a large acute bleed on a specific occasion, but don't often bleed slowly and insidiously. I am unsure if this clinical impression has been properly established by an epidemiological survey. Nowadays there are clear and agreed guidelines about the need to investigate the whole of the gut when iron-deficiency anaemia is diagnosed.

Epidemiology

Duodenal ulcers, though very common, have been declining slowly in incidence for many years. Some estimates suggest that 10–15% of men in many parts of the world have suffered from them. Women have usually been less affected, though after the menopause the sex difference disappears. There is notable geographic variation in the UK. People in Scotland and the north of England are more affected than people in the south. Smoking and high alcohol drinks are highly provocative factors, as are NSAIDs (see above).

There is some suggestive historical evidence that duodenal ulcers were rare in Western Europe until the beginning of the twentieth century. Since we now know that a specific bacterial infection underlies 95% of duodenal ulcers and about 70% of gastric ulcers, it is tempting to suppose that the infectious agent responsible for peptic ulcers might have been introduced into Europe at about this time. The role of infection in the causation of peptic ulcers has only been recognised in the last two decades, DU having been thought of during most of my own career as some sort of stress disorder. There are still large gaps in our knowledge of its natural history and epidemiology.

Genetics

The late Iain Aird observed that there were proportionately more people with Blood Group O having surgical operations for duodenal ulcer than people with other blood groups. This points strongly to some genetic predisposition to peptic ulceration, perhaps in the way that the stomach responds to local infection. I have always admired this observation. It is an elegant example of an important observation being made simply by the retrospective examination of hospital notes – since candidates for DU surgery necessarily have their blood groups analysed and recorded.

Cause

One way to discover the cause of a disease is to study it in animals. Unfortunately this doesn't work for peptic ulcers. They are unknown in animals, even though many animals have stomachs which secrete digestive enzymes in a strongly acid stomach juice. It is possible to produce acute peptic ulcers in animals by rubbing off the protective mucous layer of the organ concerned by various traumatic manoeuvres. This produces acute peptic ulcers similar to those which are seen in human beings after traumatic events. Bleeding from acute stomach ulcers is familiar to staff in Intensive Care Units looking after people who have suffered extensive trauma or burns, e.g. from road traffic accidents. But acute ulcers of this type soon heal after the initial trauma has ceased, when patients are at rest and not in pain.

So why do acute ulcers only become established, i.e. 'chronic', in human beings but not in animals? Obviously this might reflect differences in the habitual diets. But there may be a simpler explanation. I recollect that many years ago, before the arrival of specific ulcer therapies of many kinds, the cornerstone of medical treatment of peptic ulcer was prolonged bed rest in addition to the obligatory milky diet. I will therefore suggest another very simple reason why animals other than ourselves do not get chronic peptic ulcers. When an animal gets an acute ulcer it presumably experiences pain. This makes the animal rest and stop walking about. He doesn't feel that he has to get to the factory or the office or get the children to school on time. He has no money worries. So his acute ulcer heals and never becomes established and 'chronic'. It would be monstrously cruel deliberately to put a dog or a cat or any other large mammal through the sort of social stresses that human beings inflict on one another. The UK Home Office would never allow the experiment. So my ludicrously simple hypothesis may never be tested. But I rest my case.

Duodenal ulcers

One contributory cause of duodenal ulcers (DU) is that the actual amount of hydrochloric acid produced by the stomach is greater, on average, in people with DU than in normal people, though there is a lot of overlap. A peak acid output greater than 50 mmoles of hydrochloric acid per hour is almost diagnostic of a DU. One below about 15 makes DU very unlikely. But since infection by the bacterium *Helicobacter pylori* can increase stomach acid secretion, it is uncertain how much of the increased acid secretion is part of someone's natural inheritance and how much is due to the additional infection. Furthermore, infection can decrease as well as increase stomach acid secretion. Different strains of *H. pylori* have different associations with peptic ulcers. This may account for some of the different views about causation. It might also help to explain why animals don't get chronic peptic ulcers. Maybe there is no need to invoke the 'social' explanation that I envisaged earlier in this chapter. Time will tell.

Overproduction of hydrochloric acid is especially notable at night in patients with DU and may relate to pain at that time. I recall that junior doctors used to measure the amount of acid produced by feeding patients a test meal of 'gruel'. Later the meal was replaced by a histamine injection and later still by a synthetic analogue of gastrin (pentagastrin), which can maximally stimulate stomach acid secretion. When acid production was found to be high the patient was given large amounts of sodium bicarbonate or other acid-neutralising drugs. Then James Black discovered the H2-blocking drugs.[6] Their effects were dramatic. H2-blockers relieved pain in most patients and allowed most duodenal ulcers to heal. These drugs were followed by still stronger ones (the 'proton pump inhibitors') which virtually switched off all acid production in the stomach. These drugs were nearly always successful in healing duodenal ulcers but they did not cure patients. All too often the ulcers recurred when the drugs were stopped.

The discovery of the infecting bacterium *Helicobacter pylori* by two Australian doctors[7] has revolutionised the way we think about the disease and the ways in which we now treat peptic ulcers. By examining stomach tissue under the microscope, they had identified curved bacteria which seemed to be present in inflamed and ulcer-prone stomachs. Marshall deliberately infected his own stomach with the stomach juices of someone with an established peptic ulcer. This produced active stomach inflammation which would presumably have led to a chronic ulcer had he not taken bismuth and an antibiotic to eradicate the infection. He was following in the footsteps of many brave and resolute scientists who have carried out important experiments on themselves. It is fascinating that bismuth compounds, introduced originally to neutralise stomach acid and which over many years have had a reputation for relieving peptic ulcer pain, also have a specific anti-bacterial effect on *H. pylori*.

After *H. pylori* had been identified, many fellow scientists, myself included, felt that the problem of causation of peptic, especially duodenal, ulcers had been solved. But the story is still complicated. *Helicobacter pylori* cannot invariably be found in patients even with DUs, although there is no doubt that the bacterium can cause ulcers and that its eradication can produce a cure.[8] It seems that the organism inhibits somatostatin secretion. It may by this means increase acid secretion by the stomach. In some parts of the world *H. pylori* infection is almost universal, though peptic ulcers are uncommon. In developed countries only about 15% of people carrying *H. pylori* get ulcers. I imagine that there are different strains of bacteria with different abilities to cause disease – attributes classified as 'pathogenicity'.

When *H. pylori* bacteria reach the stomach they become attached to the mucus-secreting lining cells of the stomach by specialised adhesion molecules which cover the surface of the bacteria. The bacteria survive in the acid environment of the stomach because they can neutralise stomach acid. Fortunately we have a rather good and ingenious test which can tell if a patient is infected with helicobacter organisms, without the need actually to sample stomach contents. This is the so-called 'breath test'. *Helicobacter pylori* produces the enzyme urease. This breaks down the nitrogenous waste product urea, with the production of ammonia and carbon dioxide. If synthetic urea containing the carbon isotope ^{13}C is fed to someone, carbon dioxide gas containing ^{13}C carbon can be detected in the breath. The severity of infection can be roughly gauged by the concentration of radioactively labelled carbon dioxide in the breath.

There are still missing pieces in the jigsaw.[9] Much further research is still needed. Unfortunately helicobacter bacteria are difficult to eradicate completely. This makes it difficult to decide what their role is and how much is contributed by a patient's diet or genetic inheritance.

Gastric (stomach) ulcers

The causation of gastric ulcer (GU) is still more complicated, though undoubtedly *H. pylori* infection can contribute to GUs as well as DUs. The peak acid output of the stomach with a gastric ulcer is seldom greater than 50 mmoles per hour, but it can be much lower and even well below the normal range. Ulcers typically develop on what is usually described as the 'lesser curve' of the stomach, which is the junction between the acid-secreting upper part of the stomach and the antrum.

Gastric ulcers definitely need acid to become 'chronic' (i.e. long-lasting). Ulcers do not develop when acid is absent – in pernicious anaemia, for example – a condition in which vitamin B_{12} is not absorbed properly because of atrophy of the stomach lining. A gastric ulcer developing in the absence of stomach acid is often 'malignant', i.e. caused by cancer. On the other hand, stomach cancer is virtually unknown in people with duodenal ulcers. The prolonged use of drugs which switch off or neutralise stomach acid may heal stomach ulcers but risks leaving the stomach defenceless against harmful chemicals, especially so-called 'free radicals'. I vividly recall one of our laboratory assistants, in whom I had found high stomach acid levels and whom I had treated successfully with H2-blocking drugs for a duodenal ulcer. He returned many years later with absent stomach acid (achlorhydria) but with an inoperable cancer of the stomach.

As a general principle, sensible physicians try to avoid interfering with the body's natural defences if they possibly can. If I had not treated this patient's duodenal ulcer (successfully) with H2-blocking drugs, he might not have later developed stomach cancer.

An unusual complication of *H. pylori* infection is a low-grade stomach lymphoma – a tumour of lymphoid cells in the stomach wall. Left untreated this would be expected to spread and in the end kill the infected individual. It is interesting, and encouraging, that total eradication of *H. pylori* seems sometimes to be able to stop this tumour in its tracks.

Summary

Peptic ulcers, i.e. chronic ulcers in the duodenum or stomach, are very common. Duodenal ulcers are often associated with the presence of higher concentrations and higher secretion rates of hydrochloric acid than are found in normal people, or in people with stomach (gastric) ulcers.

'Peptic' ulcers were at one time believed to be not only associated with stresses in patients' lives, but also caused by such stresses. We now recognise that infection by the bacterium *Helicobacter pylori* plays a major part. If this infection can be eliminated, peptic ulcers can not only be healed but also cured, even without the use of acid-neutralising and acid-suppressing drugs. Whether infection causes a peptic ulcer in a specific patient or not depends on the bacterial strain and on the patient's genetic susceptibility, environment and diet.

Other factors, especially the consumption of non-steroidal anti-inflammatory drugs, cigarette smoking and excessive alcohol consumption are also aggravating factors.

11

BILE AND GALL BLADDER DISORDERS

In classical and medieval times the human body was thought to comprise mixtures of four 'Humours' – Blood, Phlegm, Choler (yellow bile) and Melancholy (black bile). These were thought to give rise to psychological characteristics such as 'red-blooded', 'phlegmatic', 'choleric' and 'melancholic'. Today we still find bile invoked when someone takes a 'jaundiced view'.

We now know what bile is and what its main functions are. It is a brown fluid made in the liver, stored in the gall bladder and concerned with the digestion of food. When food is eaten the gall bladder contracts and expels bile into the gut through the common bile duct. The liver of an adult is a large solid organ weighing 3–4 lbs ($1\frac{1}{2}$ – 2 kg). It lies in the upper abdomen on the right side, behind the lower ribs. The gall bladder is a small sac (a cul-de-sac) some 2 inches long, attached to the common bile duct and lying below the right lobe of the liver (Fig. 16). The common bile duct leads into the duodenum and joins up with or runs close to the pancreatic duct from which pancreatic juice is released. Coordinated release both of bile and of pancreatic secretions is under the control of the nervous system and of chemicals (hormones) circulating in the blood.

Bile is alkaline because it contains sodium bicarbonate – known in the kitchen as baking soda. This is also present in the alkaline secretions of the pancreas. Together, bile and pancreatic juice neutralise the acidity of the stomach contents when they are squirted into the duodenum by stomach contraction. This allows the powerful pancreatic digesting enzymes, notably trypsin, to start breaking down proteins and other food components. These enzymes do not work effectively in an acid medium, hence the importance of the fluid contents of the duodenum being alkaline.

Adults produce about $1\frac{1}{2}$ –2 quarts (700–1200 ml) of bile daily. It is recirculated some 6–10 times daily. After its secretion into the duodenum, 95% of its contained water and bile salts are absorbed through the walls of the intestine and get back to the liver via the bloodstream. The brown colour of bile comes from 'bilirubin', the main bile pigment. This is the breakdown product of the red oxygen-

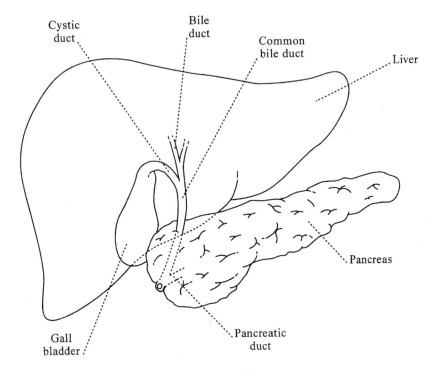

Cystic duct

Bile duct

Common bile duct

Liver

Pancreas

Pancreatic duct

Gall bladder

Figure 16 Diagram of the liver, gall bladder and pancreas.

carrying protein 'haemoglobin', which is contained in the red cells of the blood. Bilirubin is not very soluble in water. It can form precipitates or actual stones (see below) which are wholly or partly composed of bile pigments.

Bile also contains 'bile acids' (sometimes called bile 'salts'). These are emulsifying agents synthesised from cholesterol in the liver by 15 successive enzyme-facilitated steps. Bile acids help to make fats soluble in water, to allow them to be broken down and taken up by the lining cells of the small intestine. Bile has been accurately described as nature's own detergent.

Obstruction to the free flow of bile from liver into the gut causes bile pigments to pile up in the body. When enough of these accumulate in the body the skin becomes dark yellow (jaundice) and the whites of the eyes (the sclera) also become yellow. The duration and severity of biliary obstruction can be measured by the blood concentration of bilirubin.

The liver-produced enzyme alkaline phosphatase and the concentration of cholesterol in the blood are also increased by obstruction to free flow of bile, though the precise reason for both these changes are at present a mystery. Bile also contains cholesterol, a fatty material synthesised in the liver. Although cholesterol is an essential component of virtually all cells of the body, it also makes up most of the white deposits (atheroma) in the walls of the larger arteries. These start to appear in middle age and are the main cause of heart attacks and strokes.

Gallstones

Most people have more cholesterol dissolved in their bile than would be expected by its relative insolubility. Bile is therefore technically 'supersaturated' with cholesterol, which can easily precipitate and form solid lumps: 'gall stones'. These are mostly composed of cholesterol, sometimes with additional pigment. One medical mystery is not so much why some people form solid cholesterol stones in their gall bladder but rather why most of us do not. Some protection against gall stone formation is due to bile acids, which help to dissolve cholesterol in the gut and keep it in solution in bile. Bile contains lecithin (a phosphate-containing lipid), and fatty acids in bile also inhibit gall stone formation.

Gall stones give trouble in two ways, by obstructing bile flow, or by predisposing to infection of the gall bladder lining, i.e. 'cholecystitis' (Greek: *chole* = bile; *kystis* = bladder; the suffix 'itis' signifying 'inflammation'). The most notable symptom of gall stones (jaundice) arises when a stone has impacted in some part of the common bile duct, usually at its end where the duct gets narrower. The jaundice is described as 'obstructive'. If there is no pain this may not cause other symptoms, though the accumulation of bile salts can make the skin itch. If it is unduly prolonged, obstructive jaundice affects the absorption of fat and of the fat-soluble vitamins A, D and K.

But more often obstructive jaundice due to gall stones is accompanied by spasms of central or right-sided upper abdominal pain. The bile duct resembles other muscular tubular structures in the body, like arteries, veins and gut. It is not pain-sensitive if squeezed or cut, but it produces severe pain if its walls are overstretched. The 'hard wiring', as it might be called, of the nerves supplying the muscles of the bile duct ensures that if outflow of bile is obstructed the constricting muscle of the bile duct behind the obstruction intermittently contracts. This helps to shift the obstruction but also causes spasms of pain known as 'biliary colic'. A gall stone may also cause spasms of pain,

119

without jaundice, when it has got stuck in the cystic duct but has not reached the common bile duct.[1]

Gall stones and gall bladder disorders affect between 10% and 20% of the world's population, but most people with stones in their gall bladder have no serious symptoms and are unaware of anything amiss. In the UK about 8% of all adults over 40 have gall bladder stones and more than 20% of people over 60 have them. Geography appears to influence gall stone formation: e.g. almost 100% of the native population of women in Chile and Peru suffer from gall stones. Whether this is due to a genetic predisposition or to differences in diet is not known. I have attended many post mortem examinations (necropsies) in which someone's gall bladder was found to be full of gall stones, but the patient's medical notes recorded no complaints which could have arisen from this cause. I have also seen several patients complaining of abdominal pain and found to have stones in their gall bladder, but whose pain was not relieved by cholecystectomy (Greek: *ektome* = cutting out). It is all too easy for a physician to find stones in someone's gall bladder, usually by an ultrasound examination, make this the main diagnosis, calling it 'cholelithiasis' (Greek: *lithos* = stone) – but then having to apologise later to the patient whose symptoms were no better after the gall bladder had been removed. Unfortunately there are many causes of upper abdominal pain. Cholelithiasis is only one of them.

Despite its occasional failure to relieve abdominal pain, cholecystectomy is a common operation because gall stones are so common. It is sometimes possible to avoid open operation by breaking up gall stones by focused sharp sound waves, though there is always the risk that small particles may later get stuck in the common bile duct and cause severe pain. Cholecystectomy can nowadays be done by a surgeon making only a tiny incision and visualising the abdominal organs by means of a laparoscope – a hollow tube with a bright light at its end. The cost/benefit ratios and the relative dangers of various methods of treating gall stones are topics of current dispute. A 'wait-and-see' policy is probably inadvisable, because about half of all patients with one attack of biliary colic get another. One third eventually need to have their gall bladder removed as a matter of urgency. But cholecystectomy is never a trivial operation.

I retain a great respect for the potential danger of bile getting into the peritoneal cavity. Bile salts are emulsifying agents and make fats soluble. The abdominal cavity is not at all well equipped to seal off bile leaks by its own resources. Many years ago I had the horrifying experience of watching my chief, an expert and very experienced surgeon, remove a stone-containing gall bladder, then close the cystic duct without inserting a 'drain' to allow any leak of bile to escape from the abdominal cavity. (The surgeon told me that he had previously done this a dozen times in his life without ill consequence.) He thought that if his sewing technique was careful and meticulous enough and there were no stones in the bile duct, he could guarantee no bile leakage. Alas, this time he was wrong. Bile spread around the peritoneal cavity causing biliary peritonitis from which the unfortunate patient died a week later, despite antibiotics and all possible supportive measures. Bile is a very dangerous fluid if it gets in the wrong place. If one day I need to have a cholecystectomy myself, I shall ask for an open operation and insist that the surgeon leaves in a drain!

Gall bladder problems arise from two causes. The first is obstruction to the free flow of bile, either along the main bile duct (caused by a stone stuck at the end of the common bile duct) or in the cystic duct (with a stone stuck at the exit of the gall bladder). Obstruction of the common bile duct causes jaundice because bilirubin in bile accumulates in the blood. It stains many internal organs as well as the skin. When obstruction has gone on for many days, there may also be itching of the skin. This is probably due to a high concentration of bile acids.

Many factors predispose to gallstone formation. Medical students like *aides mémoires*. They all remember that the typical patient with

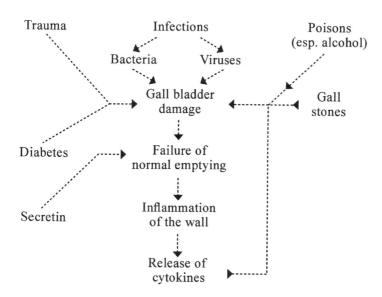

Figure 17 Factors contributing to cholecystitis.

gall stones is a female who is 'fair, fat, forty and fertile'. This can certainly be true, but is misleading as often as not. Obesity certainly is associated with gallstones. There may also be an association with a sedentary lifestyle, because of links between physical inactivity, abdominal adiposity, slow intestinal transit of food and excessive insulin production.[2]

The second complication of gall stones is infection, which is especially likely to arise if the cystic duct is obstructed (Fig. 17). If infection gets in (either through the bloodstream, or by ascending from the gut) the gall bladder can become inflamed: this is cholecystitis. This may present itself as a patient with symptoms resembling appendicitis, though the pain is more typically in the upper rather than the lower abdomen.

Cause of gallstones

Since both cholesterol and bile pigments are usually technically in a supersaturated solution in bile, any small 'nidus' (Latin: nest) could start the process of crystallisation and initiate the production of a stone. The late Lord Moynihan was impressed by the thought of bacteria beginning the process. He produced the aphorism 'every gallstone is a tombstone to the bacteria buried within it'. In recent years other ideas such as disordered mucus secretion by the gall bladder lining have also been invoked.

Slow transit of food through the gut appears to favour stone formation, presumably because the gall bladder is less regularly emptied of its contained bile. Another stone-promoting factor is the synthetic drug 'octreotide' which chemically resembles the anterior pituitary gland hormone somatostatin. It is used in the treatment of certain pituitary disorders. Octreotide inhibits gall bladder contraction and gall stones are one of the recognised complications of octreotide therapy.

An obvious possible cause of gall stones is increased synthesis of cholesterol by the liver. Seven different genes are known to influence cholesterol synthesis. Although it is easy to envisage that increased cholesterol production might cause gall stones, this sequence can only be incriminated in about a quarter of victims. Clearly gall stones have many other causes.

Bile acid therapy reduces cholesterol hypersecretion in bile and increases cholesterol solubility. Ursodeoxycholic acid (a natural bile acid) has proved popular as a treatment to prevent or dissolve gall stones. Non-steroidal anti-inflammatory drugs (NSAIDs) also help to prevent recurrence of gall stones but the reasons are not at present clear.

Primary biliary cirrhosis

Middle-aged women who become jaundiced are sometimes wrongly suspected of having gall stones stuck in their main bile duct when in reality they are suffering from an entirely different condition: 'primary biliary cirrhosis'(PBC).[3] The yellow skin colour may be the first sign of the illness, but other symptoms caused by retained bile acids, such as itching of the skin, may also bring the disease to light. Sometimes the disease is discovered accidentally in the course of health screening by routine liver function tests on a blood sample: e.g. by abnormal elevation of alkaline phosphatase and gamma glutamyl transferase enzymes in a blood test. As its name suggests, the end stage of PBC is scarring and eventual failure of liver function, during a course which (untreated) lasts about 10 years from first symptom to death. About 40% of sufferers die from liver failure, others from diseases like bronchopneumonia which are associated with loss of appetite and general enfeeblement. Lack of bile can interfere with the absorption of fat and particularly of the fat-soluble vitamins A,D and K. Lack of vitamin A leads to night blindness. Lack of vitamin D can cause undue softness of bones (osteomalacia: p. 323) and consequent pain and risk of fracture. The associated muscle weakness can cause difficulty in walking. Lack of vitamin K can impair blood clotting.

PBC has a worldwide distribution and currently affects at least 100 million people. More than 90% of these are women, usually between the ages of 40 and 60. There are known to be 20–30 million female sufferers in the USA, Canada, Australia and Japan. Current prevalence is 23–66 per million population in developed countries. Curiously PBC is almost unknown in Africa, India and most parts of Asia, though it does occur among the Hong Kong Chinese. Such huge differences might be genetic. One estimate is that first degree relatives of sufferers have about a 400 times higher chance of getting the disease than those without a family background. But this does not rule out a major contribution from an environmental cause such as infection[4] or diet. An important environmental cause could well operate within family groups, independently of genetic factors. Vegetarians have a 50% lower incidence of the disease than non-vegetarians. Clustering of cases has been noted. Both these observations suggests an environmental rather than a genetic cause.

Microscopical examination of the liver in PBC shows that the small bile ducts are infiltrated with lymphocytes and other cells associated with tissue destruction, but polymorph white cells are absent and pus does not form. The diagnosis of PBC can usually be made by the blood tests, mentioned above, and by finding antibodies against mitochondria (present in 95% of cases). Liver biopsy is then not essential. But as well as confirming the diagnosis, biopsy helps to identify the stage which the disease has reached. Staging has also been done by a complex mathematical index incorporating a patient's age, symptoms, serum albumin and bilirubin, and blood clotting factors (the 'Mayo index').

Cause of primary biliary cirrhosis

Primary biliary cirrhosis has all the characteristics of an 'auto-immune disease' (p. 69). Certainly it seems that the disease is kept going by the release of antigens from bile duct destruction. But what starts the disease off? Why should it continue its inexorable and eventually lethal course unless the initial trigger factor is still operating? Normal gut bacteria such as *E. coli* and various common viruses have been suggested as trigger factors, but there is no convincing evidence for these so far.

The extraordinary epidemiology of PBC is quite fascinating to someone, like me, working in an Institute of Preventive Medicine. PBC seems best explained by infection with an agent present only in some parts of the world and not in others, or by damage from an agent perhaps only present in certain particular foods. Unfortunately no infectious agent has yet been found. Infection of adults with the Epstein-Barr virus causes glandular fever and immunological changes not dissimilar to those in PBC. That virus has been observed sometimes to lead to malignant change (lymphoma). There are also many similarities between chronic hepatitis C (HC) infection (p. 256) and primary biliary cirrhosis. HC virus causes a slowly developing illness involving the liver. It does not usually clear up on its own and it leads to slow deterioration over many years. The similarities between HC infection and PBC are obvious.

So it seems most likely that PBC is due to infection with a virus which has not yet been identified. I recall that decades passed before the virus of hepatitis C (HC) was finally recognised as a cause of what was previously categorised as 'non-A, non-B' hepatitis. Indeed, at the present time HC virus has not even been cultured. My best guess at present about the cause of primary biliary cirrhosis is that it is due to an infection with an ubiquitous virus which is unevenly distributed throughout the world.

There is certainly involvement of the immune system. Auto-immune diseases commonly can accompany PBC. They can be seen in up to 80% of cases: e.g. thyroid disorders (Chapter 6) and – less commonly – myasthenia, Addison's disease, vitiligo and systemic lupus erythematosus. Chronic fibrosing alveolitis, particularly the 'sicca' form with dry eyes and mouth (due to inflammatory infiltration of the lachrymal and salivary glands) is present in about 50% of cases. Antibodies directed against liver mitochondria and the pyruvate dehydrogenase complex are present in the blood in 96% of cases and may be present before there is any clinical manifestation of disease. Activation of complement and specific T-lymphocytes are also commonly found. The latter surround the small bile ducts within the substance of the liver and may play a part in the destruction of the bile ducts which characterises the disease.

PBC is at one end of the spectrum of auto-immune liver diseases. Another is the mis-named 'lupoid' hepatitis. In this disease chronic active auto-immune hepatitis becomes frankly 'cirrhotic' (i.e. it scars the liver). Other auto-antibodies (e.g. against smooth muscle) are found. There are also intermediate disorders. Accurate diagnosis is important because steroid drugs help in chronic active hepatitis but are useless in PBC.

A number of empirical treatments for PBC have been tried but most have failed. The first of many therapies to be discredited was penicillamine. Currently ursodeoxycholic acid is being tried because it increases bile flow and has been reported to help. It has at least the advantage of being harmless. Steroids are often given and can make patients feel better but do not influence the course of the disease. They are no longer used. Although transplantation of a whole liver from someone recently dead (e.g. in a traffic accident) is hazardous it is the only treatment which can relieve all the symptoms and signs.

Summary

Bile is necessary for the emulsification and ultimate digestion of dietary fat. Its alkaline nature helps to neutralise stomach acid and hence activate the powerful pancreatic digestive enzymes. Bile also contains residual pigment from the breakdown of haemoglobin in red blood cells. Gall stone formation must inevitably be facilitated by the (apparent) supersaturation of bile with cholesterol and bile pigments. Both of these can participate in gall stone formation. Stones may remain in the gall bladder, causing no symptoms other than a propensity to infection (cholecystitis). Small stones may also leave the gall bladder and pass down the cystic duct into the common bile duct and lodge at the sphincter at its lower end. Obstruction produces spasms of pain (biliary colic) and obstructive jaundice.

An obstructive type of jaundice can also be produced by disease of many small bile ducts within the substance of the liver – a situation which obtains in various types of liver scarring, including the mysterious disease: primary biliary cirrhosis.

12

PANCREATITIS

The pancreas of mammals is an abdominal gland concerned with the digestion of food and also with the control of blood sugar by its secretion of insulin. In English butchers' shops the pancreas from cattle is known as 'sweetbreads'. Some people reject it as unfit to eat. Others, myself included, regard it as a delicacy.

The human pancreas lies in the upper abdomen behind the stomach. It is a soft flattened structure about 6 inches long and $1\frac{1}{2}$ inches wide, with its larger end (the 'head') closely applied to the inner curve of the duodenum (Fig. 18). Part of its structure comprises an exocrine[1] gland which synthesises and secretes powerful digestive enzymes that can break carbohydrates, proteins and fats down to their constituent molecules, making them capable of being absorbed in the small intestine.

The pancreas of adults produces between a pint and pint and a half of pancreatic juice (500–900 ml) daily. Like bile, it is alkaline. Most of its water and contained salts are reabsorbed through the walls of the intestine and thus returned to the body. Pancreatic juices are secreted in a controlled fashion in response to food entering the small intestine. Pancreatic juice can also be secreted in response to psychological stimuli. These could be the sight, smell or taste of food, or even an enthusiastic description of some mouth-watering menu. Secretion is switched on through the nerve supply of the pancreas, but may also be stimulated by two chemicals (hormones) circulating in the blood and produced by cells lining the walls of the small intestine. One of these is 'secretin', the other is 'pancreozymin/cholecystokinin' (PZ/CK: p. 107). Both make the pancreas secrete its juices and start digestive processes in the gut. PZ/CK also makes the gall bladder contract and eject bile.

An average day's European diet contains about nearly a pound's weight (400 g) of carbohydrate, mostly starch and sugar. Starch itself is a complex molecule, a polymer of glucose. Digestion of carbohydrates begins in the stomach whose juices contain enzymes collectively known as amylases (Greek: *amylon* = starch). Digestion really gets going in the small intestine when food meets pancreatic juice which

127

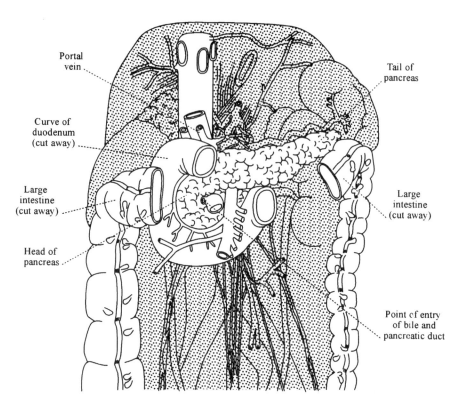

Figure 18 Position and appearance of the pancreas seen from the front, after cutting away the stomach, small intestine and transverse colon (part of the large intestine). The head of the pancreas is lying within the curve of the duodenum.

also contains amylases. Further breakdown of carbohydrates takes place in the lining cells of the small intestine. The end products are mainly the simple sugars glucose and galactose, which are absorbed into the bloodstream by specialised chemical transport systems.

Proteins in food are initially attacked by hydrochloric acid and by the enzyme pepsin, both of which are present in gastric juice. Most later protein digestion takes place in the duodenum and upper part of the small intestine. Proteins are broken down into their constituent amino-acids by a set of powerful enzymes contained in pancreatic juice. These include trypsin, chymotrypsin and elastase. All of them need to be activated by another enzyme (enterokinase) which is secreted by the cells lining the small intestine. Thus until food reaches the small intestine, when the powerful protein-digesting enzymes of the pancreas can be activated by pancreatic juices making contact with the

128

walls of the small intestine, the enzymes remain inactive. Digestion does not begin.

Fats are made up of fatty acids combined with glycerine (the correct chemical name is 'glycerol'). They are broken down by enzymes known as lipases. With the additional aid of bile acids, fat products become water-soluble, in the form of covered fat droplets known as 'micelles'. These can directly enter the absorbing cells of the small intestine.

Certain vitamins, salts and essential minerals such as calcium and iron are absorbed from the gut by specific chemical transport systems located in the gut walls. All these transport systems use energy. This is supplied by the oxidation of foodstuffs in mitochondria, which generates adenosine triphosphate (ATP). This is in effect the body's favourite rechargeable battery (p. 464). Water follows mainly by simple diffusion across the concentration gradients created by the active transport of many food constituents.

Endocrine function of the pancreas

The tapering tail of the pancreas also contains the 'islets of Langerhans'. These are small multiple ductless (endocrine) glands secreting insulin into the bloodstream from specialised cells (the 'beta-' cells). A smaller number of 'alpha-'cells in the pancreatic islets produce another hormone (glucagon), most of whose chemical actions are the opposite of those of insulin. Glucagon raises rather than lowers blood sugar concentration. Insulin and diabetes are discussed further in Chapters 14 and 15.

Pancreatitis

Inflammation of the pancreas[2] is an uncommon but alarming and dangerous condition, for the very obvious reason that all the structural tissues of the body are held together by proteins. These can be rapidly broken down and dissolved by the enzymes (themselves proteins) contained in pancreatic juice. Each of us has within our body all the ingredients required for an unpleasant vicious circle. Any form of pancreatic damage may release into the bloodstream powerful digestive enzymes which have the potential to break down proteins in pancreatic cells, thus releasing more enzymes. Figure 19 shows the interrelationship between some of the factors causing acute pancreatitis.

Once these processes have got under way they can progress with

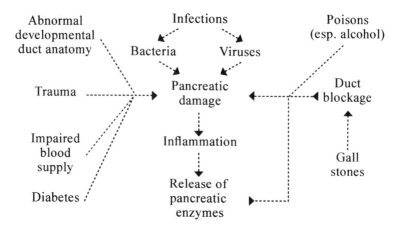

Figure 19 Factors potentially involved in causing pancreatitis.

horrific speed. About 10% of first attacks of acute pancreatitis are fatal within a few days. I have seen two patients, one a previously fit man in his thirties, progress from the sudden onset of central abdominal pain to circulatory collapse and death, within 48 hours. More often the condition slowly gets better after a few days. The healing processes often result in the generation of a lot of tough fibrous tissue in the pancreas. This can then protect against further sudden overwhelming attacks of acute inflammation, but it may also lead to chronic (i.e. longstanding) pancreatitis, with symptoms of inadequate pancreatic digestive function.

Self-digestion of the pancreas releases its enzymes into the bloodstream where they can be chemically measured. A high level of the enzyme amylase in the blood is often used as a diagnostic test for acute pancreatitis. Breakdown of fat tissue in the body releases fatty acids which combine with calcium in the blood. This reduces the blood concentration of calcium, which may even cause 'tetany' – a tight contraction of hand muscles. Blood calcium concentration has been used to gauge the severity of an attack of acute pancreatitis. A very low blood calcium concentration has been found to predict a bad outcome. When pancreatic self-destruction involves the islets of Langerhans in the tail of the gland, insulin secretion may also be affected, with consequent diabetes. Many other complications of an attack of acute pancreatitis result from damage to the inner linings of blood vessels in many organs.

The many different manifestations of acute pancreatitis make the condition difficult to diagnose. I have seen one victim not diagnosed until post mortem examination revealed the reason why a previously healthy middle-aged man should have suffered sudden severe abdominal pain, collapse and unexpected death. He had, not unnaturally, been misdiagnosed as suffering from a heart attack.

Chronic pancreatitis

Permanent damage to the pancreas may result in scarring with a lot of fibrous tissue replacing the secretory part of the gland. Small solid lumps of calcium phosphate mineral are often found in a damaged pancreas. Chalky calcium deposits in the pancreas often come to light unexpectedly when an X-ray of the upper abdomen is examined. When enough of the pancreas has been destroyed a state of chronic pancreatic insufficiency may result. This can interfere with food absorption so badly that a patient may lose weight and develop fatty stools (faeces) through inability to digest fat. The medical name for this condition is 'steatorrhoea' (Greek: *stear* = tallow, resembling fat; *rhoia* = flow). In addition several complications may result from deficiency of fat-soluble vitamins, notably of vitamin D causing osteomalacia (see Chapter 30). Permanent Type 1 diabetes (Chapter 14) can follow destruction of the pancreatic insulin-secreting cells. Sometimes recurrent attacks of pancreatitis can only be prevented by a surgical operation. This has commonly involved making a new connection between the head of the pancreas and the duodenum, sometimes with excision of some part of the diseased organ.

Epidemiology

Acute pancreatitis is increasing in incidence in most urban communities. It can occur at any age, in either sex, but in most surveys men in their fourth and fifth decades have been its main victims. There is clear evidence that a high intake of alcohol is a causal factor, though the reason for this is not known. Smoking is well known to be associated with cancer of the pancreas and is probably also a cause of acute pancreatitis. Gall stones are also associated with pancreatitis. Lack of fresh fruit may be a significant factor. Some individuals have an abnormal anatomy of the duct system of their gland. Anomalies of pancreatic and bile duct anatomy are often found in people who have had an attack of acute pancreatitis. Blockages and perhaps occasional backward flow of pancreatic juice may sometimes occur and predispose to local inflammation, even in the absence of actual infection.

Causes of pancreatitis

Epidemiological studies are few because acute pancreatitis is uncommon and unpredictable. Since the pancreas is effectively a bag of powerful digestive enzymes which only need a small amount of a catalyst to activate them, a damaged pancreas can easily start to digest both itself and adjacent organs once its contained enzymes have been activated. Inappropriate activation of the digestive enzyme trypsin seems to be the first step and may become self-sustaining. As I have emphasised, this can happen in acute inflammation of the pancreas (pancreatitis) with devastating speed. Acute pancreatitis can occur in several situations. In many of them it seems that an abnormal anatomy of the pancreatic duct system may have allowed activated enzymes to flow backwards into the body of the pancreas.

Impaired blood supply (ischaemia) of the gland is another important factor. This has been regarded as a rare cause of pancreatitis, but may be commoner than generally thought. Ischaemia followed by reperfusion has been suggested as a factor causing acute pancreatitis in a number of situations.[3] One of these is cardio-pulmonary bypass – the technique commonly used to allow operations to be performed on the coronary arteries while the heart's beating is temporarily stopped. Transplantation operations on the pancreas and sudden severe blood loss from accidents may also precipitate acute pancreatitis because of pancreatic ischaemia. Acute pancreatitis is much more common in HIV-infected people than in the general population,[4] though we do not know why.

> A severe attack of acute pancreatitis involves interaction between cytokines (especially IL-1 and tumour necrosis factor), auto-immune mechanisms and the complement system. In animals (rats) reduction of pancreatic inflammation has been recorded following the intravenous administration of antagonists of both IL-1 and TNFα.

There are a lot of mysteries surrounding pancreatic diseases. Indeed, the more one finds out about the anatomy and digestive function of the pancreas, the more extraordinary it seems that most people's digestion works so well and so seldom goes wrong. The rarity of acute pancreatitis makes it a particularly difficult disease to study. We do not know whether particular foods are provocative or causal. Do all victims have congenital abnormalities of pancreatic duct anatomy (as some people have suggested)? Or are deficiencies in pancreatic blood supply significant? Is there a particular virus or bacterial pathogen which starts the disease off? Why is alcohol overindulgence often associated with the disease?

Rare but interesting cases of hereditary pancreatitis have been identified. Most appear to be associated with genetic mutations affecting the activation of trypsin[5] Activation is normally inhibited by a protein called SPINK1, which is lacking or defective in hereditary pancreatitis. Other studies suggest that some sporadic attacks of acute pancreatitis may be linked to other gene mutations, but the relative rarity of the condition makes large-scale epidemiological investigation extremely difficult.

Chronic pancreatitis is a frequent accompaniment of cystic fibrosis, the common but serious genetic disease that mainly affects children's lungs. Although the two diseases are genetically quite distinct, there is some evidence of genetic interactions between cystic fibrosis genes and an individual's liability or resistance to chronic pancreatitis.

Summary

The human pancreas is a medium-sized gland lying at the back of the upper abdomen, surrounded by the duodenum. It has two functions: an 'endocrine' one, to synthesise, store and secrete the hormone insulin, and an 'exocrine' one, to secrete digestive juices.

The tail of the pancreas contains the 'islets of Langerhans'. These are small groups of specialised cells, most of which synthesise and secrete insulin, whose action will be described in Chapter 14. Insulin lowers the concentration of glucose, the main sugar present in the blood. A smaller group of cells secretes the hormone glucagon, which has main actions opposite to those of insulin.

The bulk of the pancreas comprises a gland which synthesises and stores pancreatic juice. This is released through its nerve supply but also by chemical stimulation provided by two hormones produced by cells in the small intestinal wall (secretin and pancreozymin/cholecystokinin). Pancreatic secretions contain powerful enzymes which break down proteins, fats and carbohydrates once their enzymes have been activated by contact with the walls of the small intestine. Normally the need for activation in this way prevents pancreatic enzymes digesting tissues outside the gut.

13

MIGRAINE

The word 'migraine' may have been derived from a corruption of '(he)micrainia' (something affecting one half of the cranium). It is a very common condition, affecting 20% of women and 15% of men at some time in their lives. It is commonest in early adult life, though first attacks often occur before the age of 10. It may be diagnosed retrospectively by talking to intelligent and observant older children. As sufferers grow up, attacks become less frequent. Migraine is rare in the elderly.

The manifestations of migraine are varied. Typically it is a specific type of episodic headache with a small set of associated neurological symptoms. Classic attacks, experienced by a quarter of migraine sufferers, begin with an 'aura' (Latin: breeze, smell or gleam of light). This usually takes the form of a so-called 'fortification spectrum', in which there appears to be a curved horizontal ridge of a zig-zag pattern in front of the eyes. The sufferer usually describes it as looking through a heat haze. The aura lasts for 20–40 minutes and may be followed by a headache lasting 12–48 hours if it is not treated. The headache is often initially confined to one side of the head. It may be associated with nausea, sometimes vomiting, and very occasionally with abdominal pain. The aura with its fortification spectrum may occur without the succeeding headache. Or headaches may occur without any preceding aura, as happens in the majority of cases. A third of migraine sufferers have experienced both types of presentation. During the visual aura there may be short-lived neurological defects, such as temporary paralysis of skeletal muscles, or curious localised changes or defects in sensation. Untreated attacks may last between 4 and 72 hours, and typically recur once or twice a month. After an attack victims may report feeling particularly well, though this is not surprising because they have previously felt so rotten during the attack.

The neurological signs accompanying the headache are normally transient. Recovery is usually complete, though a severe attack of 'hemiplegic migraine' (migraine accompanied by paralysis down one side of the body) may leave a permanent disturbance of function. One of my patients, a man of 19, had a well-marked partial spastic paralysis on one side of his body which persisted for many weeks after he had otherwise recovered from a particularly severe attack. It is not too surprising, therefore, that very occasionally migraine sufferers have experienced persisting disturbances of movement, balance, vision or hearing. These presumably reflect actual damage either to a brain pathway, or to the eye or inner ear during an attack.

The extraordinary and rare condition of transient global amnesia is thought to be a manifestation of migraine. Its cause is unknown but an attack clears up completely and seldom recurs.

Epidemiology

Prevalence of migraine is remarkably constant in developed countries. Symptoms typically begin in the teens and diminish in frequency and severity after middle age. In people with active migraine, attacks typically come every two to three weeks and last about a day. Migraine attacks are often related to the menstrual cycle in women, but usually remit during pregnancy. Head trauma has often led to precipitation of attacks of migrainous headaches which can usually be treated effectively by anti-migraine drugs. Diet has often been invoked as a precipitating cause of migraine, usually through an allergic response to certain foods.

Treatments for migraine

It is worth reviewing briefly the currently available treatments, for the light this might throw on the nature of the disease. Migraine is initially managed with aspirin or paracetamol, perhaps with an anti-vomiting drug. More powerful and specific treatments fall into two main groups: relievers and preventers. For relief, the first really effective one has been sumatriptan, which is a selective serotonin receptor agonist, i.e. a drug which mimics the effects of the natural hormone serotonin and constricts blood vessels in the brain. It works best when given by injection under the skin, though is also moderately effective by mouth. Several similar compounds such as naratriptan and zolmitriptan are available. 'Triptans' are thought to act on specialised serotonin receptors in brain artery walls which when activated produce constriction of those arteries. These drugs work quickly and provide fast relief of headache for 80% of sufferers in 2–4 hours. Although serotonin itself is a small simple chemical molecule, it can react with many different

136

receptors and perform many different functions. At least seven major types and eight sub-types of serotonin receptor have already been identified within the central nervous system. It seems certain that many other drugs will be introduced in the future.

Triptans also block the release of calcitonin gene-related peptide (CGRP) from the terminals of the sensory nerves supplying the face and scalp. CGRP is a potent dilator of brain blood vessels, and during a migraine attack the local concentration of CGRP in the brain increases. Blocking CGRP receptors with CGRP antagonists has proved effective in relieving migraine attacks.

'Preventer' drugs include pizotifen (Sanomigran) and methysergide. 'Beta blockers', like propranolol, are thought to work by stabilising cerebral blood vessels. They occasionally induce a permanent cure after several courses of treatment.

It is difficult for today's patients and their doctors to imagine the suffering brought about by severe attacks of migraine, before medical treatments were available. One of my former colleagues, a respected and conscientious chest physician who had bad migraine attacks about once a month, told me that his whole life was split into the days when he was able to work normally and attack days when he was unable to do any work at all.

Genetics

About 70% of migraine sufferers have a first degree relative (parent, sister or brother) who also has migraine. But migraine is so common anyway that many apparent examples of heredity may simply be due to chance. The disease does not occur in any simple 'Mendelian'[1] fashion. The shared environment of family members could be as important as inheritance. This may be specially relevant in families whose migraine is not associated with an aura. Such cases may sometimes be best classified as 'recurrent tension headache' rather than true migraine. A large study of adult twin pairs in Finland compared the coincidence of migraine in identical and non-identical twins. This allowed the genetic contribution to migraine to be accurately estimated. It varied between 34% and 51% for different migraine types. There is some evidence to suggest that migraine accompanied by an aura is specially strongly genetically determined, with first degree relatives having a four-fold risk of the condition in comparison with people unrelated to a migraine sufferer. A specific chromosomal mutation has been identified in 25% of Japanese sufferers from this variety of migraine. Migraine attacks without an associated aura may be fundamentally different from classic migraine; it is notable that spouses of sufferers are often affected.

One identifiable biochemical difference between people with the two types of migraine has been observed. Superoxide dismutase (SOD) is a natural cellular enzyme. It is found in many places, but particularly in the blood platelets, where it may give protection against damage by oxidising agents. In typical classic migraine with aura, the blood concentration of SOD is reduced. This is not observed in migraine without accompanying aura.

A marker for the rare condition of familial hemiplegic migraine[2] (an autosomal dominant condition) has been found in two thirds of cases on chromosome 19p3. A minor faulty gene on the same chromosome could perhaps contribute to the inheritance of other types of migraine, though such a link has only rarely been reported. The mutation causing familial hemiplegic migraine seems to involve a gene coding for voltage-sensitive 'calcium-channels' in brain cells. These have been categorised as of the 'P/Q' type and are distinct from those involved in blood vessel function.

Changes in cerebral blood flow

The entry of calcium into cells through sub-microscopic calcium channels is a trigger which switches on many cell functions. Familial hemiplegic migraine (see above) seems to be associated with a sudden reduction in blood flow starting at the back of the brain. An imaging technique known as 'positron-emission tomography' (PET) can non-invasively quantify local blood flow and also the local rate of consumption of glucose by brain cells. The technique known as 'single photon emission computerised tomography' (SPECT) allows the rates of blood flow in different parts of the brain to be compared. Yet another technique, 'functional magnetic resonance imaging' (fMRI), allows measurement of the local oxygen content of different brain areas.

Cause

The two main current hypotheses of the causation of migraine are (1) the vascular spasm model, and (2) the spreading cortical depression hypothesis. Most researchers believe that the aura of migraine has a different cause from the headache. Certainly the two can occur separately, as I can testify from my own experience. I have had several episodes of typical visual aura (a fortification spectrum), each lasting about 30 minutes, but I have never had any succeeding headache.

Most people believe that migraine headache is due to dilation of some of the main brain arteries, which grossly look like Figure 20. But this may be wrong because headache can occur at the same time that blood flow to the brain cortex is reduced. The aura was traditionally thought to be caused by arterial constriction reducing local blood flow; but this view may also be incorrect. The aura may rather reflect some abnormal electrical excitation of neurones, without any corresponding reduction of blood flow.[3] The striking relief of headache by sumatriptan – a drug which selectively constricts blood vessels in the head – does not necessarily mean that there must be locally increased cerebral blood flow in migraine attacks. Nerve pathways and nerve

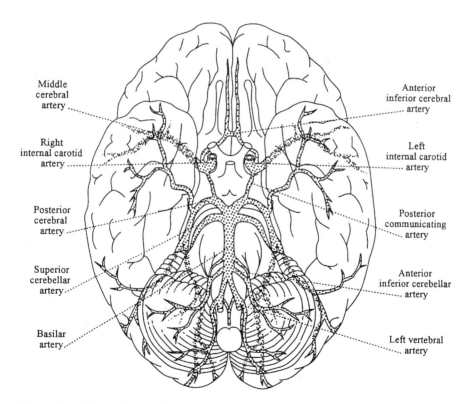

Figure 20 The main arteries at the base of the brain, viewed from below after removing the brain from the skull.

centres in the brain stem are involved in a migraine attack. This is probably the case when pain is felt over one side of the head, in the distribution of the fifth cranial nerve (the trigeminal) on that side. Some defect in the control of the entry of calcium into the muscle cells surrounding brain arteries might lead to the changes in brain blood flow which may accompany a typical migraine attack.

A point in favour of 'vascular spasm' sometimes causing reduced local cerebral blood flow perfusion is that there have been well-documented cases of intermittent blindness in one eye leading – after many years of attacks – to permanent blindness of the affected eye, accompanied by reduced calibre of all the retinal arteries. 'Infarction' (death of tissue caused by inadequate blood supply) of the retina of the eye has been occasionally seen in migraine. This has apparently been caused by temporary closure of the central retinal artery. Observations such as those of mine on the young man with long persistence of a spastic hemiplegia (cited above) can only reasonably be explained by severe local reduction of blood flow to some area of the brain.

If an attack of migraine can be precipitated or at least accompanied by constriction of brain arteries, it is natural to ask whether there is any evidence of circulating constrictor chemicals in the blood of migraine sufferers. Cytokines such as 'substance-P' and 'neurokinin-1' have been looked for, but have yet to be assigned a definite causal role. Neither has serotonin, even though sumatriptan (a drug with serotonin-like actions) is an effective treatment for the migraine headache. It can reduce cerebral blood flow in some conditions in which it is abnormally increased.

Constriction of blood vessels could also be due to reduction in the concentration of the simple gas, nitric oxide. However, nitric oxide is more likely to be relevant in migraine as a potential dilator chemical causing headache. Its antagonist (LNMMA) has been reported to alleviate migraine headache. Another minor point in favour of a vascular explanation for migraine is that freestyle ice skaters who spin a lot get more frequent migraine attacks than ice dancers, who don't spin.[4] The recent discovery of a link between migraine and a hole connecting right and left sides of the heart also supports a vascular theory.

It is remotely possible that the first thing that happens in an attack of migraine is local dilation of brain arteries. But if so, why should this sometimes lead to examples of semi-permanent damage apparently due to a local *reduction* of blood flow? Could excessive arterial dilation at one site lead to a reduction in local blood pressure and hence flow at another site? We need more surveys of local brain blood flow distribution during the migraine aura, to see whether there is simply a

140

reduction in overall cerebral blood flow, or whether there is evidence of unequal excess perfusion in one area causing underperfusion in other areas.

Evidence of a primary alteration in nerve activity comes from many sources. An association between epilepsy and migraine has been firmly established and is not due to shared genetic susceptibility. In between attacks, migraine sufferers have been reported to have increased electrical excitability of their brain surface, though there is no agreement about its cause. Fits or seizures (actual epileptic attacks) are due to uncontrolled electrical excitation spreading over the brain. One subject of hot debate is whether migraine might result from similarly spreading electrical excitation, soon succeeded by 'spreading cortical depression'. There is some evidence that the brain stem as well as the brain cortex may play a part in initiating migraine attacks – although a clear causal link between neuronal excitation and brain stem blood flow changes has yet to be firmly established.

Electrical excitability of the brain has been measured in an interesting way through the intact skull, by magnetic stimulation. Michael Faraday discovered that changing magnetic fields generate currents in electrical conductors. So if a powerful magnetic field around the head is suddenly switched on, or suddenly changes direction, small electric currents are generated in conducting tissues in the brain. When the nerve tissues stimulated in this way control externally-visible muscle movements, an objective measurement can be made of the electrical excitability of the brain surface.

Major epileptic fits can be caused by a number of single gene mutations in ion channels or excitation receptors which increase the electrical excitability or instability of the brain surface. In addition, focal epilepsy may be triggered from a small previously damaged area of the brain surface.

Other hypotheses[5]

One hypothesis is that vascular spasm and spreading cortical depression might be linked through a vicious circle perpetuated by a local rise in the concentration of potassium, an ion specially concerned with electrical activity in nerves. Cortical depression might be initiated either by intense localised inhibitory nervous activity or by a transient reduction in local blood flow to a small area of the brain cortex. A local rise in potassium concentration might cause spasm of small arteries and local reduction of blood flow, thus starting a vicious circle.

Blood platelets, the sticky elements of blood, are concerned in blood clotting but have come under suspicion of being involved in migraine attacks. Temporary aggregation of platelets is well established as a cause of the so-called 'transient ischaemic attack' (TIA) – a sort of temporary stroke. However, aspirin, which reduces platelet stickiness and gives some protection against both coronary artery thrombosis and TIAs, gives little protection against migraine, though it gives some relief of the headache.

The trigger which switches on a migraine attack has been looked for but has not so far been convincingly identified. There is suggestive evidence that gut infection with the bacterium *Helicobacter pylori*, an organism associated with peptic ulcer, may be a trigger. Some protection against recurrent migraine attacks has been reported to follow eradication of this bacterium from the gut.

One possibility, which might account for the initiation of some attacks of migraine, is that they might be caused by an 'axon reflex'. This term describes the situation in which nerve impulses are flowing in a reverse direction because they have been initiated at an abnormal site. This site might be the dura (the tough membrane covering the brain). Such possibilities arise because nerves conveying sensation to the brain sometimes have many branches. A sensory signal coming from one area can get routed backwards in another nerve branch to inflame a different area. This bizarre situation is well recognised in the skin. Impulses running backwards in nerves ordinarily conveying sensation can cause inflammation and a red flare in undamaged areas of skin surrounding a damaged area. Migraine has often been noted to be associated with sinusitis and with dental disease, either of which could be sending signals up branching sensory nerves to the brain, creating the possibility of an axon reflex causing pain. When nerve impulses go down sensory nerves in a reverse direction, they can liberate cytokines at the ends of the nerves. These chemicals can damage capillary blood vessels and make them leak protein. This has been shown to occur in the dura of rats after an episode of induced spreading cortical depression.

Summary

Migraine is an extremely common condition which usually appears in early adult life and gets less common later. Classic migraine has two well-defined phases. One is associated with loss of function, most probably due to spasm of arteries supplying affected parts of the brain. This is associated with a sensory aura, usually visual. The later phase comprises a headache, typically covering one side of the head only. This phase is almost certainly associated with, and probably

142

caused by excessive dilation of arteries. The best treatment remedies are those which mimic the constrictor effect of serotonin, a natural chemical which acts on brain arteries. It is not known at present whether recurrent otherwise inexplicable headaches, not accompanied by an aura, are the same disease as classic migraine.

Although the migraine aura has for years been thought to be due to spasm of brain arteries, and the succeeding headache to dilation of the same arteries, attention is now being increasingly focused on electrical activity of nerve cells, especially in the brain stem. There is a relation between migraine and epilepsy. This may be related to changed electrical excitability of nerve cells in the brain, associated with changes in cell membrane properties in respect of ions of certain chemical elements, especially potassium. We do not know whether or not an attack of migraine starts with a spreading electrical excitation followed by depression over the brain surface. This sequence of events could produce first a consequent increase in local blood flow which would be followed by a decrease. Alternatively, the whole sequence of events might be triggered by initial spasm of certain brain arteries. Fortunately many of these questions are at present being comprehensively answered as the techniques for non-invasive investigation of brain function improve.

Although understanding of migraine is advancing with increasing speed – chiefly because of better methods of imaging and localising the electrical activity of nerve cells in the brain – many mysteries still remain.

14

DIABETES – TYPE 1

The Greek word 'diabetes' means 'a passing through'. This describes the major symptom of the disease: the production of large quantities of urine. Doctors sometimes further categorise the disorder as 'mellitus' (Latin: honey), because the urine tastes sweet. This is because it contains glucose (also known as dextrose). Glucose is the body's main sugar. The much sweeter cane sugar which is sold in grocers' shops is a different substance (sucrose). This is a compound of glucose and a related sugar, fructose. When someone eats sucrose, the body converts it all into glucose.

Diabetes mellitus is completely different from the much rarer disease 'diabetes insipidus',[1] in which the urine is tasteless. In regular common use the word 'diabetes' always implies diabetes mellitus.

The presence of glucose in the urine has the undesirable effect of turning the urine into a good culture medium – the term used to describe a solution used in a laboratory to grow bacteria. Thus one common effect of diabetes is liability to infection of the urine. This causes pain on passing urine, frequency of passing urine and other more general symptoms. The bacterium *Escherichia coli* is always present in abundance in the large bowel (the colon and rectum). It often infects the urine, especially in females, because the rectum opens close to the opening of the urethra, which conveys urine from the bladder. Males are better protected by their anatomy, but urinary tract infections are not uncommon in men with diabetes. (Note that I do not say 'in diabetics'. Many patients resent being described as 'diabetics'. They regard themselves as normal people who happen to have diabetes.)

An excess of glucose in the urine betrays an unduly high concentration of glucose in the blood. One criterion for the diagnosis of diabetes is that someone with appropriate symptoms can be classified as having diabetes if a random plasma glucose sample is equal to or above 11.1 mmol/litre (200 mg/100 ml), or if the concentration of glucose in the blood of someone who is fasting is equal to or above 7.8 mmol/l (120 mg/100ml). If the samples are of whole blood rather than of plasma (the liquid part of whole blood) the criteria for the diagnosis of diabetes are lower: 10.0 and 6.7 mmol/litre.

Although vast quantities of fluid, containing vast amounts of glucose, are filtered out of the blood plasma through the kidney glomeruli (p. 354) each day, normal people's kidney tubules are able to reabsorb all the glucose into the blood. There is a threshold of plasma glucose concentration of 10 mmol/litre (180 mg/100 ml). When this threshold is exceeded, no more glucose can be reabsorbed. Glucose then appears in the urine. This interferes with the absorption of water and salt from the kidney tubules[2] and increases the volume of the urine. 'Polyuria' (too much urine) causes inconvenience, as does 'nocturia' (having to get up at night to pass urine). But excreting too much salt (sodium chloride) can lead to a serious shortage of salt and water in the body and a reduction in the volume of circulating blood. This in turn can reduce blood pressure and lead to a rise in concentration of waste products in the body. This can cause vomiting and lead to further depletion of salt and water. To extract my patients from this situation – a positive feedback vicious circle – I have several times in my life had to put up an intravenous drip and infuse a salt solution to prevent fatal circulatory failure. But, as I shall discuss later, this complication is only commonly seen in people with diabetes when they have an absolute deficiency of insulin.

A high concentration of glucose in the blood dilates the 'arterioles' (small arteries, e.g. $\frac{1}{50} - \frac{1}{100}$ mm diameter) which take blood from the main renal arteries to the kidneys' filters (the glomeruli). Each glomerulus comprises a ball of capillaries (Latin: *capillus* = a hair) – very small blood vessels without muscular coats, with a diameter $\frac{1}{100}$ – $\frac{1}{50}$ mm (Fig. 45, p. 354). Dilation of the small feeding arterioles raises the pressure in the capillaries of the glomeruli. A high glomerular capillary pressure is well established as a prime cause of kidney damage in diabetes. It is present in about 25% of patients. Doctors looking after people with diabetes regularly test the urine for the presence of protein. When more than trace quantities are present in the urine it suggests that the glomerular capillaries have been overstretched and damaged, and have become leaky.

An excess of protein in the urine is always a worrying finding. It signifies some structural damage to the kidneys. But kidney failure is not a common cause of death in people with diabetes. Such people more often die prematurely from heart attacks and strokes. The blood pressure is above normal for age and sex in 50% of all people with diabetes and is known to be specially associated with strokes (Chapter 34).

A high concentration of glucose in the blood has other damaging effects. In the short term a sudden rise in blood glucose concentration

146

changes the refractive index of the eyes, which temporarily lose focus. In the longer term diabetes is associated with excess production of a polypeptide chemical known as angiogenin. This increases the density and number of the minute blood vessels in the retina at the back of the eyes, impairing vision.[3] Diabetes can cause blindness in this way if left untreated. A curious but rare complication of diabetes (whether or not it is associated with insulin deficiency) is diabetic amyotrophy, in which there is pain and muscle weakness lasting some 6–12 months, but eventually recovering. Its cause is a mystery.

Diabetic eye disease is the commonest cause of blindness in the working population in most developed countries. One of the most important things that any doctor looking after people with diabetes needs to do is to ensure that the eyes are inspected regularly by an expert so that new growth of retinal blood vessels is detected and damage prevented. Protection is achieved by burning away (with a laser beam) the outer parts of the retina, which are less important for vision than the central ones. This reduces the vascularity (number of blood vessels) of the retina as a whole and prevents the important light-sensitive nerves from being unduly obscured.

Other ill-effects of 'hyperglycaemia' (too high a level of glucose in the blood) are more subtle. But there is no doubt that hyperglycaemia increases the amount and severity of atheroma, the white cheesy deposits of cholesterol which block arteries and predispose to thrombosis. This is a major cause of heart attacks and strokes, as I shall describe in Chapters 20 and 34. Diabetes is also thought to increase the chances of atheromatous plaques in large arteries cracking or rupturing.

A single measurement of blood glucose concentration says almost nothing about the adequacy of control of diabetes because blood glucose concentration is constantly changing, especially after meals. A better assessment takes advantage of the fact that circulating glucose becomes loosely combined with the oxygen-carrying pigment haemoglobin, inside red blood cells. The percentage of 'glycosylated' (sometimes called 'glycated') haemoglobin present in the blood is a good measure of how well-controlled the blood glucose concentration has been over the preceding few days, though the necessary (electrophoretic) analytical methods are difficult. Physicians treating diabetes aim to achieve a glycated haemoglobin concentration (HbA_{1c}) of 7% or less in their patients. There is a strong positive relation between an elevated HbA_{1c} percentage and long-term diabetic complications of the eyes and kidneys.

The role of insulin

The simple protein insulin plays a cardinal role in the causation, prevention and treatment of every variety of diabetes. Indeed, one definition of diabetes is that it is a 'state of diminished insulin action due to its decreased availability or effectiveness, in varying combinations'. Insulin was first introduced into medicine in 1921 and had a huge practical and emotional impact on medical practice. The well-known British physician RD Lawrence was rescued from the point of death in 1921 by timely injections of insulin. He lived to become one of the best known physicians specialising in the disease, and wrote a classic textbook.

Insulin has another first to its credit. It was one of the first proteins to be 'sequenced' – i.e. to have its exact chemical structure determined. It was also the first protein to be crystallised. It is now possible to synthesise insulin in the laboratory, sometimes using living bacteria, without having to get it from an animal. Since it is both formed and stored in the pancreas (a large gland at the back of the upper abdomen), much commercially available insulin is still extracted from the pancreas glands of animals. Despite its vital function in preventing diabetes, the main function of the pancreas is not the synthesis of insulin but rather the digestion of food. The pancreas secretes into the duodenum (the first part of the small intestine) alkaline pancreatic juice. This contains powerful digestive enzymes like trypsin, which break down food proteins into their component amino-acids (Chapters 11 and 12) and lipase, an enzyme which breaks down fats.

Insulin is formed and stored in small groups of ('beta') cells in the tail part of the gland. These are the 'islets of Langerhans', named after the man who first discovered them. The pancreas normally contains about 200 'units'[4] of insulin, which can only meet the body's needs for a fortnight, or less.

Langerhans cells synthesise a polypeptide chain compound of 51 amino acids, called proinsulin. This is then split into two smaller polypeptide chains (A and B) which later link together in a different configuration to form insulin proper. Insulin aggregates appear as granules in the islet cells. Each granule contains about 4000 molecules of insulin.

Insulin is structurally very similar to another small protein called insulin-like growth factor 1 (IGF-1). If this material is infused intravenously, it reduces the insulin requirements of someone with diabetes by about 50% and evidently possesses similar chemical affinities and actions.

The rate of synthesis of insulin is mainly dependent on the concentration of glucose in the blood passing through the gland. Insulin has many actions in the body, but it notably lowers the concentration of glucose in the blood and accelerates the synthesis of proteins and fat. If the blood sugar concentration rises, more insulin is released, and vice versa. The nerve supply of the pancreas is probably not very important for the control of insulin secretion. The negative feedback control system for insulin is mediated chemically. So the brain need not intervene to send nerve messages telling the islet cells to switch the secretion of insulin on or off.

Adequate insulin is important in seriously ill patients, whose prospects of survival are much improved by insulin therapy.[5] The blood glucose-lowering effects of insulin are increased by alcohol. This can produce dangerously low levels of glucose with consequent mental disturbances and even loss of consciousness in patients whose blood sugar is normally well controlled by insulin injections.

Specialised ('alpha') cells in the pancreas produce another hormone: 'glucagon'. This has many functions which are the opposite of those of insulin. It increases the rate of breakdown of fat and protein, and raises blood glucose concentration. It has been used as an antidote for people who have inadvertently taken too large a dose of insulin.

Metabolic effects of insulin

Fat is the body's main energy store. It is built up when food is abundant and broken down to supply energy when food is scarce. Life can be sustained for only about 3 hours by the breakdown of circulating glucose and amino-acids and for only about 15 hours by the breakdown of glycogen, a kind of stored starch. So fat is literally vital. After a meal, insulin secretion is the main message sent to fat tissue to increase the rate at which glucose crosses cell membranes and enters fat cells. This provides the energy for fat synthesis. Glucose is the chemical precursor of 'triglycerides', the building blocks of fat. Insulin also reduces the rate at which fat breaks down. In muscle and in liver insulin enhances protein synthesis and also promotes the conversion of glucose into glycogen.

Insulin is known to act at the surface of cell membranes. There is a story that a Harvard undergraduate once caused consternation when he said that he had discovered that glucose travelled faster across synthetic cellophane membranes when insulin was present than in its absence. This suggestion was soon disproved, but something of a mystery remains. Much of insulin action certainly takes place at the surface of cells, but there are probably additional actions within cells.

149

Infused insulin can lower blood glucose concentration very rapidly. This leads to adverse symptoms (confusion and odd behaviour) at levels below about 2.5 mmol/litre of glucose. People can lose consciousness even at higher levels, e.g. 2.8 mmol/l. The body's protective mechanisms are automatically switched on at somewhat higher levels. The hypothalamus, a small region in the centre of the brain (Fig. 7, p. 45) is the detector. When the blood passing through it has an unduly low glucose concentration, various mechanisms act to raise blood glucose again. These are mainly the secretion of adrenaline by the adrenal medulla gland in the abdomen, secretion of glucagon by the pancreas, and activation of the 'sympathetic' nervous system, which forms part of the so-called 'autonomic'[6] nervous system. Both these actions have opposite effects to insulin.

Insulin also has a direct action on blood vessels and the brain. When infused into a vein insulin mimics the effects of adrenaline, activates the sympathetic nervous system and constricts small arteries (arterioles) in most organs. But insulin is also itself a direct dilator of arterioles. The two actions usually cancel out, so that infusion of insulin into a human volunteer produces little overall effects on blood vessel resistance or on blood pressure.

Insulin's physiological effects are strangely similar to those of carbon dioxide gas. I am fascinated by the possibility that the effects of both insulin and carbon dioxide on blood vessels might work through the same final common path, although I have not examined this possibility further. I have documented elsewhere[7] the powerful blood-pressure-lowering effect of carbon dioxide inhalation in someone whose sympathetic nervous system has been blocked by drugs.

Epidemiology of diabetes

Type 1 diabetes is a major cause of human morbidity and mortality. In the world there are more than 20 million sufferers. Even so, Type 1 accounts for only about one tenth of the total number of people with diabetes. The remainder are mostly classified as having Type 2 disease, which will be described in the next chapter. Taken together, both type of diabetes are currently calculated to cost the National Health Service 9% of its entire budget: over £100 million per day.

The abbreviation 'IDDM' (Insulin-Dependent Diabetes Mellitus: doctors often talk about 'iddum' for short) is often used for Type 1. This distinguishes it from Type 2 (Non-Insulin-Dependent Diabetes Mellitus: 'NIDDM' – pronounced 'niddum'). Since absolute degrees of insulin dependency can be difficult to determine in borderline cases,

150

most physicians prefer to classify patients with diabetes as Type 1 or Type 2, without necessarily implying that they either need or do not need to take insulin.

It seems that numbers of both types of diabetes are steadily increasing. The peak incidence of Type 1 diabetes is in children of 5–15 years, although some people think that many older people who seem to have Type 2 really have mild Type 1. The incidence of Type 1 falls dramatically after the age of 15. People in different parts of the world have a vastly different incidence of Type 1 diabetes, e.g. 0.1 per 100,000 population per year in one part of China, and 40 per 100,000 per year in Finland. Some of the difference is certainly genetic, but there must be enormously important environmental factors. We have no idea what they are. There is no clear relation to ambient temperature, for example – which has a huge influence on the incidence of multiple sclerosis (Chapter 3).

The observation that new cases of Type 1 diabetes seldom appear after the age of 15 is fascinating. It might suggest that an environmental influence disappears at about that time. Alternatively, perhaps by age 15 potential subjects have had time to develop resistance to an infection, e.g. by developing antibodies. Some 80% of children who will develop Type 1 diabetes by the age of 15 have already developed recognised antibodies by age 5. This strongly suggests (to me) that a major precipitating trigger factor causing Type 1 diabetes is probably an ubiquitous childhood virus infection such as measles, mumps and chickenpox. But if so, it still awaits discovery.

Sufferers from Type 1 usually need insulin injections, because insulin by mouth would simply be digested and almost none would enter the blood unchanged. People with Type 1 can become seriously and rapidly ill if they miss out on their insulin injections or if their requirements for insulin go up suddenly because of an infection. Not only does the blood glucose concentration go up, with the ill consequences I have listed, but in addition the metabolism of so-called 'ketone bodies' (β-hydroxybutyric and aceto-acetic acid) is impaired. These accumulate in the blood and make it unduly acid. Indeed, the terminal event in uncontrolled Type 1 diabetes is 'keto-acidosis' when the pH[8] of the blood may fall below 7.0, with fatal consequences for many enzyme functions.

Possible causes of insulin deficiency

Everyone knows that lack of insulin causes diabetes. There is no immediate mystery why the pancreas of people with diabetes doesn't produce insulin normally. When it is examined under the microscope the islets of Langerhans are reduced in number, infiltrated with mononuclear cells, fibrosed or even absent. But why does this happen? It has been clear for many years that the problem is misbehaviour of the body's own immune protection system.

I was lucky to receive tutorials in the immunological causation of Type 1 diabetes from the late Andrew Cudworth while we were drinking beer after our weekly games of squash. Andrew had made use of the extensive and carefully documented records of diabetic families compiled by John Lister in Windsor, and by others in East London and in Oxford. Some people deride epidemiological studies as intellectually not demanding enough to be taken seriously as 'research'. This is a misguided attitude. There are innumerable examples of great discoveries being made by unexpected relationships and associations coming to light in large epidemiological studies. The careful collection of large population databases is nearly always necessary at some stage to allow possible causes of diseases to be systematically examined.

Investigation of many potential patients by assay of circulating antibody chemicals has revealed that Type 1 diabetes does not start suddenly. Before blood sugar starts to rise there is often evidence of the slow production, over months or even years, of circulating antibodies to pancreatic islet cells or to some of their constituent parts. This gives yet another possible handle on causation. HLA genetic status (p. 474) can be strongly associated either with resistance to or undue susceptibility to infections, by both bacteria and viruses. Could Type 1 diabetes be initiated in a susceptible subject by an infection, or by exposure to some noxious agent in the environment? Such studies also raise the possibility of treating potential sufferers from Type 1 diabetes before they became ill, perhaps by using immunosuppressive drugs. Also, if an infective agent can be identified, prophylactic vaccination might be a possibility.

Unhappily so far the results have been disappointing. No definite or generally accepted trigger factor or initiating infection has been identified, though there have been intensive studies of many viruses (e.g. coxsackie and cytomegalovirus). The long-term effects of immunosuppressive drugs, though they may delay or even arrest someone's progress towards Type 1 diabetes, have usually been judged to be worse than the disease itself. The whole situation for patients suffering from Type 1 would be transformed if insulin could be given by mouth. Digestive juices break oral insulin down to such an extent that almost none remains to be absorbed. But work is in progress to maximise the absorption of insulin, whether it is inhaled, swallowed or squirted into the mouth. Our current understanding of structural protein chemistry is already so extensive that it would not be surprising if within the next (say) 20 years an oral drug was developed to mimic the effects of injected insulin.

Patients with Type 1 diabetes develop circulating antibodies directed against several targets: (1) pancreatic islet cells or some of their contained protein constituents, notably insulin itself; (2) the enzyme 'glutamic acid decarboxylase' (GAD); (3) another protein called IA-2. At one time GAD seemed to be the answer to the $64,000 question. Was either GAD, or perhaps IA-2, the main body constituent which triggered damaging immunological destruction of the islet cells of the pancreas?[9] (The molecular weight of GAD just happens to be 64,000!) Certainly several parts of the GAD molecule are able to initiate immune reactions in susceptible people. If a non-diabetic individual is found to be carrying circulating antibodies against GAD, he or she is almost certain eventually to develop Type 1 diabetes, although this may not happen for a long time, even as long as 16 years. A large international study is under way, to find whether vaccinating potentially susceptible children against GAD may prevent them later acquiring auto-immunity against GAD. (Better still, of course, would be to find the presumptive infective agent or toxin which stimulates the human body to make GAD antibodies.)

Additional damage may be due to T-lymphocytes. Treatment of newly diagnosed Type 1 diabetic individuals with an antibody directed against certain specific T-cells may slow down the progress of the disease. More emphasis recently has been put on circulating antibodies produced by B-lymphocytes. But typical immune-mediated type 1 diabetes has been recorded in a patient who could not generate any circulating antibodies at all because of an inborn lack of B-lymphocytes.[10]

A curious aspect of the GAD story is that discretely different antibodies to GAD are also found in another entirely different condition, a rare neurological disorder which causes painful muscle spasms and rigidity and is associated with impaired transmission of nerve impulses.[11] Only about half such patients also have Type 1 diabetes. Unusually, the disease has not yet been given a complex Greek or Latin name. It is known simply as 'stiff man syndrome'.

Genetics

By determining the human leucocyte antigen (HLA) inheritance of patients and family members, Cudworth and others had observed that the chances of people developing Type 1 were strongly influenced by their HLA inheritance (note 9, p. 474). Another way of identifying potential victims before they had developed the disease was to study the identical twin of someone who had already developed diabetes but was currently well. There is only about a 50% chance of an identical twin developing Type 1 diabetes over a lifetime if his or her identical twin has it. This remarkable observation tells us that genetics is only part of the story. There must be very important environmental influences which start the disease off. As I pointed out earlier, these probably operate in early childhood.

> Type 1 diabetes can arise from mutations in either nuclear or mitochondrial genes.[12] HLA class II genes DQ and DR are important. Some confer protection against disease, but others make auto-immune islet-cell destruction more likely. One gene at fault is on chromosome 6 in the HLA complex[13] but other genes can contribute, including one on chromosome 11p which codes for the insulin molecule.

Other causes of Type 1 diabetes

There are several types of (hereditary) haemochromatosis, in which the pancreas is damaged by undue accumulation of iron. These are described in Chapter 26. When the consequential diabetes is severe, there is an absolute requirement for insulin injections. In severe forms of chronic pancreatitis the whole pancreas is severely inflamed and may be auto-digested by its own enzymes. Such a process can also incidentally destroy the islets in the tail of the pancreas and thus cause Type 1 diabetes.

I have seen one elderly man who got insulin-requiring Type 1 diabetes when he developed cancer in the tail of his pancreas. Diabetes is a recognised, though rare, occurrence in this situation. Another curious category is 'tropical' diabetes, which accounts for 5% of Type 1 diabetes in the tropics. There is T-cell infiltration of the pancreas but no GAD antibodies. I imagine that this must be due to an infection with a tropical pathogen which has not yet been identified.

Other aspects of auto-immune disorders associated with diabetes

A curious observation has been made in an animal model of Type 1 insulin-requiring diabetes. This is the inbred mouse strain known as NOD. This mouse, left untreated, will develop most of the signs and symptoms of Type 1 diabetes, with antibodies directed against its own pancreatic islets. But if young animals are deliberately infected with a gut parasite, auto-immune destruction of the pancreas is prevented. (I should add that this is only one of a very large number of methods of preventing diabetes developing in the NOD mouse!)

There is a suspicion that the increasing amount of Type 1 diabetes seen in developed countries may be due to unduly careful protection of young children against odd infections in the home. My younger daughter (herself a GP) never stops her own small daughter eating food that has fallen onto the floor. Is she protecting our grand-daughter against later development of auto-immune disease by ensuring that the child encounters a huge variety of different chemicals and potentially infectious agents which may perhaps exercise and stimulate the immune system? I don't know: but on balance I think she may be right. There has been a recent report that exposure of children to farm stables and farm milk in early life confers strong protection against asthma and other allergic disorders of sensitisation.[14]

There is a category of auto-immune diabetes which was previously classified as Type 2 but is now recognised to be a particular variant of Type 1. This is the 'Latent Autoimmune Diabetes of Adulthood' ('LADA'). This disease is recognised in about 10% of people with Type 1 diabetes. It occurs mainly in adults, as the name suggests. Such people notably have circulating antibodies to the enzyme 'GAD' and often have DR3 and DR4 HLA antigens.

A potentially very exciting new development is the administration of a peptide with the commercial name 'DiaPep277'. This development was first worked out in NOD mice (see above). The apparent protection against auto-immune destruction of the pancreas conferred by infection with a gut parasite has been recently found to relate to a change in T-cell function. This concerns a change in a specific (heat shock) protein called hsp-60 from a T-helper-1 (Th1) pro-inflammatory mode to a T-helper-2 (Th2) anti-inflammatory mode. Preliminary observations suggest that part of the hsp-60 protein, a peptide called 'p277', may be able to make this change in man, and thus delay or even prevent the development of Type 1 diabetes in predisposed humans. Trials so far look promising.[15]

Summary

Type 1 diabetes is due to an absolute lack of insulin, a small protein produced and stored in the tail of the pancreas, a gland at the back of the upper abdomen. Insulin is made in specialised cells which are found in small groups known as the islets of Langerhans. These are entirely separate from most of the glandular pancreas which secretes powerful digestive juices into the gut. In Type 1 diabetes the islet cells are degenerate, reduced in number, and infiltrated by lymphocytes.

Type 1 diabetes is a classic example of a disease associated with both genes and environment.[16] Both seem of equal importance, but in different situations and in different ethnic groups one or other may predominate. Susceptibility is mainly mediated by differing inheritance of Human Leucocyte Antigens (HLA); but disease development also requires a trigger factor to initiate the development of antibodies to pancreatic islet cells, or to some of their components. Many trigger factors have been suggested – mainly enterovirus infections – but none has so far been either proved or generally accepted as the main cause of type 1 diabetes.

15

DIABETES – TYPE 2

In the last chapter I summarised current knowledge about the causes of Type 1 diabetes, which occurs typically in children or young adults. In that disease there is an absolute deficiency of insulin, usually due to inflammation or destruction of the insulin-secreting cells in the tail of the pancreas gland in the upper abdomen. The patient has usually lost weight, passes a lot of urine, is liable to keto-acidosis, and usually needs insulin injections to get well and to avoid diabetic complications.

Ten times as many people have diabetes classified as Type 2 as those classified as having Type 1. Sufferers from Type 2 are typically female, middle-aged and usually overweight, although the disease also occurs in males, and in children. Excessive abdominal fat is characteristic and overweight is the single most important predictor of the later development of Type 2 diabetes. Smoking is also a predictor. On the other hand, regular exercise and the consumption of small amounts of alcohol lessen the chances of developing Type 2 diabetes.[1]

Type 2 diabetes develops insidiously over months or years. Treatment bringing adequate control of high blood glucose concentrations (hyperglycaemia) lessens the incidence and severity of complications. But it has not yet been convincingly shown to retard the slow progression of the disease. Type 2 diabetes is not a clearly-defined disease but rather 'a complex of risk factors for diseases of heart and arteries'. So strong is this association that it has even been described as 'a condition of premature cardiovascular disease'.

Hyperglycaemia in Type 2 patients can usually be controlled either by modifications of diet, or by drugs which can be given by mouth. Patients are not commonly at risk of keto-acidosis and seldom need insulin. Long-term studies suggest that good control of Type 2 diabetes (measured by a glycated haemoglobin concentration no higher than 7%) reduces long-term complications, though adequate control of hypertension and unduly high blood cholesterol are more important. I used to believe that all Type 2 diabetic patients could be controlled adequately by diet alone and that giving drugs, especially insulin, to reduce blood glucose would simply increase body weight without doing any real good. I was cured of this misapprehension by

Andrew Cudworth, who drew my attention to several early trial results which showed that hyperglycaemia is fundamentally bad for you and that reducing blood glucose by almost any means is beneficial. This view is now firmly established and accepted by all doctors, although it can only be proved for Type 2 diabetes. The blood-sugar-lowering drug metformin has been proved to reduce long-term complications of Type 2 diabetes.

Type 2 diabetes substantially reduces life expectancy. How much of this is due to the associated obesity and how much to high blood glucose concentrations is difficult to determine. Between 50 and 75% of deaths in people with Type 2 diabetes are due to diseases of the heart and arteries, classified collectively as 'cardiovascular' diseases. Some 40% of newly diagnosed people with diabetes already have recognisable cardiac and arterial disease when the diagnosis is first established. Their blood concentrations of harmful low density lipoprotein (LDL) cholesterol and triglycerides (fat precursors) are abnormally high. Conversely, their blood concentrations of high density lipoprotein (HDL) cholesterol (which seems to be protective against arterial disease) are unduly low. Treatment by lipid-lowering drugs such as 'statins' can slow the progression of arterial disease. So also can changes in life-style, particularly by increasing someone's level of physical exercise.

The risk of stroke is increased in Type 2 diabetes independently of associated hypertension: i.e. high blood pressure and diabetes have additive effects on the risk of stroke. As I mentioned in the last chapter, insulin stimulates the sympathetic nervous system. The increased concentrations of circulating insulin in most patients with Type 2 diabetes may account for some of the increased heart rate and blood pressure.[2]

Perhaps Type 2 diabetes is best described as a syndrome of abnormally increased resistance to the metabolic effects of insulin in muscle, fat and liver. This may be followed by failure of pancreatic beta cells to compensate adequately for this resistance, despite increased insulin secretion. In many human populations more than half the excess risk of coronary heart disease is associated with increased resistance to the actions of insulin. Furthermore the effects of insulin may be interfered with by circulating insulin antagonists or by damage to the chemical receptors with which insulin combines and acts. There has been some recent excitement in the identification of a newly identified hormone secreted by fat cells called 'resistin'. This has been suggested as a possible link between insulin resistance, obesity and Type 2 diabetes. So far the genetic links do not seem to be very strong.[3]

Epidemiology

About 4% of the entire world adult population has diabetes. In different countries the prevalence of Type 2 – much commoner than Type 1 – has been between 2% and 6%. The worldwide incidence of Type 2 is steadily increasing. In the USA the incidence of Type 2 diabetes in children and adolescents increased ten-fold during the 1980s. At present about 16 million Americans have the disease. In Europe three new cases of Type 2 diabetes are found every minute. In the UK there are 1.5 million people with diabetes, but it is estimated that there are another one million not yet diagnosed. About 10% of 65-year-old white people living in the UK have Type 2 diabetes, but the prevalence in UK Afro-Caribbean and Asian populations is higher still (between 15% and 20%). Type 2 diabetes costs the National Health Service about 2 billion pounds each year. This will increase to 10% of the UK health budget and is predicted soon to reach an annual 3 billion. Most of the cost arises from treatment of the cardio-vascular complications, predominantly heart attacks and strokes.

In developed countries about 4 in every 1000 children have the disease. But in adolescent Pima Indians, who are notably grossly overweight, the prevalence is 51 per 1000. It is interesting that exclusively breast-fed Pima Indians have a lower rate of diabetes than those exclusively bottle-fed.[4] The incidence of Type 2 in Japan is rising rapidly and is also associated with worsening overweight. Since it has been reckoned that about 20% of children in the USA are overweight and because the proportion has been steadily increasing, we can expect the incidence of Type 2 diabetes also to increase steadily with time.[5] Type 2 diabetes is specially prevalent among people acclimatised to eating high levels of fats and carbohydrates but taking little exercise. Diabetes is common among Australian aboriginals even when they are not overweight, suggesting that their inheritance may have evolved towards being able to take a highly calorie-rich diet appropriate for high levels of exercise, but inappropriate for a sedentary lifestyle.

Type 2 diabetes is commoner amongst poor people than amongst rich ones; but we do not know how much of the difference is due to richer people having a better diet, or to paying greater attention to their weight.

Genetics

A basic test to find to what extent a disease is genetic is to examine twin pairs. As I mentioned in the last chapter the concordance between identical twins with Type 1 diabetes is only around 50%. But for Type 2, given similar degrees of overweight, the resemblance and diabetic status (assessed by impaired tolerance of a glucose load) between identical twins with Type 2 diabetes is 90% after 15 years. So although the inheritance of Type 2 is complicated and confusing it is undoubtedly strong.

> Recently a search for susceptibility genes in Mexican Americans located a gene on chromosome 2 designated NIDDM1. This gene codes for an enzyme called 'calpain 10', the expression of which seems to confer resistance to the action of insulin. It increases susceptibility to Type 2 diabetes in elderly people.[6] Other possible markers have been reported on chromosome 1 (1q21-23) and on chromosomes 5, 8 and 10.
>
> In addition to chromosomal abnormalities predisposing to Type 2 diabetes, some 42 different mutations in mitochondrial DNA have also been recorded. One such is maternally inherited diabetes and deafness (MIDD), a kind of Type 2 with an onset usually before age 40.

Although the exact genetic causes of most cases of Type 2 diabetes have yet to be discovered, extensive studies have been made in rodents[7] When recalling the story of the discovery of the hormone 'leptin' (described in the next chapter) I am encouraged that intensive study of animal examples (models) of Type 2 diabetes in rats and mice may lead the way to identifying and classifying the many genes responsible for Type 2 diabetes in man. When this has been done it may become possible to devise more logical treatments than we have available at present.

Maturity-onset diabetes of the young

The six types of Type 2 diabetes categorised as 'maturity-onset diabetes of the young' (MODY) fall half-way between Types 1 and 2 Patients are mostly obese and sometimes have high blood pressure and lipid or cholesterol abnormalities.[8] Diabetes is typically diagnosed between the ages of 25 and 40. MODY is reckoned to account for 2% to 5% of all Type 2 diabetic patients. Antibodies to GAD (p. 160) are not present. In the first described type of this disease there is defective but not complete lack of function of the beta cells of the pancreas. The situation thus resembles an intermediate stage of Type 1 diabetes, described in the last chapter. It has only recently been recognised as having a different cause.

> Other varieties of MODY have other causes: e.g. MODY2 appears to be due to an inherited defect in the detection of blood glucose level by the

pancreatic beta cells, so that blood glucose concentration is set at too high a level. The inheritance of MODY is in an autosomal dominant mode. Several mutations have been recognised, affecting different pathways of glucose metabolism within cells. MODY can be due to mutations of chromosome 20 (MODY1), but also to mutations affecting chromosomes 7, 12, 13 and 17 – causing diseases which are classified as MODYs 2, 3, 4 and 5 respectively.

Cause

It is evident from what I have already summarised that Type 2 diabetes is, in part at least, a self-inflicted disease. Indeed a recent review concluded that the majority of cases of Type 2 diabetes could be prevented by the adoption of a healthier lifestyle – i.e. by reducing weight, taking more exercise, stopping smoking, eating a diet high in cereal fibre and polyunsaturated fat and taking a regular small amount of alcohol daily. Unhappily most of this excellent advice conflicts with human nature – except, perhaps, that for alcohol. A doctor's job is certainly to ensure that patients know the facts about the cause of their disease. But then the doctor must accept that most of us have weak wills. Fortunately, even if Type 2 diabetes cannot be prevented, many drugs can reduce its ill effects.

Immune mechanisms

The evidence for an inflammatory and possible auto-immune basis for Type 2 diabetes is not strong, but suggestive: e.g. the blood concentrations of C-reactive protein (a marker for inflammation somewhere) are on average twice as high in people with Type 2 diabetes as in a control population without diabetes. Minor changes in some inflammation-producing cytokines (p. 18) have also been reported.

Insulin resistance

Claims have been made that a polypeptide other than insulin – 'amylin' – might be a main cause of Type 2 diabetes, by antagonising the actions of insulin. Amylin is co-secreted by and extractable from pancreatic islet cells. Thus Type 2 might logically be treated by drugs specifically antagonising amylin. This approach has unfortunately proved to be a blind alley. But the story of the decline and fall of interest in amylin is a fascinating one which has been described in the pages of the journal *The Lancet*.[9]

Another hormone derived from and produced by fat cells ('resistin') has been found to reduce the metabolic effects of insulin. It increases 'insulin resistance' which is strongly associated with overweight.[10] This recent discovery has stimulated a great deal of work. Attempts are being made at present to design chemical antagonists to resistin in the hope that such drugs might be useful both in treating Type 2 diabetes and also perhaps in helping patients reduce weight.

Another aspect of insulin resistance is its association with so-called 'non-alcoholic fatty liver disease'[11] which is strongly associated with obesity, especially in children. In adults it is the commonest cause of abnormal results in blood tests for liver function. There is no single cause for this condition, although weight reduction may improve liver function tests as well as reducing insulin resistance.

Aspects of treatment

Extensive evidence links good diabetic control (normal blood glucose levels) with a decreased incidence of complications, although there is some worry about the sulphonylurea drugs. Some drugs reducing cholesterol (notably the 'statins') may protect against complications in Type 2 diabetes independently of blood glucose control.

A few years ago a new class of orally-effective drugs (the 'glitazones') was introduced into diabetic therapy. These drugs act mainly on fatty tissue and in some way sensitise fat cells to the effects of insulin by acting on specialised receptors in fat cell nuclei. Current clinical trials are comparing their effectiveness with standard therapy. It already seems that although glitazones are not a cure for Type 2 diabetes and probably do not slow down the rate of progression of the illness, they can successfully reduce blood glucose concentrations. This will surely give some long-term protection against cardiovascular complications, unless they prove to have some unanticipated damaging side-effect (such as liver or muscle necrosis, which has been observed with one of the drugs).

Insulin resistance has probably many different causes which may involve protein kinase C and beta3-adrenoreceptors in fat tissue. Resistance to all drugs lowering blood glucose tends to increase with time, as the disease itself progresses because of pancreatic beta cell failure. The so-called ACE inhibitors are believed to slow progression of disease even in people with no obvious involvement of the kidneys. Some authors feel that the cardiovascular risks of gross obesity (body mass index ⩾35) in someone with Type 2 diabetes are so severe that surgery may be justified.

Summary

A definition of Type 1 diabetes was given in the last chapter. In that condition there is a true deficiency of the blood-glucose-lowering chemical 'insulin' because the islets of Langerhans in the pancreas gland are destroyed or non-functional.

Type 2 diabetes is different because insulin is usually present in normal or even above-normal concentrations, but its effects are diminished by resistance to it in most organs and tissues. There are very strong genetic factors predisposing both to Type 2 diabetes and to obesity. There may also be circulating insulin antagonists. Resistance to insulin actions is greatly dependent on the amount of fat in the body.

Cardinal therapeutic objectives in treatment are reduction of body weight, blood glucose, blood pressure and smoking, together with dietary or drug treatment to improve cholesterol and lipid levels.

16

OBESITY

Who is 'overweight', 'obese' or 'too fat'?

We all have different ideas about which of our acquaintances can be realistically and fairly described as overweight, fat or too fat. Fortunately there is an internationally recognised measurement which usefully defines overweight and obesity in human adults. This is the Body Mass Index (BMI), which is calculated from the body weight in kilograms, divided by the height in metres, squared. (For those scientists who consistently use S.I. units for everything except everyday life, Fig. 21 shows body mass index calculations in terms of pounds, feet and inches!) The criteria are somewhat different for children. A generally acceptable normal weight for an adult is a BMI which lies between 18.5 and 24.9,[1] i.e. in the shaded area of Figure 21. A healthy man should have less than 20% of his body weight as fat tissue and a healthy woman not more than 25%. All these measures are obviously arbitrary. They are strongly influenced by prevailing fashions.

Someone with a BMI between 25 and 30 would usually be regarded as 'overweight', someone with a BMI above 30 as 'obese', and one above 35 as 'grossly obese'. This classification is widely accepted and has been used in many studies to predict the risk of heart attacks and strokes, both of which happen more often in obese than in lean individuals. For those without weighing scales and calculators, waist circumference is almost as good a predictor as BMI. Men with a waist circumference greater than 36 inches (90 cm) should be classified as overweight and those with waists greater than 40 inches (100 cm) should be classified as obese. In women the equivalent measurements are 33 inches (83 cm = overweight) and more than 37 inches (93 cm = obese). In England a decade ago 13% of men and 16% of women were classed as obese. These proportions have now risen to 16% for men and 17.5% for women. In the USA the overall prevalence of obesity rose from 12% to 18% over a recent 4 year period of observation.[2] In the UK about £$\frac{1}{2}$ billion of health-care costs and £2 billion other costs are attributable to obesity. The same applies in the USA,

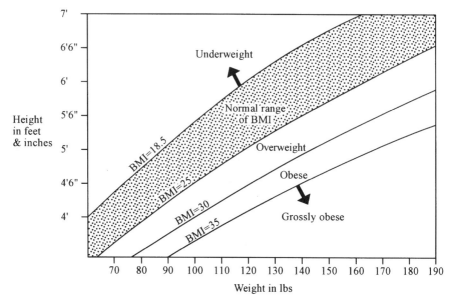

Figure 21 Chart relating height and weight (in 'traditional' units) to body mass index (BMI). The shaded area indicates the generally accepted normal range of BMI (18.5–25) for adults of different heights and weights. People whose height and weight takes their BMI above 30 can be regarded as obese; those above 35 could be described as 'grossly obese'.

in which the percentages are even higher. Drug treatments for obesity are approved for people with a BMI greater than 27.

Overweight is an important cause of diabetes, high blood pressure and arterial disease. With fair certainty we can place female fertility on a weight-dependent scale. Women's periods stop when their weight drops below about 40 kg but their fertility is also impaired by gross obesity. People's suitability for occupations other than reproducing their species will depend on whether they are weightlifters, sprinters, fashion models, Channel swimmers or Japanese Sumo wrestlers. Should we choose fitness for our chosen occupation or sport as the criterion for assessing body weight? Do we choose sexual attractiveness – in which case, to whom? And what about longevity?

The ill effects of obesity

Many of the ill effects of obesity are obvious, e.g. reduced exercise capacity, wear and tear on weight-bearing joints and psychological distress from a perceived unaesthetic body image. But there are many more ill effects which are not so widely known. Obesity is associated with an increased volume of circulating blood as well as with increased blood pressure.[3] The blood pressure of obese people is higher than that of people the same age but who are not overweight. Regardless of other factors, this increases the risk of a stroke. There is a tendency for the amount of sugar in the blood to increase, partly due to resistance to the actions of the hormone insulin. In grossly obese people the blood sugar concentration may get so high that glucose comes out into the urine, as discussed in the last two chapters.

Surprisingly, overweight individuals have been observed to have significantly increased chances of getting most varieties of cancer. A recent calculation suggests that in the USA 90,000 deaths per year from cancer would be prevented if men and women could maintain normal weight.[4] Coronary artery disease, varicose veins, gall stones, constipation, ankle swelling, menstrual irregularities, skin irritation and poor wound healing are all more common in fat people than in lean.

Human weight regulation

A very simple animal such as the sea slug from Tenerife has two activities in life: searching for and eating food, and copulation. Each of these two activities is brought about by the secretion of one of two circulating chemicals (hormones). The chemicals concerned have been identified and made synthetically. A sea slug injected with the appetite-stimulating chemical eats more and gets fatter, while the one injected with the sex hormone stops anything else it is doing and starts copulating. Human beings have more complex control systems! To understand obesity it is obvious that we need to know what controls human appetite.

Clearly obesity must be due to an imbalance between the energy taken in as food and that expended in all bodily activities. This applies to lower animals as well as ourselves. Although the laboratory rat living in an artificially constant environment maintains a constant body weight over months and years, it can easily be made obese if it becomes a family pet and is given large amounts of the foods it likes. Our own cat at home is lazy and getting fatter each year, no doubt because she is frequently given appetising titbits from the kitchen. During the evolution of other mammals as well as man, eating up to a tolerable limit and perhaps even beyond it may have been advantageous as a buffer against later food scarcity. Greed may thus have had a survival advantage.

To ensure that no reasonable opportunity should be lost in stocking up food when it is available the human race has evolved the genetic behaviour pattern that we call appetite. Some people make a distinction between hunger (a desire for any food) and appetite (a desire for a particular food), but the distinction is blurred. Most discussions use 'appetite' as a useful general term. From animal studies and from occasional inadvertent human experiments (mostly from bullet wounds) we know that appetite and its control resides in in the hypothalamus, which lies in the centre of the front part of the brain (Fig. 7, p. 45). The central parts of the hypothalamus produce chemicals directly diminishing appetite and have nervous connections with other parts of the brain which also depress appetite. On the other hand, the parts of the hypothalamus at either side stimulate appetite. Damage to these areas causes loss of appetite. Animals with such lesions may even starve to death when food is available. Damage to the central hypothalamic structures increases appetite and reduces the production of heat within the body, by reducing the activity of sympathetic nerves supplying brown fat. Such changes lead to obesity both in man and animals.

Many studies have been made of energy balance in man, adding up the total calorie value of each item of food consumed and comparing this with the energy expended. The total energy in any particular food can be calculated by burning it up in a 'bomb calorimeter' which accurately measures the quantity of heat produced. More conveniently, the energy equivalent in the diet is calculated from tables showing the calorie value of each food item eaten, adding it all up to get a grand total. Some foods present difficulties. For example, fresh mushrooms contain little energy, but when fried they can contain a lot because fat has replaced the water which has been driven off.

Studies in obesity

Many people imagine that fat people are fat and remain fat because they eat more food than slim people. This is roughly correct, but the situation is more complicated. Someone's energy expenditure from the metabolism of food is proportional to their lean body mass, i.e. the mass of body tissue excluding fat. But lean body mass goes up in parallel with fat mass, though not so rapidly. Someone whose weight is greater than that of someone else with similar body build must necessarily be eating more, providing that medical conditions such as thyroid hormone deficiency have been excluded.

Obviously an individual's level of habitual physical activity is very important. Gareth Williams once put it to me dramatically: sitting brain dead in front of a television set uses up about one calorie per minute, whereas kicking a football around outside consumes about seven times as much. So a young man would gain about 20 pounds weight (9 kg) in a year simply by being brain dead for half an hour each day instead of kicking a football around for half an hour – a dramatic way of looking at childhood obesity! Some of the sums are a bit depressing. Eating an apple a day is reputed to keep the doctor away. But an apple contains 70 kcalories, equivalent to 7 grams of fat. Over 10 years this practice would increase body weight by 16 kg (35 lbs)!

It is interesting that although obesity may certainly be a family trait, body proportions in childhood may bear no relation to adult body build. Fat children can become slim adults and the tiniest children tend to have the highest risk of adult obesity. But as we can all observe, fat parents often have fat children. Everyone knows families who seem to have inherited a tendency to obesity. It can be difficult to be quite sure about this, because of the effects of the environment. If your parents, especially your mother, are fat, there may be psychological pressures to conform with a pattern of eating in the family which encourages obesity. Parental obesity is the most important risk factor for childhood obesity. Most twin studies comparing obesity inheritance in identical and non-identical twins show that between a quarter and a half of the differences in weight between individuals is genetic, though a few larger estimates have been made. The remaining variation is environmental.

There is a lot of current interest in 'fetal programming' – i.e. the possibility that nutrition of the fetus in the womb during pregnancy may have a life-long influence on body build and bodily functions in later life.[5] Most of this work has been done in rats. It is difficult to transfer or interpret much of the work to a human scale. Published reports about the long-term effects on women pregnant and starved during notable wartime sieges (e.g. of Stalingrad) suggest that the long-term effects of fetal undernutrition are surprisingly small. Several epidemiological investigations suggest that malnutrition in childhood may predispose to later obesity, but there are so many possible confounding factors, related to the availability of money and food choices, that it is difficult to decide what is most important. Personal observations suggest that obesity is most common among low socioeconomic groups.

The story of leptin

The discovery of leptin is one of the most remarkable and exciting recent advances which have followed intense study of a genetically obese rat. In 1961 Lois and Theodore Zucker described a strain of rat with a voracious appetite. Zucker rats become grossly obese from an early age. They get diabetes, with the expected complications, and are resistant to insulin.[6] The Zuckers called the defective gene 'fatty'. They found that it behaved as an autosomal recessive[7] character (p. 480). Rats with the *fa* mutation failed to respond to a circulating hormone which normally damps down appetite. A rat which has inherited this receptor defect from both its parents continues to eat even when it is grossly obese. It has a much shorter life-span than an average laboratory-bred rat and eventually succumbs to degenerative disease of heart and arteries. The gene concerned with the defect was present in normal rats, but when it was deficient or defective it resulted in obesity.

The responsible protein in humans which normally combines with the receptor discussed in the previous paragraph has been given the name 'leptin' (from Greek: *leptos* = thin). Leptin has turned out to be a circulating chemical produced by fat cells all over the body. Since the rate of production of leptin is directly proportional to the total mass of fat in the body, the way seems open to characterise a plausible negative feedback system which might underlie long-term regulation of human body weight (Fig. 22).

The discovery of leptin immediately led to the hope that leptin or a related compound might be the answer to human obesity. Alas, this has not proved to be the case. An obese human family was soon identified whose members were truly leptin deficient. They had a mutation in the leptin gene known as *ob*. Another obese human family

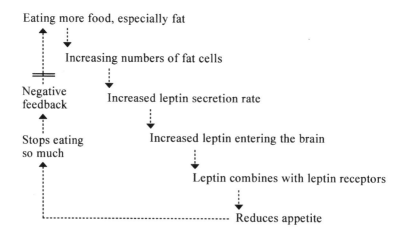

Figure 22 Components of a possible negative feedback system involving leptin, which could keep body weight constant over time.

had members (like those of the original Zucker rat strain) who lacked the chemical receptor with which leptin combines. In people with leptin deficiency, injections of leptin can successfully reduce both appetite and weight. Unfortunately it soon became clear that true leptin deficiency is very rare. Most fat people have the expected amounts of circulating leptin in their blood, corresponding to their extra amounts of fat tissue. The fatter they are, the more leptin they produce.

Although leptin deficiency is only very rarely the cause of human obesity, the discovery of leptin has created tremendous interest.[8] Recent work all tends to the conclusion that most human obesity results from the combined effects of many genes which control appetite and determine whether excess food will be stored in the form of fat or not. Zucker genes are not the only ones involved. Variations in the gene which codes for the leptin receptor are commoner than mutations in the leptin gene itself. Minor changes in the receptor genes may comprise some of what have been described as 'polygenic influences on the nutritional environment'.[9]

Since leptin is synthesised in and released from body fat cells the concentration of leptin in the circulating blood is normally increased in direct proportion to an individual's obesity. It has even been regarded as 'one of the best biological markers reflecting total body fat'. Leptin also has a role to play during the development of puberty, in the menstrual cycle, in pregnancy and during lactation. It has even been regarded as a critical link between fat and the reproductive system. Undernourished individuals or those with chronic conditions such as heart failure have low leptin levels in the blood. But despite all the current interest in leptin, it appears that leptin is probably a less important controller of body weight in man than it seems to be in the rat.

It is fascinating that recent Japanese work has reported a link between leptin and taste preference for sweet tasting food. Obese *fa/fa* mice lacking the leptin receptor prefer sweet-tasting food. This appears to be because they possess a 'sweet-receptor gene' known as T1R3 which is selectively expressed in the taste cells of the tongue and mouth. When given leptin, *fa/fa* mice lose their sweet-taste preference. The authors suggested[10] that the taste organ is a natural peripheral target for leptin. Minor degrees of leptin deficiency could obviously act together with other obesity-predisposing factors (see below).

Other factors influencing appetite

For most of the population the inheritance of obesity is 'polygenic': i.e. it depends on many genes. There is no single gene or inherited characteristic the presence of which determines whether someone will be fat or not. But there are a few rare human genetic defects involving a single gene. Several have been found so far in addition to leptin. It is worth considering some of these because of their intrinsic interest and because they might suggests new ways to control appetite.

In addition to leptin, fat cells (adipocytes) synthesise, store and release a hormone which might contribute to obesity, either by stimulating appetite or antagonising other factors which normally depress appetite. To give a proper impression of the complexity of the factors which influence appetite and weight, I have summarised in the paragraphs that follow the main factors so far identified. To avoid confusion I have referred to most of these by their abbreviated chemical nicknames. It is quite certain that the story is by no means complete! Many of these chemicals are now targets for the pharmaceutical industry because most fat people have enormous difficulty in controlling their appetite. They are quite prepared to spend huge amounts of money to reduce their weight by taking drugs which can avoid them having to produce an effort of will.

Other appetite-controlling hormones and neuropeptide-Y

Sympathetic nervous system influences are important. Many of the drugs which have been used in the treatment of obesity are related to the adrenal gland catecholamines (p. 150). Serotonin and noradrenaline inhibit feeding, but adrenaline and dopamine stimulate it. Sibutramine inhibits the re-uptake of serotonin and noradrenaline and thus prolongs their actions and effects. It has been approved by the UK Government's regulatory body for treating obese adults in whom simpler treatments have failed.

Apart from leptin, peptides produced by genes implicated in obesity include those which code for the production and secretion of many chemicals, including the most active of all, 'NeuroPeptide-Y' (NPY). This is released from the terminals of sympathetic nerves together with noradrenaline. It shares many actions of noradrenaline, including constriction of blood vessels and is found in high concentration in the brain and in many other tissues. NPY is a key regulator of energy storage. The molecule of NPY contains 36 amino-acids. It is synthesised everywhere in the brain of man and of rodents, especially in the hypothalamus. When injected into the ventricles of the brain or into specific regions of the hypothalamus it increases food intake, reduces heat production and stimulates release of insulin. On repeated injection into animals it can cause obesity. Antagonism of NPY by artificially-created NPY-antibodies reduces food intake. An important role of NPY is to restore

172

energy stores after food restriction and starvation. High concentrations of NPY are found in the blood of people with heart failure (Chapter 21) but we do not know why.

Several chemicals related to NPY combine with it. Technically speaking they are 'receptors' for it. Six different ones have been identified. They are tempting drug targets to reduce appetite. A Y5 blocking compound (found only in the brain) looks to be a good target as an anti-obesity drug. An important recent discovery is that when food enters the gut its lining cells release into the bloodstream a hormone known so far as peptide YY_{3-36} (PYY). When its role has been finally established it will doubtless be given a trendier name. Its secretion is proportional to the total number of calories ingested and it acts on Y2 receptors in the central parts of the hypothalamus to reduce appetite. It seems well suited to play some part in a negative feedback path to control body weight. Its blood concentration has already been reported to be reduced in obese subjects and it might prove a useful human appetite suppressant.[11]

Antagonists to several other appetite-stimulating peptides have been examined by the drug industry. There is current interest in the 'hypocretins' (otherwise known as orexins), also found in the hypothalamus. There is additional recent interest in these peptides because deficiency may cause the mysterious sleep disorder known as narcolepsy. Genetic or acquired deficiency in any of the known appetite suppressors (including CRF, CART, CCK, GLP-1) could all contribute to obesity. Related compounds are being actively investigated as possible appetite-suppressing anti-obesity drugs.

One of the most potent feeding inhibitors is 'α-melanocyte-stimulating hormone' (α-MSH). A genetic lack of α-MSH may account for a few cases of genetic obesity manifest in childhood. Another rare genetic cause of childhood obesity is failure of normal suppression of another peptide (AGRP), which may be an anti-obesity target. Recent success has been reported for rimonabant, a drug which blocks the cannabis-related receptors which combine with natural morphine-related appetite stimulants.

'Melanocortins' (MC) are hormones closely concerned with reproduction and with the onset of puberty. They also suppress appetite. Mutations in a receptor with which MC combines (MCR4) are at present the commonest known dominantly-inherited single gene causes of human overeating and obesity. Though rare, they are much commoner than leptin deficiency. The melanocortin-4 (MC4R) receptor gene may be inadequately expressed in some obese individuals.[12]

Interesting new work has identified a peptide called 'ghrelin' made by specialised cells in the stomach wall. It stimulates eating when injected into rats or mice and makes them fat. It also stimulates the release of growth hormone. Injected into human beings it makes them hungry. So far there is no evidence that ghrelin overproduction is a cause of obesity[13] – indeed, ghrelin secretion is inhibited in obese individuals.

The human body can synthesise and release many other appetite-stimulating chemicals, including TNFα, IL-6, neurotensin, bombesin, GLP-1, galanin and CRF. Many different factors influence the storage of fat in fat cells, including 'peroxisome proliferator activator receptors' (PPARs).[14] Yet another hormone, 'gastric inhibitory polypeptide' (GIP), influences the storage of dietary fat in fat tissue and determines whether or not it is consumed as fuel. Its release is triggered by absorption of fat or glucose by the intestine.

Why do people get fat?

There are many factors which can determine whether someone gets fat or not: the amount of food eaten, the rate of turnover of that food inside the body, the proportion used to generate heat and the size of the body fat stores.[15] Exercise affects food consumption and food metabolism. Although most adults living in the developed world get slowly fatter as they grow older, at least until their sixties or seventies, the long-term stability of most people's weight is really remarkable. People talking about stabilising systems which work on the principle of negative feedback often forget one necessary component of any such a system: it must have a fixed set point to hold long-term stability.

Many years ago, when I was working full-time in a physiology laboratory, I built many pieces of electronic apparatus using war surplus material from aircraft radar equipment. The long-term stability of many of these devices required a power supply of constant voltage. To get this I soon learnt that it was necessary to incorporate as a reference a constant voltage source with which the output voltage of the power supply could be continuously compared and continuously readjusted. My best pieces of equipment at that time (in the 1950s) contained a 'neon stabiliser'. This used a two-element neon-filled glass tube which, once the neon tube had 'struck' (lit up) and was conducting electrons, had the property of maintaining a constant voltage across it despite wide changes in the current passing through it.[16] By continuously comparing the output voltage of the power supply with the reference voltage available across the neon tube it was possible to create a power supply with a steady output voltage despite changes in current load.

Even if you can't immediately identify it, any stabilising system using negative feedback must have a fixed reference point if it is not to drift slowly in one direction or another. Ancient steam engines had a 'governor' comprising two steel balls which were whirled round higher and higher as the engine speed increased. The governor was connected to the steam valve so that steam was shut off when the balls reached a certain height. In this case the fixity of the reference point was obtained by the fixed mass of the whirling balls acting against gravity.

I do not apologise for labouring this point – *the absolute necessity of a fixed reference point for any stabilising system* – because it is so often forgotten by people describing biological systems. They feel that they have fully described the system when all that they have described is the relation between input and output. Such thoughts are highly relevant to the study of obesity. Is the problem the lack of a fixed reference point? If so, where or what is it? How is it that some individuals manage to maintain a virtually constant weight, or one appropriate to their habitual physical activity, whereas others seem powerless to stop themselves getting gradually fatter? Are the media so powerful in stimulating people to do more of what they like doing anyway that they can persuade otherwise intelligent people to override all the controls on body weight which the human race has acquired by evolution over millions of years?

What is the link between the level of habitual and regular exercise and food intake?

This question is one of the most interesting of our current medical mysteries. Obviously we can, within limits, control the amount of exercise we take. We know that we can either accept or ignore the signals that our bodies tell us about the amount and kind of food that we should eat. We also know that most of us are made (in the words of the Bible) of flesh that is 'weak'. The human race is bound to have evolved a link of some sort between physical exercise and appetite. We all recognise that people who habitually take a great deal of exercise are usually a bit under average weight, seldom above it.

It is tempting to suggest or hypothesise that physical exercise might reduce appetite by increasing the rate of production of leptin from fat cells. Indeed this could be thought of as a very appropriate design which would explain why people taking a lot of exercise rarely put on excessive weight. Although initial studies based on single measurements of leptin before and after exercise failed to find any supporting evidence, better studies have confirmed a weak link.[17] Quantitatively it does not seem to be of great importance. But I confidently expect that many other links between exercise and appetite-controlling chemicals will be discovered.

Treatments for obesity

In addition to approaches by blocking the action of appetite-stimu-lating drugs and enhancing the action of appetite-inhibiting drugs, other approaches have been tried, but so far with only modest success. None the less, one interesting completely different approach to human weight control is to interfere with fat absorption, e.g. by orlistat. This is a drug which inhibits lipase, an enzyme secreted in pancreatic juice. Lipase breaks down fats, rendering them better absorbed. Orlistat is well tolerated and has achieved some success in a careful clinical trial.[18]

The success or failure of anti-obesity treatment is highly dependent on psychological factors, as we all know. Some of these are financial. I recall an enormously obese man in charge of a betting shop. He was threatened with dismissal by his employer unless he got back to a more normal size – which he promptly did. I have come across many similar examples.

Summary

Overweight is defined by a body mass index (BMI) greater than 25, and obesity by a BMI greater than 30. In studies of populations, obesity has been shown to shorten life-span and to predispose to arterial disease, diabetes and cancer. Although a few individuals have rare single gene defects causing obesity, in most cases it is due to the gratification of an appetite which is excessive and inappropriate for the body build. If the energy taken as food is greater than that expended by physical exercise, the excess energy will be stored as fat. Since appetite is controlled by the brain's hypothalamus, intensive research is currently concentrated on chemicals produced by or reacting with nerve cells in that organ.

One recently identified chemical is leptin, produced by fat cells. This inhibits appetite, but when either leptin itself, or the receptor chemical with which it normally combines is missing, the individual becomes obese. Similar defects have been recognised in inbred rat strains. Many other chemicals have been identified which either increase appetite (e.g. neuropeptide-Y, the hypocretins and ghrelin) or decrease it (e.g. serotonin, noradrenaline and melanocortins). Human obesity in most cases is polygenic. It results from the integrated effect of many genes and also of many psychological factors. Exercise tends to reduce appetite, but we do not know why.

Partial success in treating obesity has come from drugs such as sibutramine (acting directly on the appetite-stimulating centres in the brain) and orlistat (which interferes with the enzymic digestion of fat in the gut). Future work is likely to concentrate on the large number of hypothalamic hormones and on the receptor chemicals with which they combine.

17

ENDOMETRIOSIS

Endometriosis (EMT) is a common but bizarre condition. It describes a situation in women in which the normal inner lining of the womb (uterus) is not confined to its normal situation. It has appeared in one or more places outside the womb, usually within the abdominal cavity, most often on the surface of the ovaries. During the reproductive years, some of this inner lining (the endometrium) is normally shed from the uterus each month, accompanied by bleeding from the vagina (the menstrual 'period'). The menstrual cycle is indirectly (via the ovary) controlled by circulating chemical substances (hormones) which are secreted into the bloodstream from the pituitary gland, lying deep inside the skull at the base of the brain. The ovarian hormones act on chemical receptors in the endometrium telling it to shed its old lining cells and regrow its lining at the end of each month, unless other chemical instructions have been given to the womb by secretions from a newly fertilised egg (ovum).

Unfortunately all these effects can be as true for endometrium outside the womb as for the normal endometrium lining the womb. Therefore a lump of endometrial tissue which has somehow got into the abdominal cavity – perhaps stuck on to a piece of the gut – may shed cells and perhaps bleed slightly each month. This can cause abdominal pain at the time of a woman's period by irritating the smooth lining of the abdominal cavity (the peritoneum). If the blood does not leak out it may be retained in the endometrial tissue itself, forming dark-coloured ('chocolate') cysts.

The cause of the pain is rather similar to the pain which some women get between periods, the well-known 'mittelschmerz' ('middle-pain'). This is produced by slight irritation of the peritoneum when a new egg breaks out from the surface of an ovary and briefly enters the peritoneal cavity on its way to one of the two fallopian tubes, which convey it to the womb. If it has been fertilised by a man's sperm it becomes implanted in the endometrium about 9 days later.

Although the pain of endometriosis occurs particularly at the same time as menstruation, for obvious reasons, it is also a cause of vague and ill-defined abdominal pain. The diagnosis can only be made for sure by inspecting the membrane lining the abdominal cavity. This can obviously be done when the abdomen has been opened surgically, but it can also be done, though with greater difficulty, by the use of a laparoscope (a slim hollow tube with a light at its end) which is inserted into the abdomen via a small incision. EMT lesions appear as superficial bluish-red patches or as 'chocolate cysts' containing old changed blood. They most commonly occur on the surface of the ovaries but can be found anywhere in the abdominal cavity: on the pelvic organs, on the inner abdominal wall, on the surface of some part of the gut, or on the surface of the liver. Patches may also be seen in unusual places, difficult to inspect, such as the lower surface of the muscular diaphragm, which separates the chest from the abdominal cavity. Sometimes actual lumps of endometrial tissue may resemble and be mistaken for a tumour mass. Occasionally lesions can occur within the abdominal wall, or even outside the abdominal cavity altogether.

Under the microscope, the tissue in endometriosis patches resembles normal endometrium, but some differences have been noted when the tissue is cultured in the laboratory. It produces two proteins which are not produced when cells lining the uterus are grown in tissue culture. In addition, it fails to produce three other proteins which normal endometrial cells produce. We do not know whether these results indicate a true difference in endometrial cells themselves, or whether their synthetic capabilities have been altered by the unusual environment.

Epidemiology

When severe enough to cause symptoms, endometriosis affects between 3% and 7% of all women between the ages of 20 and 45 in developed countries. In the USA it has been reported in about 70% of adolescent girls complaining of chronic pelvic pain. Overall prevalence in the general female population has been estimated as 10%. Prevalence increases with age in pre-menopausal women. It is also associated with shorter (and therefore more frequent) menstrual cycles. There have been useful reviews both of possible causes and current methods of treatment.[1]

The prevalence of endometriosis in undeveloped countries has never been reliably evaluated. African women are generally believed to be relatively unaffected. This seems to be borne out by the paucity of case reports from Central Africa. I have been able to find only one such report published in the last 30 years.[2] It might be relevant that the five women reported in this paper were professionals: two were nurses, one a pharmacist, one a school teacher and one a secretary, i.e. all were highly educated. I could find no published survey of naturally-occurring abdominal endometriosis in Indian women. In terms of publications about endometriosis during the last 30 years, there have been 1200 from the USA, about 250 from the UK, but none from Saudi Arabia and only the one (already mentioned) from Central Africa. Either the condition is very rare in these parts of the world, or doctors there do not report it in medical journals.

Genetics

There is some evidence of genetically determined susceptibility to EMT, but no clearly defined Mendelian (p. 480) pattern of inheritance. When the disease is extensive it is associated with infertility. It is sometimes said to be a *cause* of infertility, but it is much more likely that infertility and endometriosis share a common cause. Treating or removing endometriosis lesions does not usually restore fertility, though a recent report has been more encouraging.

Cause

The simplest explanation (the 'transplantation theory') for endometriosis is that one or more of the small lumps of endometrium which are shed each month from the lining of the uterus find their way through (up) a fallopian tube into the abdominal cavity, and lodge there. This idea, best described as the 'retrograde menstruation' hypothesis, was first put forward by John Sampson in the 1920s. It is supported by the frequency with which EMT deposits are found on the surface of the ovaries, close to the open ends of the fallopian tubes. Figure 23 illustrates the relationship between the abdominal cavity (lined by the smooth peritoneum), the two ovaries, the two fallopian tubes, the uterus, and the vagina.

Experiments in rats have shown that when a lump of tissue from the wall of the uterus (the endometrium) is brought into contact with the lining of the peritoneal cavity, the lining itself disappears. The new tissue appears to be joined seamlessly to the old. This happens in most experiments within 18–24 hours. The new tissue has in effect become part of the lining of the abdominal cavity (the peritoneum). This very convincingly verifies that transplantation is both feasible and highly likely to occur on most occasions that a piece of endometrium comes into contact with the peritoneum.

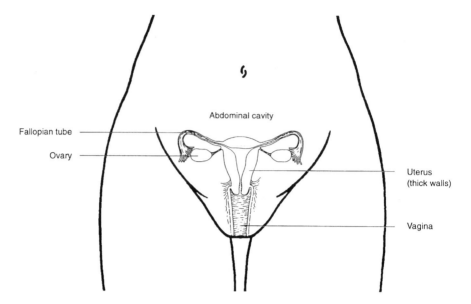

Fallopian tube

Ovary

Abdominal cavity

Uterus
(thick walls)

Vagina

Figure 23 Diagram of the spatial disposition of the internal female organs of reproduction.

The normal function of the fallopian tubes is to convey an egg,
newly liberated from an ovary, from the peritoneal cavity to the inside
of the womb. The complicated arrangement normally gives good
protection against infection from outside the body getting into the
abdominal cavity. The neck of the womb, the cervix (Greek: neck) is
normally closed, though it opens to let out the menstrual blood and
shed endometrium once a month. It is also negotiable by sperms
deposited in the vagina. These can swim upstream, like miniature
tadpoles,[3] into the cavity of the uterus. If they encounter an egg in a
fallopian tube, or perhaps in the uterus itself, the egg can be fertilised.
The cavity of the uterus connects with the abdominal (peritoneal)
cavity via the two uterine (fallopian) tubes (Fig. 23) which end closely
adjacent to the two ovaries. Each tube is about 4 inches (10 cm) long.
The opening of the tubes into the uterus is very small, the thickness of
a bristle. The complex anatomy may have evolved to provide the
maximum protection against infection getting from the uterus up into
the fallopian tubes. This can cause 'salpingitis' (inflammation and
infection of the fallopian tubes) or even infection of the peritoneal
cavity ('peritonitis').

Current techniques of treatment unfortunately give few clues about
the cause of endometriosis. One obvious and generally accepted line of

treatment is to interfere with the hormones which control the menstrual cycle and endometrial bleeding, though inevitably this impairs fertility. Removal of the ovaries usually produces complete cure and relief of symptoms, but inevitable sterility. The preferred conservative treatment of severe cases in many centres is careful and accurate destruction of the aberrant endometrial tissue. This can conveniently be done with a laser light beam, either at open operation or via a laparoscope (see above). Active lesions absorb light energy on their dark surfaces. The controlled light beam does not penetrate deeply enough to damage the normal organ beneath the EMT tissue. Laser treatment of the lesions themselves is effective in relieving pain even though it does not improve fertility.

According to the transplantation theory, the probability of a woman developing endometriosis can be regarded as quantitative and dependent on the interplay of various factors:

1. sufficiently large amounts of endometrial tissue somehow getting into the abdominal cavity;
2. the inherent ability of tissues in the pelvis to nourish and support the transplanted tissue;
3. a combination of (1) and (2).

> Other possibilities have been considered. One is that the lining membrane of the abdominal cavity (the 'mesothelium') changes its character and forms typical endometrium-like glands and tissue. This situation is described as 'c(o)elomic metaplasia'. Another suggestion is that the lining of the womb is not itself transplanted but that chemicals are produced by endometrial tissue which make tissues in other places turn into endometrium. This rather improbable theory suggests that perhaps the body's immunological defence system somehow encourages endometrium to appear in abnormal sites.

Retrograde menstruation

It seems to me, as it has seemed to many others,[4] that the Sampson theory of implantation of menstrual endometrium is far the best explanation for endometriosis. The suggestion has been made that retrograde menstruation is common, perhaps nearly a universal occurrence. This implies that instead of all the endometrial lining tissue shed each month passing out through the cervix into the vagina, some gets back through the fallopian tubes into the peritoneal cavity, perhaps helped by muscular contractions of the uterus. Living endometrial cells have been identified in fluid in the abdominal cavity in about 50% of all pre-menopausal women.[5]

Previous pelvic infection makes endometriosis more likely and more severe, presumably because of obstructed passage of menstrual material through the cervix. Could the use of tampons by women in developed countries be a cause of retrograde menstruation and hence predispose to endometriosis? Although tampons are loose-fitting, might they partially obstruct free menstrual flow? A survey by the American Endometriosis Association showed that rates of tampon use by women with endometriosis were similar to those of the population not using tampons, though women with endometriosis had started to use tampons earlier in their lives than those without the disease. In a small survey of tampon use, comparing 100 users with a similar number of non-users, long-term tampon users (14 years or more) were 3.6 times more likely to have endometriosis than non-users of tampons. The 'confidence intervals' for this ratio were wide (1.05–13.5) and thus only barely significant.[6] So tampon use might have a small effect encouraging endometriosis but it cannot be a major factor. The subject would clearly repay further epidemiological research.

The outstanding mystery which needs explaining is why endometriosis is not much more common than it is. This intellectual difficulty accounts for the current interest in a possible immunological cause, such as deficient protective 'T-cell' lymphocyte function. This theory supposes that the peritoneal lining membrane which surrounds the abdominal organs is immunologically protected against bits of endometrium grafting themselves on to some part of the abdominal organs or onto the peritoneal lining membrane. I do not think much of this theory. In several animals grafted endometrial tissue has been shown easily to attach itself to abdominal organs and grow there. Various rather unimpressive differences in immune function have been reported between women with endometriosis and women without. But the obvious way to test this theory is to look for the same condition in animals.

Endometriosis in animals

Rodents lack a menstrual cycle and don't get spontaneous endometriosis. Rabbits lack the so-called 'luteal' phase of the human menstrual cycle. Thus animal research on EMT has only proved feasible in primates. The closest animal model of the human disease is the baboon. This has a 33-day menstrual cycle which continues throughout the year, even in captivity. In a survey of baboons examined under anaesthesia only 4 out of 52 (8%) previously unoperated baboons of proven fertility had a few small plaques of endometrial tissue in the abdominal cavity, outside the uterus. The lesions were mostly small white plaques with pigmented spots, unlike the appearance of human EMT lesions, though occasional typical blue/black cysts were seen. Furthermore, baboon endometriosis was not seen on the surface of the ovary, where it is commonest in women. Surgical opening of the abdominal cavity in baboons leads later to a great increase in the number and extent of endometriosis lesions.[7] Rather similar though more limited observations have been made in other primates. Endometriosis has been produced consistently, though to a variable extent, by putting lumps of endometrial tissue into the abdominal cavity of cynomolgous monkeys – an operation which must acutely lower intra-abdominal pressure. Consequent reduction in fertility was related to the extent of endometriosis. 'Spontaneous' endometriosis has been reported in rhesus monkeys, most of whom had been exposed to surgical operations. Endometriosis can be induced in female rhesus monkeys whose immune system has been damaged by long-term dioxin exposure. Since this toxin affects ovarian function it may alter oestrogen levels, which could be important.

For the tissue to establish itself in the abnormal situation certain key steps are required: (1) the new tissue needs to adhere to the basement membranes of cells of the host tissue; (2) local dissolution of protein has to clear a path for growth; (3) the endometrial tissue cells need to migrate into the colonised host tissue; (4) the grafted tissue needs to acquire new blood vessels if it is to get larger than one or two millimetres in diameter. Despite these difficulties, most experimental work suggests that lumps of endometrium are easily able to survive, integrate with the host tissue, and grow – outside the womb.

Partial obstruction of the cervix is associated with endometriosis. Previous pelvic infections, leading to fibrous adhesions keeping the fallopian tubes open rather than flat shut, should also be a risk factor, as it has been reported to be. If the non-pregnant uterus contracts and raises its internal pressure, the conditions for retrograde (reversed) flow of uterine contents could exist, but only if the uterine/fallopian tube junction does not contract at the same time. My guess is that the entry of a few individual endometrial cells into the peritoneal cavity is trivial and harmless. But if a small lump of endometrial tissue – not just a single cell or two – gets into the peritoneal cavity the tissue could stick onto the peritoneal lining membrane and grow. A lesion of endometriosis would then have appeared. When this bleeds at the time of menstruation it would cause pain, the outstanding symptom of endometriosis.

The animal results seem to me to speak rather powerfully against any immunological theory. If bits of endometrium can easily be induced to stick onto and grow on abdominal organs in normal non-human primates whose female pelvic anatomy closely resembles human female anatomy, why don't all women get endometriosis if retrograde menstruation is as common as most people say it is? One obvious requirement for transplanted endometrium to survive is a blood supply. As I have discussed elsewhere (p. 75), diffusion can only supply oxygen and nutrients over a distance of 1–2 mm. Angiogenic growth factors, discussed in Chapter 7, might be the missing factors which determine whether EMT deposits can get large enough to cause symptoms. So far they have been little studied. But I would like the reader to consider a completely different explanation for endometriosis.

How can we make sense of a confusing situation?

A particular interest of mine has always been pressures in blood vessels, a topic to which I shall return in Chapter 31 and in succeeding chapters. It is thus natural for me to see the uterus as having two valves in series: the cervix and the junction between uterine cavity and fallopian tube. A rise of pressure in the abdominal cavity (e.g. from straining at stool) will preferentially close off the thin fallopian tubes, because the thick-walled uterus will more strongly resist external pressure. Any material in the tubes will therefore be forced in towards the uterine cavity. But when abdominal pressure falls again, the pressure in the cavity of the uterus will be briefly higher than that in the abdomen, so that any unattached contents will tend to move up the fallopian tubes and into the abdominal cavity. In particular, if the intra-abdominal pressure has been raised for many hours (rather than perhaps just for a few minutes' straining during defaecation) the pressure inside the cavity of the uterus would be expected to be about the same as that in the abdominal cavity. Such a situation would be expected in any woman wearing a corset or any other tight constricting garment which raised the average pressure in her abdominal cavity.

I have envisaged the following scenario, illustrated diagrammatically in Figure 24. The normal situation is shown in A, in which there is a uniformly distributed low pressure which is about 5 mmHg above the surrounding atmospheric pressure. During longstanding abdominal constriction all these pressures would be increased, as at B. Immediately after taking off a constricting abdominal garment the pressure within the thick-walled uterus would not be expected to fall back to normal until some of the uterine contents had been expelled. This might lead to a situation such as in C, in which there could be a substantial and prolonged pressure gradient favouring movement of

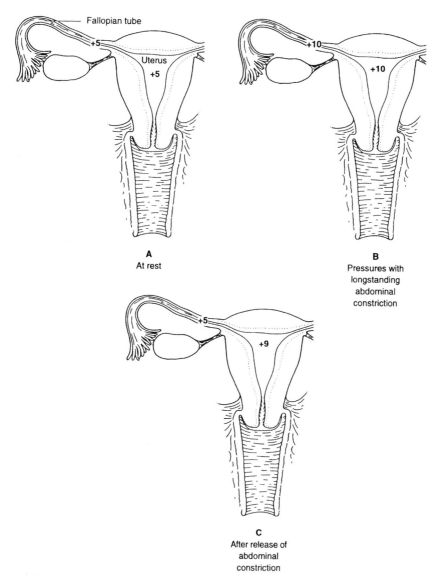

A
At rest

B
Pressures with
longstanding
abdominal
constriction

C
After release of
abdominal
constriction

Figure 24 Gross anatomy of the uterus and fallopian tubes, indicating the probable relative pressure (in mmHg) at different sites. The normal situation is shown in A. All solid tissue pressures and the pressure inside the uterus are the same, about 5 mmHg above atmospheric pressure. B shows the situation which would be expected during the application of a tight constricting abdominal garment, during which all intra-abdominal pressures are increased to the same extent (e.g. to 10 mmHg). C shows the hypothetical but plausible relative pressure values immediately after removing a garment constricting the abdomen (see text). Unless the thick muscular wall of the uterus relaxes completely, the pressure inside it will not fall back to its normal level until some of the contents of the uterus have been extruded either through the cervix (into the vagina), or up the fallopian tubes.

187

some of the uterine contents up the fallopian tubes and towards the peritoneal cavity.

This line of reasoning makes me hazard a guess that what garments a women wears while she is menstruating could be important. In particular if the garments produce a sustained rise of intra-abdominal pressure by being tight-fitting, I suspect that retrograde menstruation could occur when the garments are taken off. I also suggest that non-human primates have little propensity to endometriosis because they do not wear constricting garments. It is rather striking that experimental animal endometriosis seems to appear in primates mainly after the abdomen has been surgically opened, inevitably thus reducing the intra-abdominal pressure. Could the almost universal wearing of loose-hanging saris by Indian women and chadors by Arab women give them protection against endometriosis? I assume that they have no need for, and do not wear, tight constricting abdominal garments.

I made a computerised *Medline* medical literature search covering the last 30+ years for 'endometriosis' to see how many of the more than 5000 references mentioned 'India' or 'Indian' in the context of spontaneous endometriosis. The answer was only one, as an aside in an article about septicaemia. I have already mentioned the single report from central Africa. I have also found no reports of endometriosis from Saudi Arabia, in which country all women wear loose-fitting black enveloping garments. It seems clear that no research doctor working in India, central Africa or Saudi Arabia has much interest or experience in endometriosis – as might be expected if my hypothesis were to be correct. I have not been able to find any epidemiological evidence about garment wearing and endometriosis. But I would predict that EMT should be rare in places where women do not wear garments which increase intra-abdominal pressure.

I must acknowledge the completely speculative nature of my suggestions. My excuse for presenting them in this book is: (1) that at present there is no general agreement between experts about a possible cause of the disease; (2) no-one has yet published any evidence which categorically disproves my hypothesis – even though *The British Journal of Obstetrics and Gynaecology* published it as a brief report.[8]

If I had appropriate investigative facilities I would try to devise means for measuring all the pressures at different points in the system. Perhaps those women who wore tight abdominal garments, and consequently maintained a high pressure in their abdominal cavity, might be relatively protected until the intra-abdominal pressure was suddenly reduced, e.g. when they took a constricting garment off. At this moment a previously high pressure surrounding both uterus and fallopian tubes would fall; but there would be a finite time gap during which the pressure inside the uterine cavity would exceed the pressure surrounding the fallopian tubes, because the relatively rigid thick-walled uterus would not immediately relax. Nor could its contents rapidly escape. The stage would be set for movement of uterine contents up the fallopian tubes. Though speculative, my reasoning is hydrodynamically plausible. It has led me to wonder whether the 'period pains' often complained of by young women in Victorian England might have had something to do with their fashionable but damaging 'wasp waists', predisposing them to endometriosis.

I have been disappointed to find that no-one has so far attempted to measure the various relative pressures in the menstruating baboon. A recent issue of the international journal *Gynecologic and Obstetric Investigation* contained 28 articles concerning experimental endometriosis in the baboon[9] – but none of them was concerned with the pressure gradients I have been discussing. A recent comprehensive American review[10] listed 167 publications which discussed immunology, genetics, hormones and environmental chemical factors. Currently no investigators appear interested in pressure gradients.

Intra-abdominal interstitial fluid pressure

The kind of pressure I am describing is easy to understand: the simple hydrostatic or solid tissue pressure exerted when the heart contracts, when an artery constricts, or when the uterus at term expels its fetus. But there exists a space between tissue cells which contains a small amount of so-called 'interstitial' fluid. Amazingly, the pressure in that fluid is normally subatmospheric, about −7 mmHg, or about −1 inch of water pressure.[11] Our bodies are being gently squeezed together by the pressure of the atmosphere above us. Dropsy (oedema) arises when the pressure in tissue fluid rises above the atmospheric pressure, thus allowing tissues to become separated by retained fluid. The fluid in the abdominal cavity is on average also held at a similar subatmospheric pressure. So there will normally always be a small pressure gradient tending to move free fluid from the vagina into the uterus and from the uterus into the peritoneal cavity. The pressures concerned are very small, but will be continually present. Whether they have any relevance at all to EMT will need some difficult measurements to determine.

Summary

Endometriosis is a common condition in which small portions of bluish-red tissue which appear to have come from the inner lining of the womb (the endometrium) are found on the surface of various internal organs, predominantly those in the abdominal cavity, especially the ovary. Similar lesions can much less commonly appear in other places. Endometriosis can cause chronic pain, especially pelvic pain, particularly at the time of the menstrual 'period'. It is associated with reduced fertility. Although other explanations have been offered, the likeliest seems to be that the cause is retrograde menstruation: that is, that some of the shed womb lining gets up into the abdominal (peritoneal) cavity and sticks on some organ or lining surface. The process may be facilitated by some immunological process, but this may not be an essential factor. Pressure changes at different parts of the pelvic organs might perhaps be of greater importance.

The possible explanation that I have envisaged has not been previously made or suggested by anyone else, as far as I am aware. I wish to suggest that if menstruating women wear tight clothing, retrograde menstruation (and hence deposition of endometrial fragments in the abdominal cavity) might occur when the tight clothing is taken off. This hypothesis has received no public support so far. Fortunately it can be examined epidemiologically and also, with much greater difficulty, physiologically. It has at least one requirement of a scientific hypothesis: it can be disproved by observation and/or experiment. Meantime, endometriosis remains one of the most fascinating and interesting current medical mysteries.

18

GLAUCOMA

A word ending '-oma' suggests a Greek origin, which may be from *glaukos* = shining, bluish-green. There is no universally agreed pronunciation of the word, but 'glore-kohma' is most often used in Britain. In the past glaucoma has been confused with 'cataract' (clouding over of the lens – another common cause of poor sight in the elderly). It may have been named by mistake. Eyes affected by cataract often look shiny. But the eyes of glaucoma sufferers are neither especially bluish-green nor shiny. Sufferers from one variety of acute glaucoma sometimes notice vivid colours as their vision fails. The cornea – the transparent membrane in the front of the eye (Fig. 25) – may look steamy. But glaucoma may show no external signs and often progresses so slowly that victims do not realise that they need treatment.

A modern textbook described glaucoma as 'a disease characterised by abnormally increased intraocular pressure, optic atrophy and loss of visual field'. This definition is misleading. Some people with glaucoma never have abnormally increased pressure in the eyeball at any time, even though in other respects they suffer the same symptoms and show the same signs as those who do. So glaucoma is a real medical mystery.

Glaucoma and age-related degeneration of the macula (the most light-sensitive central part of the retina at the back of the eye) are the two commonest causes of blindness in the developed world. Old people often don't realise that their failing eyesight is not necessarily an inevitable part of growing old. At present there is no effective treatment for age-related macular degeneration. But treatment can slow down or even partly reverse the progression of glaucoma. So making the diagnosis is very important. In industrialised countries between 1% and 2% of people over 35 have glaucoma. Worldwide about 67 million people have it. Some 7 million of these will become permanently blind because of irreversible damage to the optic nerves, which connect the eyes to the brain. In the UK 12% of people registered as blind have glaucoma, but the poor vision that many people with early or mild glaucoma have is not counted in present-day statistics. Even in devel-

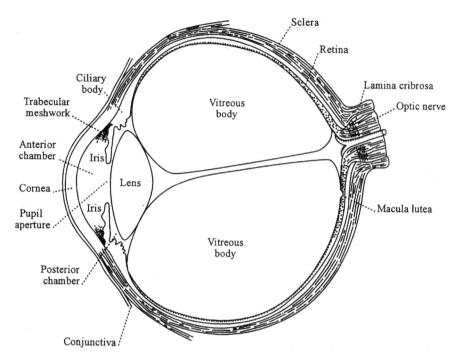

Figure 25 Longitudinal section through the human eye, seen from the side, showing the relative positions of cornea, lens and retina. The aqueous humor fills the anterior chamber. It is secreted by a ring structure behind the lens (the ciliary body). The fluid flows forward through the central opening in the iris (the aperture of the pupil) to the anterior chamber. It leaves through the trabecular meshwork, in the angle between the cornea and the lens, and empties into the ocular veins.

oped countries surveys have shown that about 50% of people with glaucoma do not seek treatment. They are not identified. The diagnosis of glaucoma can only be made by specially trained staff. Not for nothing is glaucoma known as the 'silent blinder'.

Typically the disease develops insidiously and painlessly, in both eyes at about the same time, even though it can (rarely) cause pain if it develops very rapidly. First there is loss of visual acuity, i.e. loss of fine detail in the field of vision. Later there is progressive irregular loss of the field of vision in each eye. Without adequate treatment the visual fields may constrict until eventually there is nothing left and the victim becomes totally blind. The outer (peripheral) field of vision usually goes first and central vision often remains till late. Patients may be unaware of partial loss of their field of vision, because the eyes are in continual motion, scanning the scene in front. Loss of part of the field in one eye may be compensated by preservation of the corresponding part of the field in the other eye.

Testing of the visual fields requires a technique known as 'perimetry' (Greek: *perimetros* = circumference). The subject is asked to fix vision with one eye on a point in front while the other eye is closed or blanked off. Then the subject is asked whether he or she can see a small object, ideally a point of light, in different parts of the visual field. The best technique uses a computer to make a tiny point of light appear repeatedly in random fashion over the entire visual field while the subject presses a button every time the light point is seen. Over a few minutes the whole visual field can be scanned in this way. The computer can then draw a map of any consistently missing areas of each visual field. Sometimes the pattern of visual field loss is so characteristic that glaucoma can be strongly suspected.

The other observation which helps to make the diagnosis is direct 'ophthalmoscopy'. The examiner looks through a small hole in an angled mirror from which light is reflected into the back of the subject's eye. The subject's own lens and cornea provide magnification of about 15 times. This allows an observer to make a close inspection of the 'optic disc' where the optic nerve passes out of the back of the eye. The disc is normally whiter than the rest of the retina and nearly level with it. But in longstanding glaucoma the disc appears excavated or 'cupped' because the optic nerve head has been pushed outwards and backwards.

When examining general medical patients I have always been worried about missing glaucoma. I have often been deceived by what seems rather a deep or wide 'cup' in the optic nerve head which proves to be within normal limits. I must confess to having needlessly referred several of my general medical patients to a consultant ophthalmologist for his expert opinion on their optic discs.

Fluids and pressures within the eye

It is possible to measure the tension in the walls of the eye globe and convert this to give an estimate of intraocular pressure (IOP). More often the hydrostatic pressure within the globe of the eye is measured by various techniques in which the cornea (the transparent membrane covering the front of the eye) is slightly indented by a graduated pressure applied with a plunger while the resulting deflection is measured. The cornea is a sensitive structure and well supplied with pain nerves. Measurements can therefore only be made after putting a drop of local anaesthetic on the corneal surface. Rough screening for intra-ocular pressure can also be done by the much less accurate non-contact 'air-puff' technique, in which the rebound pressure of a harmless puff of compressed air directed at the corneal surface is measured by a pressure-sensing membrane in the instrument. Measurements of IOP by these techniques suggest that the average pressure distending the globe of the eye is about 14 millimetres of mercury (abbreviated to 'mmHg'). This is equivalent to the pressure which would be exerted by a column of water about 8 inches high. The normal range of IOPs in the whole population is 10–22 mmHg. Such estimates have been checked against uncomfortable and hazardous direct pressure measurements made after pushing a needle connected to a manometer directly into the globe of the eye.

Most of the eyeball, behind the lens, is filled by about 4 ml (a large teaspoonful) of a visco-elastic transparent jelly – the 'vitreous humor' (Latin: *vitreus* = glassy; *umor* = fluid). The globe of the eye maintains its spherical shape and is prevented from collapsing by the continuous active secretion into it of small amounts of watery fluid – the 'aqueous humor' – at a rate of about two thousandths of a millilitre per minute. This fluid is produced behind the iris at the edge of the lens by a ring-shaped structure called the ciliary body. The fluid travels forward in front of the lens, driven by a small pressure gradient. Then it passes through the central hole of the iris (the pupil) into the front (anterior) chamber and reaches the trabecular meshwork (Latin: *trabecula* = beam, strut). This structure has a consistency similar to that of a bathroom sponge. The aqueous fluid eventually reaches collecting tubes in the anterior chamber of the eye, from which it is returned to the bloodstream. The total volume of fluid at the front of each human eye, in front of the lens, is very small (about $\frac{1}{4}$ ml, around $\frac{1}{10}$ teaspoonful).

The transparent cornea is a thin membrane composed of living cells. Like all living cells, corneal cells need oxygen and other dissolved nutrients to survive. Circulating red blood in the front of the eye would impair vision. So in the course of evolution the cornea has become nourished not by a blood circulation but by circulation of the aqueous humor. This fluid has an interesting and substantially different composition from the fluid part of the blood. It is not simply a filtrate of blood plasma. Notably it contains about 25 times as much vitamin C (ascorbate) as the blood. Vitamin C has two normal functions in the eye. The first is to give some protection against damage to the lens and retina by absorbing ultraviolet light. Animals living in the dark have very little vitamin C in their aqueous humor. Secondly, vitamin C helps to neutralise potentially damaging oxidising chemicals.

The intraocular pressure maintains the spherical shape of the eyeball because the intraocular pressure is always greater than atmospheric pressure. The contents of the eyeball are therefore pressed against its tough, fibrous lining (the sclera). But there is one weak area. This is at the back of the eye – the 'optic disc' – where the fibres of the optic nerve coming from the light-sensitive retinal cells emerge from the back of the eyeball to make their connections with the brain. This is a vulnerable region because compression of nerve fibres can interfere with nerve impulse conduction. In a similar way, we have all experienced loss of sensation or abnormal sensations in part of our hand and fourth and fifth fingers through a blow to or pressure on the ulnar nerve at the elbow (hence the name 'funny bone').

The vulnerable region of the eye, the optic disc, is supported by a strong fibro-elastic perforated structure called the lamina cribrosa (Latin: *lamina* = thin plate; *cribrum* = sieve). This is continuous with the sclera (Fig. 25). Small bundles of optic nerve fibres pass through the perforations. The fibrous sieve structure prevents them being bent or compressed. The lamina cribrosa is also partly elastic. This has been nicely demonstrated in life by an observation made on traumatic bleeding into the eyeball. This caused a sharp rise of IOP which pushed the optic disc backwards, causing it to appear typically 'cupped'. At the same time, the bending and compression of the optic nerves caused blindness in that eye. But after a needle had been pushed into the eyeball to allow blood to come out and to lower intraocular pressure, all the changes reversed. The optic disc became flat again and vision was restored.[1] Observations such as these prove that the lamina cribrosa has some elasticity as well as structural rigidity.

Cause

In two thirds of all people with glaucoma the IOP is consistently greater than 22 mmHg. An intraocular pressure greater than 32 mmHg is almost diagnostic of glaucoma. Most experts agree that the physical changes of glaucoma – 'cupping' of the optic disc and reduction in the extent of the visual fields – are actually caused by the raised intraocular pressure.

Unfortunately the ganglion cell bodies of the retinal nerves find out in some way (probably from a rise in fluid pressure in the nerve axons, which are hollow tubes) that onward transmission of nerve impulses is impaired. When any nerve cell discovers that it can no longer continue to work properly because onwards conduction of nerve impulses is blocked, the process known as 'apoptosis' is switched on. This leads to a quiet non-inflammatory death of the affected nerve cell (p. 97). This is probably what happens when the optic nerve fibres remain for some time (perhaps days) squashed or rucked up because the nerve head has been pushed back by a rise in intraocular pressure (IOP). Unfortunately, once apoptosis of ganglion cells has taken place the loss of vision is irreversible.

Open-angle glaucoma

This most common type of glaucoma with raised intraocular pressure affects about $\frac{1}{2}$% of people aged 40 and about $2\frac{1}{2}$% of people over 70 in most populations. It is commoner and more severe in black races than in white. In this situation the aqueous humor is produced as usual by the ciliary body, behind the iris. It runs freely forward through the pupil into the anterior chamber of the eye, but its absorption is blocked at the trabecular meshwork, at the angle between cornea and iris. The trabeculae and the drainage canal are fragmented and thickened by deposits of the structural fibrous protein 'collagen' and by defects in the elastic properties of the trabeculae. When looked at from the side the angle between cornea and iris appears to be of normal size – hence the description of this disease as 'open-angle' glaucoma. Diagnosis requires both perimetry and measurement of IOP.

There is no general agreement about the cause of this disease. After reviewing all the evidence it appears to me that a primary cause could be deterioration of the elastic fibres in the trabecular meshwork. Elastin can store energy in large scale deformations and spring back without loss or damage. As I mentioned in Chapter 1, elastin is synthesised during fetal development from its precursor (tropoelastin) in a structure which assembles itself automatically into a linear polymer, a long elastic molecule. Elastin is unique by comparison with other structural proteins such as collagen. Once formed it is neither repaired nor replaced during life. Some loss of the elastic function of the protein 'elastin' seems to be just the consequence of ageing. Although elastin genes can be switched on in adult life to make more elastin, this simply forms disorganised clumps (elastosis).

An interesting small study has described, in 20 normal men and 20 with open angle glaucoma, the effects on intraocular pressure of wearing a tight necktie. In both groups, wearing a tight necktie increased IOP slightly but significantly, by about 1–3 mmHg.[2] The authors commented that this could not only lead to a faulty assessment of glaucoma but might even contribute towards optic nerve damage. Physiologically the reasoning seems plausible to me. When intraocular fluid has drained through the trabecular meshwork it enters the episcleral veins. If venous pressure is raised for any reason, e.g. by compressing the jugular veins, intraocular pressure would also rise. Whether this could be a significant factor contributing to optic nerve damage in open-angle glaucoma will require further observations. Meantime it seems sensible for any man not to tie anything tight round his neck and leave it there for any long time!

Certain races seem especially liable to glaucoma. Elderly American black people are about four times more likely to have glaucoma than white people. First degree relatives of sufferers have 3–9 times the risk of developing the disease than the general population.

Several genes can confer susceptibility to glaucoma, e.g. GLC1A on chromosome 1 and GLC1B on chromosome 2. At least 4 other genetic susceptibility genes have been located by studying large families.[3] Degeneration of elastic tissues in the eye is a particular feature of a not uncommon type of open-angle glaucoma, known as the 'pseudoexfoliation syndrome', in which small whitish deposits of fibrillar/granular material appear in the front chamber of the eye. This also appears to have some genetic basis, with maternal inheritance suggesting a mitochondrial defect.[4]

Angle-closure glaucoma

A considerably less common cause of glaucoma is described as 'angle-closure'. This is usually associated with a disease or defect in the iris. The iris becomes thickened and lumpy and blocks the exit of aqueous humor through the pupil into the front chamber of the eye. It is specially liable to occur in long-sighted people because their cornea is relatively less curved than in normal people and makes a narrower angle with the edge of the cornea. The angle can be measured and diagnosis made by a specialised technique known as 'gonioscopy' (Greek: *gonia* = angle).

There are great differences between different racial groups in their liability to different varieties of glaucoma. Inuit and Chinese are especially liable to the angle-closure type of disease. There is is a strong hereditary element. You are some 10–20 times more likely than the average person to develop angle-closure glaucoma if you have a first degree relative with the condition. As people get older their lens enlarges and the globe of the eye gets smaller. Both changes increase the chance of angle-closure glaucoma. Symptoms can come on suddenly and (rarely) can even cause pain and vomiting as well as visual disturbances – vivid colours and haloes round lights. Intraocular pressure may rise to high levels, e.g. 50–60 mmHg. The sudden onset of this form of glaucoma results from a vicious circle:

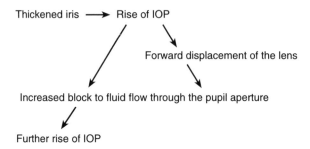

Angle-closure disease can also be caused by infection, or by any inflammatory process which sticks the back of the iris to the front of the lens.

Low-pressure glaucoma

In some 30% of people with the signs and symptoms of glaucoma, including optic disc cupping and visual field loss, the intra-ocular pressure and its changes during the day remain within normal limits at all times.[5] This situation is described as 'normal pressure' or 'low pressure' glaucoma. An individual with this condition is sometimes said to have an IOP which is too high for that individual. This unhelpful description of normal pressure glaucoma distorts ideas about the cause or causes of the disease. We do not know what is going on and whether changes in IOP are primary, or secondary to some entirely different process such as inadequate blood supply. The defects in the trabecular meshwork, especially loss of elastin, are the same as in open-angle glaucoma with raised IOP. Rare patients have been reported with an autosomal dominant inheritance.

Why should high intraocular pressure damage the eye?

High intra-ocular pressures, even as high as 32 mmHg (equivalent to a pressure head of 18 inches of water), are most unlikely directly to damage the retina and its contained cells. The problem arises from the poor structural design of the human eye. If an engineer had been starting from scratch he would have put the light receptor cells in the front of the retina and the ganglion cells behind. The nerves connecting the retina with the brain would then pass straight through the sclera (Greek: *skleros* = hard) – the tough capsule surrounding the globe – and join up on its outer surface to make up the optic nerve. Instead, the way the eye has evolved over millions of years as a bud from the brain means that light has to pass through the large ganglion cells and a network of nerves before reaching the light-sensitive receptor cells. This necessarily diffuses the light falling on the specialised light-receptor cells and makes visual acuity less than ideal.

Nerves from the ganglion cells have to get out of the globe somewhere. They are gathered up into the trunk of the optic nerve, which passes backwards through holes in the lamina cribrosa. This is the weak point of the whole system. Each of the (approximately) one million fibres in each human optic nerve are minute fluid-filled tubes which resist stretching. But they have no structural strength to resist bending or compression along their length. Any undue rise of intraocular pressure will tend to push the delicate nerve fibres backwards and ruck them up. The tough lamina cribrosa provides some support but cannot prevent nerve damage if the IOP gets too high.

Degeneration of elastin in the lamina cribrosa has been found in all eyes in which glaucoma has been diagnosed. The large confluent elastin aggregates of irregular and varied shape (elastosis) must necessarily interfere with the normal elastic recoil of the lamina cribrosa.[6] It is interesting that elastin and other proteins which make up the structures of the trabecular meshwork and of the lamina cribrosa are chemically and structurally virtually identical. 'The trabecular meshwork and the lamina cribrosa, two ocular tissues intimately linked to the pathogenesis of primary open-angle glaucoma, display remarkable similarity in protein expression. This finding may have implications for the molecular etiology of glaucoma.'[7]

I wonder whether degeneration of elastin in either the trabecular meshwork or in the lamina cribrosa might underlie several different types of glaucoma and be a major causal factor. It might be possible to examine epidemiologically whether there was any relation between glaucoma and aortic aneurysm, in which loss of elastin is almost certainly a main cause of weakness and dilation of the blood vessel. As far as I can find, this potential relationship has never been examined.

Implications for treatment

There are many ways of lowering intraocular pressure, which has been shown to give some protection to people with glaucoma. This applies even in so-called 'normal tension' glaucoma. Many different drugs have been tried.[8] I shall not discuss their relative merits and disadvantages here. In what appears mainly to be a mechanical or hydraulic defect it seems obvious that mechanical or hydraulic treatments might be best. Indeed in most trials a surgical approach to reduce intraocular pressure has done better than drug treatment. In angle-closure glaucoma the increased pressure behind the iris can usually be relieved by cutting a hole in the iris – 'iridotomy' (Greek: *tomos* = cutting). In open-angle glaucoma attempts are made to free up the flow of aqueous humor from the pupil outwards into the trabecular meshwork. The operation of 'trabeculectomy' (making extra holes or channels in the trabecular meshwork) remains popular. It might be described as the standard surgical procedure. In addition, new drugs to lower IOP are being introduced at high speed, but good clinical trials comparing different treatments for glaucoma are becoming increasingly difficult to arrange.

Summary

There are many varieties of glaucoma, which is a major cause of defective vision and actual blindness, mainly in the elderly. A common finding in all cases of glaucoma is that the optic nerve head, containing all the nerves passing from the light sensitive retina to the brain, appears to have been pushed backwards, causing the appearance known as 'cupping' of the optic disc. Pressure on the fragile nerve fibres impairs conduction of impulses and can eventually lead to apoptosis (i.e. programmed death) of ganglion cells in the retina.

In most cases cupping is due to an unduly high intraocular pressure, greater than the normal 10–22 mmHg, though it can also occur even with intraocular pressures in the normal range. In this latter case there is probably weakness in the fibro-elastic perforated platform (the lamina cribrosa) which holds the optic nerve head from moving backwards to a damaging degree. Reduction of intraocular pressure may relieve symptoms, but is often disappointing.

Glaucoma remains an obscure condition, but there is some evidence to suggest that common to most varieties is an age-related failure of function of the elastic protein 'elastin', defects of which have been identified both in the anterior chamber of the eye but also in the elastic support of the lamina cribrosa.

19

ALZHEIMER'S DISEASE

Alois Alzheimer, a German psychiatrist, gave a lecture in Tübingen in 1906 in which he described a 51-year-old woman who had hallucinations with progressively impaired memory and social relationships. He watched her for 5 years, eventually reporting the post mortem (necropsy) findings. There were plaques and fibrillary tangles in the brain and arteriosclerotic changes in cerebral blood vessels. He said that the condition was a characteristic, peculiar and serious disease of the outer layers of the brain (the cerebral cortex). The disease which Alzheimer described, which now bears his name, has since been recognised as probably the commonest cause of 'senile dementia'. (This term simply means 'lack of mind in old age' but sounds more scientific.) Two thirds of people with senile dementia are suffering from Alzheimer's disease (AD), which commonly begins over the age of 65. It is curious that most of what we now know about the disease comes from study of the early onset type of disease (which Alzheimer's original patient must have had) even though it makes up only about 10% of all cases.

The typical sufferer first experiences memory disturbances, finding it especially difficult to learn new things and to speak coherently and sensibly. Loss of so-called 'episodic' memory for recent events and episodes is disquieting, but erosion of someone's whole database of knowledge ('semantic' memory) is devastating. Episodic memory seems to depend particularly on the more central parts of the temporal lobe of the brain, technically the 'amygdala/hippocampus' complex (Fig. 26). The consolidation of a memory into someone's database of knowledge seems to depend particularly on those parts of the temporal lobes closest to the brain surface. The left side seems more important than the right, at least in right-handed people.[1]

The cost of Alzheimer's disease is not only personal and social. The total annual costs of the disease in the USA have been estimated to approach 70 billion dollars.

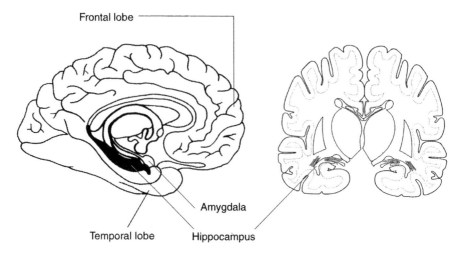

Frontal lobe

Amygdala

Temporal lobe   Hippocampus

Figure 26   On the left is a diagram of the left half of the brain, viewed from the midline after removing all the right half of the brain together with the cerebellum and the brain stem. The frontal lobe of the brain lies behind the brow (the frontal bone). The diagram on the right is the brain as it would appear if it was sliced across from top downwards by a 'coronal' section. Both views emphasise the central position of the hippocampus, which makes a curved ridge about 2 inches (5 cm) long, lying in the floor of the lateral ventricle of the brain.

Changes in the brain

Sequential scans of the brain using magnetic resonance imaging (MRI) show a gradual shrivelling up of those parts of the brain connected with memory, especially the amygdala/hippocampus complex. Later there is more general loss of brain tissue. Special imaging techniques show that there is loss of chemical energy provision in the affected areas. The fluid-filled ventricles of the brain enlarge and the surrounding brain cortex gets thinner.

With the loss of semantic memory the victim loses his or her personality, has difficulties in recognising people and behaves in an irresponsible and childish manner. Usually 5 years or so after the mental deterioration of Alzheimer's disease has been noticed, the sufferer becomes mute, immobile, rigid, unresponsive and eventually incontinent. Death usually results from accidents or infections, mainly pneumonia. Curiously, the 'sensory-motor cortex', that part of the brain concerned with physical sensations and with the initiation and control of muscle movement, is spared until late in the disease. The victim can often still walk about despite being severely demented. The

202

changes of Alzheimer's disease develop to different degrees in different parts of the brain, but those parts concerned with higher mental functions like memory and intellectual reasoning are much more affected than those concerned with coordinated muscle movement.

Under the microscope the classic hallmarks of Alzheimer's disease are basket-like microscopic tangles inside nerve cells (neurofibrillary tangles) and the building up of flat lumps of structureless starchy material (so-called 'senile plaques'). There is some evidence that plaques appear earlier than tangles. There is actual loss of brain cells. Tangles are also seen in glial cells (Greek: *glia* = glue), which lie close to nerve cells and intervene between them and their blood vessels (p. 463). Some tangles and even starch-like 'amyloid' plaques (Greek: *amylon* = starch) can be found in brain cells of some non-demented elderly people, but are much more frequent in AD brains.

Metabolic defects

In adults the simple sugar glucose, carried in the blood, is the brain's main fuel source. Its energy-producing metabolism is impaired in AD. PET scanning shows that there is a reduction in glucose consumption, especially in the hippocampus (see Fig. 26),[2] that part of the brain specially involved in memory. The most likely reason for this is that the nerve cells themselves are not working normally and therefore use less glucose. It is also possible that a defect in energy supply comes first and that other changes, such as the deposition of neurofibrillary tangles, are actually caused by the energy supply defect. This seems to me rather unlikely. Although neurofibrillary tangles are sometimes seen in the brains of people dying from strokes caused by blockage of arteries, they are much less frequent or obvious than in Alzheimer's disease. But it may be unfair to make a comparison with strokes, which are sudden events. Perhaps slow strangulation of the blood supply to the temporal lobe could yet be the underlying fault in Alzheimer's, though the progressive relentless involvement of other parts of the brain is difficult to fit with this idea.

A deficiency of the chemical neurotransmitter acetylcholine is characteristic of AD, but is not always found in the same places where glucose consumption rate is reduced. There is also current interest in the finding of reduced concentrations of the excitatory neurotransmitter glutamate in cortical nerve cells.

It is difficult to distinguish early Alzheimer's disease from the normal expected decline in nerve function with age and from other causes of dementia such as furring up of brain arteries by atheroma (cerebral arteriosclerosis). All the changes in the brain which are characteristic of AD have been seen, to a much smaller degree, in other varieties of dementia. Brain scans show overlap between Alzheimer's disease and two other conditions which can be associated with dementia: Parkinson's disease (Chapter 28) and motor neurone disease (Chapter 42) – though the microscopical findings in brain cells are different in each of these conditions.

> In all three conditions, abnormal microscopic particles ('inclusion bodies') may be seen inside nerve cells. So-called 'Lewy bodies' are specially characteristic of Parkinson's disease and 'Bunina bodies' of motor neurone disease. All these inclusion bodies contain 'ubiquitin', a protein which when combined with waste proteinaceous material marks it down for later removal by cell complexes called proteasomes.[3] Lewy bodies without any other abnormalities are also found in 'dementia with Lewy bodies', a disease which is the third most common cause of dementia in old age. It has yet to find a simpler name. Its symptoms and pathological findings overlap with those of Alzheimer's disease, though the outer layers of the brain (the cortex) are mainly affected.

Epidemiology

Alzheimer's is a very common disease in the elderly. In the whole population of men and women over 65 the lowest estimate of prevalence of Alzheimer's disease I have seen is 1%, but most investigators reckon that it is probably much higher, e.g. 5–10%. By the age of 85 a careful survey has suggested that almost 50% of the population is affected, although some authors would regard this as an overestimate. There is an exponentially increasing prevalence of Alzheimer's disease with age, in both sexes.

Current estimates are that about 600,000 individuals in the UK are suffering from Alzheimer's disease. US President Ronald Reagan and UK Prime Minister Harold Wilson were both said to have suffered from AD, doubtless accounting for their eventual memory loss and failing powers of concentration. Difficulties with memory afflict most of us as we get older. But someone like Wilson, who had a phenomenal and celebrated memory, must have found it especially distressing if he realised what was happening to him. At present there is no completely reliable way to diagnose Alzheimer's disease except by examining a small piece of brain tissue under the microscope: i.e. by brain biopsy. This obviously makes it impossible to carry out large population studies.

Genetics

The multiplicity of genetic risk factors, carried on different chromosomes, makes it difficult to envisage a comprehensive unifying hypothesis to account for Alzheimer's disease. The difficulties seem to be increasing with each newly identified risk factor. The disease may not be a single entity but rather the end stage of a number of different processes by which brain cells can be damaged.

In about 10% of cases Alzheimer's disease seems to be genetic and behaves as a dominant inherited characteristic. Some 50 different mutations have already been identified on chromosome 14 for the so-called 'presenilin' gene PSEN1, and two on chromosome 1 for the presenilin gene PSEN2. Other important genes for AD have been found on chromosomes 21 and 17. In most families with dominant inheritance the disease starts earlier in life than in the sporadic form, e.g. between 35 and 60. The mutations responsible may be connected with the production or function of the amyloid-precursor protein (APP) and with excess production of the 42–43 amino-acid fragment Aβ (see below). All currently known mutations associated with Alzheimer's disease increase the rate of production of toxic Aβ.

One genetic factor has been definitely linked with late onset sporadic disease. This is the gene responsible for a particular (fat + protein) compound known as apolipoprotein E-epsilon-4 (APOEε4), the genetic code for which is carried on chromosome 19. People with this genetic marker have been known for several years to have a higher than normal risk of developing AD. They also develop the disease at an earlier age. People unlucky enough to inherit two copies of this gene – one from each parent – will almost invariably develop Alzheimer's disease at an age which will be less than 70. But those who inherit favourable genes (e.g. a APOEε2/APOEε3 combination) have an average age of onset of AD greater than 90.

It is curious that the APOEε4 gene was first identified as a possible marker for premature arterial disease with atheroma (Chapter 20). This gene has since proved to have a much closer association with Alzheimer's disease. There also seems to be a link with smoking, which greatly increases the risk of people carrying the APOEε4 gene developing AD. The suggestion has been made that the increased risk which this gene provides is mainly, perhaps exclusively, associated with an infection or recrudescence of infection with herpes simplex virus 1 (HSV1), even though neither the particular variety of apolipoprotein, nor HSV1 infection alone, are notably associated in themselves with Alzheimer's. If this observation is confirmed (and it is disputed) finding APOEε4 in the blood will unfortunately not be specific enough to be useful in diagnosing AD. The same applies to another marker gene for Alzheimer's risk carried on chromosome 12. Another genetic mutation of a neurotransmitter protein (BCHE-K) can apparently multiply the risk of AD 30 times.

The genetic instruction code for cells to make amyloid precursor protein lies on chromosome 21. This is the chromosome which is reduplicated in individuals with the well-known common congenital abnormality known as 'Down's syndrome'. It is therefore not surprising that Down's individuals, who carry three copies of chromosome 21 instead of the normal two, have an increased risk of Alzheimer's disease. Presumably they make more than normal amounts of amyloid precursor protein.

Cause

'Attempting to understand the cause of AD from the postmortem brain is like looking out on a battlefield after the war and trying to work out how it all started'. But perhaps we can get some information from the shell cases and other debris left behind. Notably, the plaques inside neurones and glial cells have been shown to be composed of a relatively insoluble protein fragment called Aβ amyloid.

The peptide fragment Aβ containing 40 amino-acids does not appear to be damaging, but the larger fragment containing 42 amino acids is found at the centre of amyloid plaques. It is tempting to see a similarity between large protein fragments causing damage to neurones in Alzheimer's disease and large protein aggregates damaging neurones in Huntington's disease. Huntington's is an inherited condition caused by a mutation which produces abnormal brain proteins. After a normal childhood and early adult life the victim gets progressive neurological symptoms and dementia. Death occurs inexorably in middle age.

Aβ amyloid protein is derived by cleavage from the 'amyloid precursor protein' (APP) by two enzymes called 'secretases'. At present there is an urgent search for drugs which might inhibit secretases and stop the production of toxic Aβ.[4] Most animal proteins will slowly dissolve in water. Gelatin is a familiar example of a soluble protein. But other proteins are more like hair or silk. Once formed they cannot easily be broken down or made soluble within the body. Aβ amyloid fragments accumulate particularly in the junctions between individual nerve cells in AD. One of the components of amyloid protein is a chemical which acts as an adhesive and joins adjacent nerve cells together, thus allowing communication between them. This protein is widespread but found particularly in brain and in platelets (the sticky elements of the blood). It seems that in Alzheimer's disease this protein breaks down in an abnormal fashion. Strong evidence for this has come from study of a rare genetic defect in the amyloid precursor protein which makes an affected individual develop typical Alzheimer's disease before the age of 65. A transgenic mouse strain has been developed into which the defective amyloid precursor protein gene has been inserted. This mouse develops plaques, tangles and neuronal degeneration in brain cells, with all the biochemical and pathological abnormalities of Alzheimer's disease.[5] Synthetic protein fragments have been identified which can induce the formation of insoluble intracellular deposits similar to those found in Alzheimer's disease.[6]

In both Alzheimer's and Huntington's diseases a polypeptide chain of more than about 40 amino acids is found in the insoluble material: glutamine repeats in the case of Huntington's and amyloid Aβ components in Alzheimer's. There is growing suspicion that the 'inclusion bodies' found inside neurones in Alzheimer's, Huntington's and motor neurone disease (Chapter 42) – comprising insoluble lumps or plaques of protein – may all represent disorders in which newly synthesised proteins fold abnormally and even become toxic to the cell in which they were originally made.[7] The abnormally lengthened individual molecules of these proteins are larger than normal. Instead of taking up a random coil-like structure, they form fibrillary amyloid structures. The effect can be reproduced by exposing normal mitochondria to proteins with pathologically long molecules containing glutamine repeats. The effect is to reduce the supply of energy to affected cells, of which neurones are some of the most vulnerable. I shall discuss protein folding and misfolding further in Chapter 42.

Another protein (currently known as AMY117) has been reported to be specially associated with Alzheimer's plaques, possibly even more closely than Aβ.[8] Proteins sometimes become 'glycosylated', that is, they combine with glucose to form a much less soluble material, known as an 'advanced glycation end-product'. Such modified proteins are not easily broken down within the body. They may even pave the way for a change in the structure of amyloid precursor protein.[9] It is worth noting that some 20 diseases, mostly affecting the nervous system, have been recognised to be associated with abnormalities of amyloid proteins.

Tau proteins

Analysis of the neurofibrillary tangles in AD has shown them to comprise two kinds of abnormal minute filaments. Most (95%) are paired helical filaments: the remainder are straight. Both are composed mainly of 'tau' protein ('tau' being the English way of writing the Greek letter τ). This is normally produced by nerve cells and found in the microtubules of their axons. In Alzheimer's disease the tau proteins contain abnormal quantities of phosphate. They do not bind to microtubules in the normal way, but bind strongly to aluminium. This metal element has been implicated in causing Alzheimer's disease, possibly by acting as a co-factor in the formation of neurofibrillary tangles.[10]

The picture is at present extremely confusing. Is the excess of phosphate in tau protein caused by an inherited or acquired metabolic fault? The reversible 'phosphorylation' of proteins (the addition of phosphate) regulates virtually all metabolic activities in cells. If the excess phosphate in tau proteins is acquired, is it a primary abnormality or (perhaps) secondary to a non-specific reduction in nerve function resulting in an excess production of adenosine triphosphate (ATP), the source of energy for virtually all chemical processes in the brain and elsewhere? Or is it due to inhibition of a phosphate-removing enzyme (a phosphatase)? Many known toxins work by inhibiting phosphatases. Perhaps a cause of Alzheimer's disease is an as yet unrecognised toxin, causing excess phosphate attachment to tau proteins and perhaps thereby changing the folding and therefore the shape of important protein molecules.

Animal models

Although gene manipulation has created a convincingly accurate mouse model of Alzheimer's disease, no one has yet managed to reproduce the brain changes of Alzheimer's disease in normal mice or rats by injecting them with ground-up extracts of human AD brains. Some protein misfolding (p. 466) may start or spread extremely slowly. Experimental animals may not live long enough for significant amounts of abnormal protein structures to cause damage. Perhaps deterioration of brain proteins may be caused or accelerated by disease of brain arteries. This would provide the link which has often been sought between Alzheimer's disease and cerebral arteriosclerosis. Extracts of AD brains have been reported to be toxic to nerve cells living or growing outside the body in tissue culture. This research avenue will undoubtedly be further explored in the future.

Implications from treatment

Research in Alzheimer's disease would be greatly helped if there was a blood test by which the diagnosis could be made. Unfortunately there is as yet no such test. A few observations of possible lines of treatment have been made and might shed some light on causation. Some unpublished evidence has suggested that patients with AD have higher than normal concentrations of a particular amino-acid (homocysteine) in their blood. This suggests that they might be deficient in the vitamin folate, which assists the metabolism of homocysteine. I doubt whether folate deficiency has much to do with Alzheimer's disease. It is inevitable that many demented patients will be eating a folate deficient diet. If so the elevated homocysteine levels could be a consequence of this.

But it is entirely reasonable to give folic acid supplements to any elderly person who is not also deficient in vitamin B_{12} – even though it probably has nothing to do with Alzheimer's disease – because folate deficiency is a recognised cause of neuropsychiatric symptoms, especially dementia.[11] I shall discuss further some of the mysteries surrounding folate metabolism in Chapter 27.

If the blood pressure of someone with AD is raised, blood-pressure-lowering treatment is worthwhile and has been reported to reduce the incidence of dementia in a multi-centre trial.

There is current interest in the possibility that 'oestrogens', the collective name for chemicals acting in a specific way as female sex hormones, may protect against mental deterioration in Alzheimer's disease. Disease of brain arteries is commonly associated with AD. Since pre-menopausal women may be partly protected against arterial disease by oestrogens, the possible beneficial effects of these drugs may be indirect.

There has been an interesting long-term study of a group of nuns relating linguistic ability in early life, assessed by personal autobiographies written by women in their early twenties, to the development of AD 50–60 years later. Poor linguistic ability was found to be a strong predictor of subsequent development of Alzheimer's disease and of poor intellectual function later in life.[12] This observation is difficult to categorise, but complementary results have been reported in another survey in which it was noted that high early educational and occupational attainment lessens the risk of developing AD later in life.[13] Are these further examples of the physiological generalisation that the more some bodily organ or function is used, the longer it lasts – and vice versa?

There is an important inflammatory element in Alzheimer's disease. Anti-inflammatory drugs such as ibuprofen and diclofenac have a place in treatment. They delay or even inhibit development of AD. All this suggests that an infection (causing inflammation) could be a trigger factor for Alzheimer's in susceptible individuals. A virus like HSV1 might act as a trigger. Another pointer to an external pathogenic factor is that there are substantial geographical differences in Alzheimer's disease incidence.[14] Unfortunately it is difficult at the bedside to distinguish AD from other causes of dementia in old age. Victims may live for many years. I have already mentioned that the disease can only be identified for certain in life by brain biopsy.

A series of observations has been made in Alzheimer patients of serial changes in brain size developing over time. If these are plotted graphically, they suggest that Alzheimer's begins in the temporal lobe of the brain at a discrete point in time, rather than being a slow progression over decades. It has even been suggested that a spirochaete, a bacterium of the same type that causes syphilis, might be involved as a trigger to set the disease off, though this has not at present been confirmed.

One of the measurable changes in Alzheimer's disease is a reduction in concentrations of the neurotransmitter[15] acetylcholine in the brain. Attempts have been made to improve brain function by giving drugs such as tacrine, donepezil, rivastigmine and metrifonate. These drugs inhibit acetylcholine esterase (the enzyme which normally rapidly destroys acetylcholine). They thus increase the amounts of acetylcholine at nerve junctions. In some trials they appear to have brought benefit. Unfortunately this tends to be only shortlasting and is reversed when the drug is withdrawn. Another problem is that these drugs are non-selective and block the action of the enzyme elsewhere, causing a build up of acetylcholine in places such as the gut, causing nausea and increased gut movements.

There is some recent interest in the neurotransmitter galanin, which appears to stimulate neuronal growth and may play some part in nerve regeneration.

Energy supply to the brain

If Alzheimer's disease slowly progresses through the accumulation of some damaging material in brain cells, it would be necessary to invoke some sort of vicious circle to explain why brain damage seems to speed up towards the end. One suggestion has been the 'excitotoxic' theory: that damage of nerve cells from any cause (e.g. impaired blood supply) might liberate excessive amounts of the excitatory neurotransmitters glutamate and aspartate. This would increase metabolic demands on the remaining living nerve cells, release more glutamate and create a vicious circle. I find such ideas difficult to reconcile with evidence that metabolic rate and glucose consumption seem to be especially reduced in those regions of brain most affected by Alzheimer's disease. Memantine (a glutamate receptor antagonist) may slow down the progression of AD.

There is some evidence for a specifically maternal inheritance of Alzheimer's disease. Surveys have shown that there is a higher than expected ratio of affected mothers to fathers among parents of people with the condition. In other words, you are somewhat more likely to develop AD if your mother was affected than if your father was.[16] This points a finger towards mitochondria, the minute energy-supplying structures inside all cells. These are outside cell nuclei and are inherited almost exclusively from the original ovum, i.e. from the

210

mother. Sperms contain very few mitochondria. As mentioned above, affected regions of the brain in AD have a lower metabolic rate and glucose consumption than normal. So perhaps predisposing chromosomal mutations depend on some defect in mitochondrial energy supply to exert their full damaging effect.

Experiments in mice have shown that these genes are intimately involved in cellular energy supplies and in the metabolism of glucose. Inheriting even a single copy of the APOEε4 gene reduces the efficiency of glucose metabolism. It has even been suggested that Alzheimer's disease is 'diabetes of the brain'!

Summary

Alzheimer's disease is probably the commonest cause of loss of mental functions in old age. It afflicts at least 1% of the population over 65, probably more. There is initial memory loss, but later all intellectual functions are impaired. The brunt of the damage falls on the hippocampal complex at the front of the brain, in which energy metabolism is reduced.

There are at least three, possibly more, different dominantly inherited mutations which determine that a person will develop Alzheimer's disease. None has yet been linked with the much more common occurrence of sporadic Alzheimer's disease. This is marked by brain neurones and glial cells accumulating fibrillary tangles and plaques containing an insoluble starchy material, Aβ amyloid. The larger form of this molecule seems to be less soluble than the smaller form and is particularly associated with Alzheimer's disease.

The disease probably starts at a discrete point in time, but the precipitating factors are not known. There have been suggestions that an infection with herpes simplex virus 1 (HSV1) might be the trigger. It seems more likely that the pathological changes diagnostic of Alzheimer's disease may be induced by several different routes in people with several different genetic predispositions. In some people with AD the cause seems to lie in their genes, but most cases are sporadic. If AD is triggered by an infection it is particularly difficult to see why sporadic cases should be almost confined to the elderly.

There are many mysteries wrapped up in Alzheimer's disease. No one has yet envisaged any single unifying explanation. The epidemiology is extraordinarily difficult. The world awaits a simple but accurate non-traumatic diagnostic test which can be applied prospectively to large populations. Such a test is needed not only for unravelling and making sense of the large number of possible causes, but also for assessing possible treatments and designing trials. There is growing suspicion that the defect in AD may involve abnormal protein folding, especially involving Aβ amyloid protein.

20

CORONARY HEART DISEASE: ATHEROMA

Everyone knows what happens in a heart attack. We have seen so many in films and on television. The victim, a burly man, has just been in a fierce argument and loses his temper. He clutches his chest, loses consciousness and quickly dies. This can certainly happen in real life if regular coordinated heart contractions stop. A heart which was previously beating regularly at, say, 80 beats/min may go suddenly into a lethal rhythm disorder such as ventricular fibrillation. Contractions at a rate of many hundreds per minute obviously cannot shift any blood. The heart valves could not open and shut quickly enough. Ventricular fibrillation is as immediately lethal as complete stoppage of the beating heart.

But it is not always like that. For some eight years I was a medical assessor for the British Medical Research Council's Coronary Prevention Trial. In this capacity I read and assessed many hundreds of medical records and post mortem reports on the circumstances of death of trial participants. Some patients had 'died in their sleep', i.e. were found dead in bed in the morning. More commonly, a man had complained to his wife of feeling ill with some discomfort in the chest, seldom with excruciating pain. A doctor or ambulance had been summoned, but the patient was dead before reaching hospital.

On the other hand, nearly a third of patients later found to have had a heart attack were not complaining of chest pain when they first presented themselves to hospital. They may have had isolated neck or jaw pain, pain in the upper abdomen or back (attributed to indigestion), or a non-specific feeling of illness, perhaps with profuse sweating. The clinical diagnosis can be difficult. I have seen two men who insisted that they had never experienced chest pain or any other symptoms at any time in their life, but yet had unmistakeable evidence of a previous heart attack in the electrical record of their heart. I have seen another man who got bouts of severe upper back pain on running. This behaved exactly like 'angina pectoris' (Latin: *angina* = pain in the throat, now used for pain elsewhere; '*pectoris*' = of the chest, breast bone). It was brought on by exercise and quickly relieved by rest. I was fascinated that, when this man eventually had a complete and established heart attack, the pain from that was also felt in the back. It was initially misdiagnosed as collapse of a bone in his vertebral column. He must have been born with an unusual wiring pattern of pain nerves coming from his heart.

In my clinical experience the most telling symptom of a severe heart attack is cold sweating – i.e. sweating with no elevation of body temperature and with a cold skin; but doubtless other experienced physicians have made different observations.

The immediate cause of a heart attack

In almost every case of a sudden heart attack the immediate cause is a clot which has blocked one of the main coronary arteries (Fig. 27) or

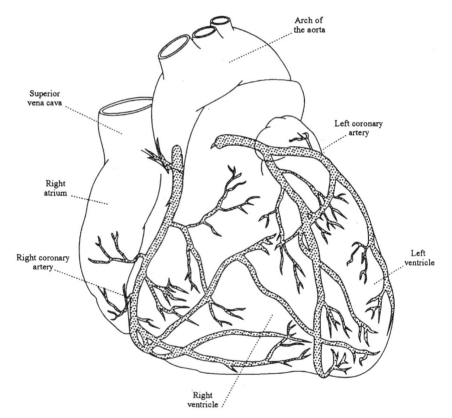

Figure 27 The heart seen from the front, showing the appearance of the main coronary arteries on the front surface of the heart.

214

one of its branches. Heart muscle contains nerves which signal the sensation of pain to the brain when its blood supply is inadequate. If heart muscle tissue actually dies – a process which takes between 1 and 6 hours after its blood supply is interrupted – the pain may get better because the nerves which signal pain sensation have themselves died. A portion of heart muscle which has died from lack of blood is technically a 'myocardial infarct'. In medical jargon this is commonly referred to as an 'MI'.

Sometimes an obstructing blood clot has come from outside the heart itself and has simply been swept in by the blood stream. It is then classified as an 'embolus' (Greek: 'patch' or 'something put in'). Sometimes it is difficult to be sure at post mortem whether a clot has formed on the particular artery which it obstructed, or whether it was an embolus. Most clots arise first on the surface of a lump of atheroma (p. 81). Plaques of atheroma are usually smooth on their surface. They do not cause trouble unless they are so large that they block the artery. But plaques of atheroma are brittle and may even contain mineral calcium. They sometimes split. The fissure exposes a rough surface to the blood flowing past it and attracts the sticky elements of blood, forming a clot.[1] This may get big enough to threaten the life of that part of the heart muscle which the artery supplies.[2]

A theoretical cause of a heart (myocardial) infarct is severe spasm of the circular muscle in the wall of an artery which supplies part of the heart muscle. There is no doubt that this can cause angina pectoris when a coronary artery has nearly closed. Volunteers have been given spasm-producing drugs. They reported angina-like pain at the same time that the coronary arteries were seen on X-rays to be strongly constricted. But I find it difficult to believe that in life spontaneous artery spasm could ever be so extreme as to cause an actual infarct. Such a disadvantageous situation should surely have been eliminated by natural selection during human evolution.

When a portion of heart muscle has died, even though it was supplied with blood by an artery which seems to be unobstructed, there is a much more probable explanation than extreme spasm. A previously obstructing clot has probably been removed by 'thrombolysis' (Greek: *thrombos* = clot; *lysis* = loosing, disintegration). Once a clot has formed in a blood vessel, circulating chemicals and scavenger cells in the blood attack the clot and may dissolve or 'lyse' it within an hour or two. This sequence of events has puzzled many pathologists in the past who have looked in vain at the time of post mortem examination for the cause of an 'infarct' (i.e. tissue death from lack of blood) in the heart, brain or elsewhere.

215

Blood clotting is brought about by a complex set of chemical reactions which are chemical amplifiers – that is, one chemical reaction produces many products, each of which in turn makes many more. Thus, clotting can be very rapid, once initiated. Thrombolysis is brought about by a set of chemical reactions which are nearly as complex as those involved in the formation of a clot, but which operate over minutes rather than seconds.

Diagnosis of heart attacks

Our diagnostic tests have become steadily more and more accurate and specific over the years. The electrical record of the heart rhythm (the electrocardiogram: ECG, or 'EKG' in the USA) is often informative enough to make the diagnosis. It can also guide management and determine prognosis.[3] Some family doctors (as well as cardiologists) even carry with them a portable ECG machine which can be used in a patient's home.

Blood tests have now become more specific and therefore more useful. In my early clinical years all hospital physicians relied on finding a rise in the blood concentration of proteins (enzymes) which were associated both with liver cell as well as with heart cell destruction (e.g. the transaminases). Later we relied on changes in more specific heart enzymes such as creatine kinase. But we now have available an index of heart muscle damage which is more specific still. This is elevation in the blood levels of the contractile proteins troponin-T and troponin-I. Troponins make up part of heart muscle tissue but are not present in muscle elsewhere in the body. Their blood concentrations remain raised for a week or two after a myocardial infarct. This makes them specific for heart muscle damage. There is now a bedside test kit for troponin-I in blood which can give results in 15 minutes.

Epidemiology

In developed countries, atheromatous plaques have been found in individuals' coronary arteries from the second decade onwards, i.e. even in the late teens. American physicians were shocked when they examined their young soldiers killed in Korea in the 1960s, often finding extensive coronary atheroma and even established myocardial infarcts. Coronary heart disease is now the leading cause of death in the UK and in all developed countries, though most victims survive their first heart attack and many get back to full normal physical activity. The current risk of death from any single myocardial infarct episode is between 12% and 15%. Myocardial infarction has recently been recognised as the leading cause of death in women, even ahead of cancer of the breast, though women get heart attacks 4 years later than men, on average. In the USA more than half a million women die of heart disease each year and twice as many people die from coronary artery disease as from all varieties of cancer. About half of all deaths attributable to coronary heart disease are in people older than 65. The presence of diabetes more than doubles the risk of a heart attack. Asians have a greater susceptibility to heart attacks than Europeans, but Caribbeans and North Africans have less.

In the early 1900s heart attacks were said to be rare, but by the 1970s they were responsible for nearly one third of all deaths in Western populations. During the time that I was a member of the Council of the British Heart Foundation, we had to take one of the main British cancer charities to task for suggesting, when appealing for funds, that cancer was the most common cause of death in Britain. It is not. Coronary heart disease is. By the age of 40, men in Western countries have about a one in two lifetime's risk of getting symptoms from coronary heart disease. Women have a one in three risk.

Although the number of cases in a given year per head of population (the incidence) is slowly rising, the death rate is falling. The risk of heart attacks has been greatly reduced in people who have been able to stop smoking. The late US President Lyndon Johnson – an extreme chain smoker of cigarettes – stopped himself smoking by a celebrated effort of will, leaving an open pack of cigarettes on his desk for the rest of his life.

Since smoking is the strongest risk factor for heart attacks, stopping smoking is the best way for smokers to protect themselves. But other measures can reduce risk, e.g. taking more exercise, losing weight, and eating a 'Mediterranean' diet.[4] Red wine may improve the viability and function of the inner layer (endothelium) of arteries. Many drugs can reduce the risk of heart attacks, e.g. aspirin, clopidogrel, anti-clotting agents, statins, angiotensin-converting enzyme inhibitors, beta-blockers, fibrates and calcium-channel blockers. Many trials have been made of these agents. The most spectacular has been an Oxford trial comparing in high-risk patients the prophylactic use of an orally active 'statin' drug to lower cholesterol (in this case simvastatin), a cocktail of protective vitamins, and an inactive placebo. Simvastatin reduced coronary events and strokes by about 15%, but vitamins had no greater effect than placebo tablets.[5]

Cause

Three main processes contribute to heart attacks: coronary artery blockage due to cholesterol-laden deposits (plaques) of atheroma in a coronary artery wall, cracks or fissures in an atheromatous plaque, and clot formation on the plaque crack or fissure.

Cholesterol

The best-known influence on atheroma deposition and arterial disease is the concentration of cholesterol in the blood. The concentration of this fatty material is determined by the genes that an individual has inherited from his or her parents and also by the individual's habitual diet. Cholesterol is a normal constituent of all cells, but is also the major constituent of plaques of atheroma in the coronary arteries of the heart. Large plaques are themselves major causes of artery obstruction. Also, if a brittle plaque of atheroma splits or cracks, it exposes clot-forming chemicals to the bloodstream.

Commercial animal food in pellet form can be soaked in benzene (benzol) into which cholesterol has been dissolved. Then the benzol can be allowed to evaporate, leaving cholesterol evenly spread throughout the feed. I have fed cholesterol in this way to rabbits and observed the widespread development of plaques of atheroma in the large arteries after a few weeks. I also noticed that any physical damage to an artery (e.g. by squeezing the aorta with forceps during a previous operation under general anaesthesia) made atheroma plaques appear in the damaged arterial wall several weeks later. The site and appearance of the lesions corresponded exactly to the place where the arterial wall had been previously squeezed. The ridges on the tip of the forceps were accurately reproduced by the atheromatous deposit.

There are many well-known genetic influences which affect blood cholesterol concentration. 'Familial hypercholesterolaemia' (FH) is the best recognised human genetic factor associated with arterial disease. It is due to mutation in the gene which codes for the low-density lipoprotein (LDL) receptor protein. Individuals who inherit even a single copy of this gene (i.e. they are 'heterozygous' for it) have about twice the normal concentration of cholesterol in their blood and suffer from premature arterial disease and heart attacks. In some populations, this genetic abnormality is present in 1% of individuals. In other populations it may even be present in as many as 20% of people who develop coronary artery disease symptoms at a young age. Other genetic traits causing premature arterial disease are associated with variants in the a5 lipoprotein E genes themselves, which code for components of LDL.[6]

Other aspects of atheroma formation

Although the lumps (plaques) of atheroma in the walls of coronary and other arteries are largely composed of cholesterol, they also contain variable numbers of muscle cells in which the structural protein collagen is synthesised, as well as white blood cells (macrophages). Atheromatous plaques may be covered by a thin layer of fibrous cells, but muscle cells are the only cells capable of making up a strong protective covering over an atheromatous plaque. If a plaque becomes covered by a thick layer of muscle cells it is better protected against cracking or rupture compared with a plaque which is mainly composed of cholesterol and therefore fragile. If flowing blood comes into sudden contact with the fatty core of an atheromatous plaque a large clot can form quickly. This often results in sudden death when it occurs in an artery which is already more than half blocked by a lump of atheroma in its wall.

There is evidence that minor damaging fractures or cracks in plaques of atheroma are very common. Muscle cells are continually being used to restore a smooth non-adherent surface over damaged atheromatous plaques. The group of zinc-containing enzymes known collectively as matrix-degrading metalloproteinases (MMPs) are involved in repair and remodelling of arterial walls as well as in the spread of tumours. They can be inhibited by tissue inhibitors of metalloproteinases (TIMPs). There is normally a balance between MMPs and TIMPs. One way of looking at plaques of atheroma in the walls of arteries is that they represent a defect in the repair and remodelling of the artery at the site of the plaque. One incidental protective effect of the cholesterol-lowering statin drugs is the inhibition of the 'stromelysin' enzymes (members of the MMP family), which may promote the rupture of atheromatous plaques.

High blood pressure (Chapter 31) is strongly associated with increased liability to atheroma, in the coronary and also in the brain arteries. There is no doubt that hypertension can directly cause atheroma, presumably by putting increased stress on arterial walls. There is suggestive evidence that lowering blood pressure may protect against this. But most of the protective effect of blood-pressure-lowering drugs comes from the protection they give against atheroma plaque rupture and also (in some cases) inhibition of blood clotting. There may be additional protection against the formation of atheroma, but this is difficult to prove.

Diabetes (Chapters 14 & 15) is also strongly associated with increased liability to atheroma formation, though we do not know exactly why. There is some evidence that good control of diabetes – i.e. by preventing unduly high levels of blood sugar – may reduce the liability to heart attacks.

The innermost layer of cells lining normal blood vessels is the endothelium. Recent work suggests that endothelial cells are formed initially in the bone marrow (like red blood cells and platelet precursor cells), circulate in the bloodstream, and repair defects in the lining of blood vessels.[7] The health of this layer of cells is important to prevent cells from the blood sticking to it and hence initiating clotting. As I mentioned earlier, red wine has been reported to improve the function of endothelial cells.[8]

A circulating chemical (homocysteine) can damage endothelial function. A dietary supplement of folic acid (a member of the B_2 class of vitamins) can lower the blood concentration of homocysteine. There is therefore current interest in the possible protective effect of folic acid in preventing heart attacks by reducing the concentration of homocysteine in the body.

In the USA folic acid in small amounts is routinely added to flour before baking, to protect expectant mothers against having babies with neural tube defects (see Chapter 27). This folate supplement may also be giving the American population additional protection against heart attacks. I am disappointed that so far the UK Government has not seen fit to follow the Americans and supplement our flour with folic acid.

After I had spent a long time reading all the published work on folic acid dietary supplements I wrote a review[9] which emphasised the beneficial effects of extra dietary folic acid and de-emphasised its potential dangers – though recognising that folic acid can aggravate the ill effects of vitamin B_{12} deficiency. I felt that the dangers of folic acid had been grossly exaggerated. This library research so convinced me of the merit of extra folic acid that I started and have continued to take 5 milligrams of folic acid daily for the last 7 years, with no obvious ill effect so far. I do not know whether it has helped to save me from premature cardiovascular disease, but faith is a great thing even if the evidence is incomplete!

A rise in the blood concentration of another chemical – 'Asymmetrical DiMethylArginine' (ADMA) – is associated with a rise in the blood concentration of homocysteine. This might increase the risk of heart attacks. In addition, ADMA is suspected of having a toxic effect on the endothelium of blood vessels. ADMA inhibits the formation of nitric oxide, a naturally-occurring dilator of arteries. It accumulates in kidney failure and plays a part in causing hypertension. ADMA is itself subject to degradation by the enzyme 'Dimethylarginine Dimethyl-AminoHydrolase' (DDAH). The two chemicals ADMA and DDAH are reciprocally affected by many factors involved in the oxidation of foodstuffs.

Inflammation and infections

There are many clues suggesting that inflammation and (presumptively) infections can make atheroma plaques develop in the walls of arteries. Indeed, a link between infections and arterial disease was first noted more than 100 years ago and has often been emphasised since.[10] Non-specific markers of inflammation – including the blood concentration of C-reactive protein, interleukin-6 (IL-6) and amyloid-A protein[11] – may be increased before a heart attack and may even have some predictive value. The number of inflammation-associated white cells in the blood may also increase. Every stage of atheroma formation is associated with accumulation of specialised white cells (macrophages and T-lymphocytes) in plaques of atheroma. We do not know for certain whether inflammation causes atheroma, although the evidence for this causal association is becoming stronger year by year. It is also possible that degenerative changes in atheromatous plaques may cause inflammation but this seems an unlikely or important cause of the association.

The strongest evidence that active inflammation in an artery wall often precedes a heart attack[12] is the rise in the blood concentration of C-reactive protein, already mentioned. A link between atheroma formation and inflammation has also been suggested by animal experiments. Soon after a rabbit has been given a cholesterol-rich diet, inflammatory cells (chiefly monocytes) stick to the inner lining of arteries (the endothelium) and accumulate in places where atheroma lesions later develop. These macrophages accumulate lipid and turn into so-called 'foam' cells which are seen in atheromatous plaques. Evidence of previous infections with cytomegalovirus, herpes, coxsackie B4 viruses or with helicobacter bacteria has been at times found in human atheroma plaques. Atheroma in the carotid artery has been reported as almost twice as common in people with evidence of previous hepatitis C infection as in people with no such evidence.[13]

Most clues suggesting that infections might cause atheroma come from experimental work in cholesterol-fed animals. Herpes virus infections can cause atheroma deposition in chickens. But no single infecting organism such as a bacterium or a virus has yet been incriminated in causing arterial disease in man. Most epidemiological studies of populations suggest that people living in the country suffer less from coronary heart disease and hypertension than those living in towns. This rather vague generalisation might suggest that respiratory infections such as those caused by *Chlamydia pneumoniae* might have something to do with the difference.[14]

Although this line of research has not yet come up with a definite answer, the problem is well worth further investigation. If a specific infectious cause for atheroma deposition could be identified, the way would be open to protect against arterial disease by directly attacking the infection with antibiotics or preventing it by vaccination. It is interesting that vaccinating elderly people against influenza has already been reported to have reduced the risk of hospitalisation and death from heart diseases and strokes.[15]

One recalls the vast changes in the management of peptic ulcer which have taken place since an infection (with *H. pylori*) was established as its main cause.

Clotting

The formation of a clot is often the final event causing a heart attack. A high level of fibrinogen in the blood (the protein precursor of the fibrous material which solidifies the clot) appears to be strongly predictive of a later heart attack. One potential ill effect of smoking is to increase the rate of fibrinogen synthesis. Stopping smoking reverses this effect within 2 weeks. Many other blood clotting factors – too numerous to itemise here – can influence heart attacks. They may account for many of the genetic influences which have been recognised.

> So it seems that fibrinogen concentration in blood must be a major determining factor for heart attacks. But this simple conclusion may be misleading because of the confounding effect of other associations. It remains possible that the presence of atheroma may in itself increase plasma fibrinogen concentrations. The apparent causal link has not yet been confirmed when the rigorous 'Mendelian randomisation' procedure has been used, to avoid confounding bias of all kinds. The fibrinogen story is an interesting cautionary tale for epidemiologists.[16]

Treatments, and prophylaxis

Drugs collectively known as 'statins' were originally designed to interfere with cholesterol synthesis and hence reduce atheroma formation. They have revolutionised the management of lipid disorders, despite having occasional ill effects on muscle.

Other therapeutic weapons have been introduced into medical

practice as knowledge of the causes of heart attacks has increased. I have already mentioned the beneficial effects of supplemental folic acid. Oily fish may improve the composition of body fat. Furthermore, the 'polyunsaturated' fatty acids in fish oils (known technically as the group of 'n-3' fatty acids)[17] actually become part of atheromatous plaques. They are thought to protect against plaque rupture.[18] Aspirin reduces the stickiness of platelets and thus reduces coronary thrombosis risk.[19] It should be used prophylactically by everyone in high risk groups who is not allergic to the drug. In his Shattuck Lecture to the USA Heart, Lung and Blood Institute, Claude Lenfant[20] recently deplored the failure of many physicians to make enough use of this cheap and effective drug.

In the early stages of a heart attack the drug clopidogrel may be slightly better than aspirin, though it is much more expensive. Thrombolysis using drugs such as alteplase can recanalise arteries blocked by clots, although such therapy – and indeed the use of all anti-clotting agents – runs the risk of causing bleeding within the brain or elsewhere. Large blocked arteries can often best be treated by surgical reconstruction.[21] Early angloplasty and stenting are becoming standard emergency treatment.

Summary

A heart attack is usually a 'myocardial infarct' – i.e. death of some part of heart muscle because of lack of an adequate blood supply. The immediate cause is usually a locally-formed clot arising on the surface of a plaque of atheroma – a porridge-like fatty material mostly composed of cholesterol. In addition, a clot formed elsewhere (an embolus) may have been swept into a narrowed segment of artery and blocked it.

A high cholesterol concentration in the blood favours heart attacks. These may be due to someone's inheritance of an unduly high cholesterol concentration, or to the inheritance of many other disadvantageous factors such as those favouring clot formation. Reduction of cholesterol concentration is spectacularly effective in reducing heart attacks, but vitamin supplements have no effect.

An active medical research field at present is the search for factors like specific infections which may cause local inflammation in blood vessel walls and eventually predispose to atheroma formation. So far no plausible infectious agent has been incriminated in causing heart attacks, but the search continues.

21

HEART FAILURE

What, exactly, does 'heart failure' mean?

While an adult is at rest the heart pumps some 10–12 pints (about 5 litres) of blood round the body each minute. During the most strenuous possible exercise a really fit man's heart might be able to pump around some seven times as much as this. A very small sick woman might just be able to stay alive with her heart pumping only a quarter of this, say, 3 pints per minute.

So with this huge difference in the amount that different people's hearts pump in different conditions of rest and exercise, how can we say what 'heart failure' is? Many authors define it as 'failure of the heart to meet the needs of the body'. But these needs are changeable and difficult to measure. Furthermore, the performance of the heart can be boosted a great deal by increasing the head of pressure which fills it. More than a century ago the English physiologist Ernest Starling observed that the output of an animal's heart was directly related to the pressure head filling it, providing that this was not too high. Figure 28 embodies 'Starling's Law of the Heart' with the sort of values which might be recorded if a human heart had been removed from the body and its performance studied in a laboratory. As the pressure head of blood filling the heart rises from point A in the diagram (zero filling pressure) to 1 inch head of water pressure (about 2 mmHg, point B) the output of the heart – the amount pumped per unit of time – goes from zero to 5 litres/min. If the filling pressure rises further, e.g. to point C ($1\frac{1}{2}$ inches head of water pressure: about 3 mmHg) the output might rise to 7 litres/min. At high filling pressures (e.g. 5 inches: nearly 10 mmHg) the output of the heart is reaching a plateau (point D) which is near its maximum performance under these conditions. Little further increase in output can be obtained however high the filling pressure. This is probably because overstretched heart valves start to leak.

But there are other influences on the output of the heart in addition to the pressure of the blood coming to it. The heart is supplied with sympathetic nerves (part of the autonomic nervous system: p. 481).

225

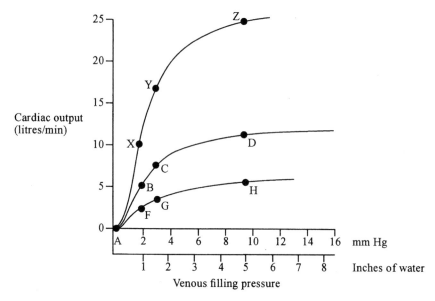

Figure 28 Various relations between the filling pressure of the heart (the pressure in the cardiac atria) and the output of the heart – i.e. how much can the heart pump in a given time. As the pressure head of blood filling the heart rises from point A in the diagram (zero filling pressure) to 1 inch head of water pressure (about 2 mmHg) the output of a normal heart – the amount pumped per unit of time – would go from 0 to 5 litres/min (point B). If the filling pressure rose further, (e.g. to $1\frac{1}{2}$ inches head of water pressure: about 3 mmHg) the output might rise to 7 litres/min (point C). At high filling pressures (e.g. 5 inches: nearly 10 mmHg) the output of the heart would be reaching a plateau (point D) which is near its maximum performance under these conditions. The upper function curve (A-X-Y-Z) represents the function curve which might be expected if the heart were being stimulated by maximum sympathetic nerve activity and maximum adrenergic hormone release. The lower curve (A-F-G-H) represents the function curve of a severely damaged heart.

These can increase the rate of beating of the heart and also increase the force of contraction at each beat. Similar changes can also be brought about by the hormone adrenaline[1] which can be secreted into the bloodstream from the central parts of the adrenal glands. The small adrenal glands lie above each kidney, at the back of the abdomen. An increase in circulating adrenaline, or an increase in the frequency of nerve impulses passing from the brain to the heart, might increase the output of the heart at 1 inch filling pressure from point B to point X (10 litres/min output) in Figure 28. The whole function curve can be shifted up, e.g. to A-X-Y-Z.

The rate of beating of a human heart which has been transplanted from someone else is no longer under the direct control of the brain because all the nerves which run from brain to heart have been cut. So the heart rate does not immediately go up with fear or excitement, although within a minute or two circulating adrenaline secreted by the adrenal glands has much the same effect as stimulation of the heart's pacemaker by its nerve supply, which uses the chemical transmitter noradrenaline. Later on, nerves grow back into the transplanted heart, which then comes partly back under nervous control by the brain.

Towards a definition of heart failure

Failure of some organ of the body to fulfil its normal function is usually easy to define and understand. The kidneys are a good example. Their main function is to get rid of the unwanted products of digestion of food. So kidney failure can be diagnosed and quantified by a rise in the concentration of various waste products in the blood. The lungs provide another example. Failure of their ventilatory function can be measured by a rise in the concentration of carbon dioxide (the waste gas) in the blood. Failure of heart function is much more difficult to quantify.

Sudden (acute) heart failure occurs if the heart stops beating altogether, or when there is rapid disordered contraction of the heart's ventricles ('ventricular fibrillation'). In either case there is loss of consciousness within a minute. Death ensues within about 4-6 minutes. But slowly-developing failure of the heart – which is what doctors mean when they say that someone is suffering from heart failure – is difficult to define and quantify. The heart's pumping function may be changing rapidly, over a wide range. It has to go up during muscular exercise and also adapt to changes in body posture. We cannot define or measure 'heart failure' simply by measuring the amount that the heart is pumping at any one particular moment in time.

Doctors use an indirect way of assessing poor heart function. They take account of certain symptoms and signs which betray the heart's inadequacy. Blood pressure may be so low that not enough blood is being pumped around – a situation which is sometimes described as 'forward failure'. Or perhaps the blood pressure is normal but an adequate output of the heart is only being achieved at the expense of an increase in the volume of the blood and a consequent rise in the pressure head filling the heart – a situation sometimes described as 'backward failure'. The heart's performance might then resemble the lower curve in Figure 28 (A-F-G-H). A cardiac output just adequate for someone at rest (e.g. 5 litres/min) could then only be achieved by a very high filling pressure (e.g. 5 inches: point H in Fig. 28). At this

227

stage an observer at the bedside would see the veins in the neck distended even with the subject sitting up. Everything depends on how rapidly the heart's function has failed.

A nice illustration of the contrasting consequences of inadequate heart function is provided by diseases affecting the pericardium, the tough fibrous membrane which envelops the heart like a bag or sack and stops it expanding too far, or bursting. Inflammation of the pericardium, e.g. by an acute virus infection, can make the lining of the pericardium pour out excess fluid. This accumulates in the pericardial sac and can prevent the heart filling properly with blood. When severe, this condition has the technical name 'cardiac tamponade'. Blood pressure falls sharply. If the condition is not treated promptly – by sticking a wide-bore needle into the pericardium to let some fluid out – it can cause death. This is a classic cause of 'forward failure'. But now I want to consider the more chronic (i.e. longstanding) common consequences of poor heart function.

Retention of salt and water

When the heart is not pumping adequately and the blood flow to the kidneys starts to fall, the kidneys may stop excreting normal amounts of salt and water. If a patient continues to eat and drink as usual, salt and water start to pile up in the body. There is then an increase in the volume of the blood and in the volume of fluid in the tissues outside the blood vessels (the 'interstitial fluid'). When any sort of heart failure has existed for more than a day or two the total blood volume increases.[2] Significant excess of interstitial fluid in the body, usually at least some 5–7 extra litres of fluid, is easy to recognise because the ankles enlarge and look puffy. They can be indented by pressing them firmly with a finger. The depression on the skin only slowly fills up again as fluid moves back from the surrounding tissues. For centuries physicians have used the word 'oedema' to describe this situation. Lay people called it 'dropsy' and the name is still sometimes used. The swelling is due to an excess of interstitial fluid accumulated between individual cells. Although oedema ('edema' in the USA) is used to describe this precise situation, *oidema* in Greek simply means 'a swelling'.

When oedema of the legs and dependent parts of the body is due to heart disease, the condition is described as 'congestive', 'systemic', or 'right' heart failure. Excess fluid not only expands the interstitial space between body cells, it also increases the total volume of blood in the circulation. The pressures everywhere in the circulation are increased. This was shown more than 60 years ago by Starr, who inserted a needle into the veins of recently dead people and observed that their veins were usually filled with blood at an average pressure equivalent to about 3 inches (6.5 cm) height of blood. But when he did the same in people recently dead from heart failure their veins were considerably more distended. The average pressure in the veins was about 7 inches (15–20 cm) height of blood.[3] The rise of pressure in the large veins is also reflected in a rise of pressure in smaller veins and capillaries. This causes oedema of the legs and of other dependent parts. Many years ago I often saw gross swelling of the scrotum in men recently dead of heart failure. This is not seen nowadays because modern diuretic drugs prevent this degree of fluid accumulation.

Increased pressure in the lung veins causes oedema of the lungs. During life this is the usual cause of breathlessness in people with heart failure. It is a particularly common complaint when there is weakness of the heart's muscular pumping function, obstruction at the region of one of the heart valves, or inefficient pumping because of leaky valves. Accumulation of fluid in the lungs is specially likely when blood is not being adequately pumped out from the left side of the heart, as is often the case after a large heart attack. This situation is often described as 'left heart' failure. Pulmonary oedema can make its victim very breathless, even at rest. The lungs become much stiffer and more difficult either to inflate or to empty. In addition, nerve receptors within the lungs[4] send a signal to the brain that the lungs are unduly congested. When this happens during exercise the nerve signals tell the brain – by creating the sensation of breathlessness – that the exercise must stop.

Many years ago I once had the horrifying experience of trying to ventilate artificially a young man dying of terminal kidney failure. He was breathless because his damaged kidneys could not excrete water properly, causing gross lung oedema. Normally it is easy, by intermittently squeezing a balloon attached to someone's windpipe, to provide adequate ventilation by moving air in and out of the chest. Squeezing the balloon pushes air into the chest. The elastic recoil of the lungs pushes it out again: you don't need suction. But my patient's lungs were so full of interstitial fluid that it was almost more than I could do to ventilate the lungs adequately by intermittently squeezing the balloon. Although a mechanical ventilator later took my place, my patient eventually died from the toxic accumulation of waste products. (This would not happen today because we now have effective ways of treating terminal kidney failure, by dialysis or kidney transplantation.)

The reflex effects of lung congestion were demonstrated to me in 1969 by Autar Paintal, in the Vallabhbhai Chest Institute in Delhi. We were studying the reflex effects of various stimuli on nerve detector elements in the lungs of anaesthetised cats (the so-called 'J' receptors). We observed that these receptors could be stimulated by nitric oxide gas, carbon dioxide, and by several drugs, as well as by lung congestion.[5] All these stimuli had an immediate relaxing effect on the resting tension (tone) in limb muscles. This powerful reflex effect can be studied in fully anaesthetised animals and is independent of consciousness. It is one of the ways in which lung congestion limits muscular exercise and athletic performance.

Paintal and I had been trying to understand the reasons why muscular exercise increases the rate and depth of breathing, so that enough extra oxygen is supplied to the body and enough extra carbon dioxide gas is removed. The natural process is exquisitely accurately tuned. One very attractive theory supposed that chemical receptors in the lungs are sensitive to carbon dioxide and signal to the brain the need to increase ventilation when extra carbon dioxide coming from exercising muscles arrives in the blood. Although 'J' receptors in the lungs are indeed stimulated by carbon dioxide, we found that neither the receptors nor their reflex effects seemed sensitive or powerful enough to increase ventilation appropriately, at least when tested in anaesthetised animals. So a good theory bit the dust. It often happens, alas! Current opinion now suggests that most of the increased breathing in exercise is an adaptation which the body has learnt, which minimises the work of breathing and minimises undue disturbances of blood-gas exchange. But I still wonder whether J-receptor stimulation might yet play a part in stimulating ventilation in conscious subjects during exercise.

The brain also receives information from nerve receptors in muscles. When muscles are working with an inadequate blood flow, these 'metaboreflex' nerve detectors make the brain switch off nervous drive to muscles. Clearly this is another system which has evolved to prevent excessive muscle activity damaging the body. I imagine that Pheidippides, the Athenian soldier who carried the news about the battle of Marathon in 490 BC (by repute running 150 miles in 2 days) must have trained himself to suppress these neurological warnings. Having delivered his message he is said to have dropped dead. I imagine that top-class athletes have to train themselves to ignore the massive input of unpleasant sensations from their lungs and from their muscles.

The breathlessness of pulmonary oedema is distressing and frightening, particularly to an individual at rest. Fortunately there are now powerful drugs available to prevent or treat severe pulmonary oedema. In days gone by the condition was often much improved by 'venesection' – deliberately letting blood out by cutting a vein in an arm or leg. Samuel Johnson – the famous wit whose Life was immortalised by James Boswell and who created the first great English dictionary – was bled several times to relieve breathlessness. We do not know how much it really helped him, because his necropsy showed gross lung disease rather than heart disease.

A definition of heart failure

With all these considerations in mind I shall propose a definition of heart failure which sounds both complicated and a bit vague, but it embraces all the conditions physicians usually describe as heart failure and excludes none:

> Heart failure exists when in the absence of deliberate fluid overload, primary failure of the kidneys to excrete enough salt and water, or obstruction of veins, there is either (1) oedema of the dependent parts together with a rise of central venous pressure, or (2) oedema of the lungs.

In both situations the essence is a rise of pressure in the venous system: predominantly in the systemic veins in right (congestive) heart failure, or in the pulmonary veins in left heart failure.

The main immediate causes of 'left' heart failure are easy to understand and classify: e.g. systemic hypertension (because of the extra work the left ventricle has to do to pump the systemic arterial pressure up to its high level); previous myocardial infarction from coronary artery disease (causing weakened contractile function of the left ventricle); mitral valve stenosis or regurgitation (because of obstruction or leaking of the valve, preventing blood from filling the left ventricle adequately); and aortic valve disease – usually regurgitation – because the left ventricle cannot cope with the extra work involved.

> When heart failure occurs in young people it is usually caused by a defect in the complex protein machinery which powers intermittent contraction of the left ventricle, with energy supplied by ATP and controlled by fluxes of calcium. The two main types of failure are 'hypertrophic cardiomyopathy' (HCM) and 'dilated cardiomyopathy' (DCM). These are dominant genetically-determined diseases. HCM is present in one in every 500–1000 people. DCM is less common, with a prevalence of about one in 2000 people. Each can result from many different single point mutations in contractile proteins.

Sometimes these disorders lead to gradual heart failure in young adults or even in children. This may clinically resemble the heart failure which in older people is caused by coronary artery disease and myocardial infarction. Both HCM and DCM can also lead to electrical instability. If a re-entrant electrical circuit becomes suddenly established within heart muscle, coordinated muscle contraction may cease and lead to sudden death. This was presumably what happened in a symptomless young soldier I once saw while I was a junior doctor in the British Army. He had been noted to have an enlarged heart on a routine chest X-ray, but he had no other signs. His blood pressure was normal. I referred him to the Army's cardiological consultant but was horrified to hear that the soldier had suddenly dropped dead a few days later, at a party.

'Right' heart failure, or just 'heart failure' commonly just follows on from one of the conditions listed above. All of them can reduce the output of blood from the left ventricle and bring into action various compensatory mechanisms which together result in fluid being retained in the body, with a consequent increase in the volume of circulating blood. In addition, any block in the free transit of blood from the right side of the heart through the lungs can cause right heart failure. I remember once being puzzled by a man of 40 admitted to hospital complaining of 'indigestion'. When I examined him I found that he had a large and tender liver. This suggested that he had acute hepatitis, perhaps caused by a virus – but I also noticed that he had distended neck veins, suggesting that the cause of the whole problem was something wrong with his heart. He had no swelling of his ankles and his breathing was not obstructed. While I was looking at the electrical heart rhythm record (the 'ECG') the man suddenly gave a gasp and died. Post mortem examination showed in his lungs one large and many small clots. These had probably been formed in his legs during a long air flight 5 days before. There had been enough time for some excess fluid to have been retained in the body and for the veins in the neck to have consequently become engorged, even though the ankles had not yet swollen.

Most recent work on the mechanisms of heart failure has involved trying to identify and quantify the contributions that each mechanism makes. There are many possible causes of heart failure, but coronary artery disease underlies many of them in middle aged and elderly adults.[6]

Epidemiology

Current estimates suggest that almost 1% of the world's population has chronic heart failure. Prevalence is increasing in developed countries, partly, of course, because the average age of their populations is increasing. Current estimates suggest that in the UK 1–2% of people between the ages of 50 and 60 have 'heart failure' as I have defined it. This estimate rises to at least 10% on average for 80 year olds. In the USA, about 40,000 deaths per year are attributable to heart failure, which is a contributory causal factor in about a quarter of a million deaths. Heart failure eventually kills mainly because congestion of the lungs with excess fluid prevents the body getting enough oxygen in.

Longstanding heart failure accounts for 120,000 hospital admissions per year in England and Wales. On average, a patient admitted to hospital with heart failure has a lower chance of survival than someone with any common cancer, apart from lung cancer. Furthermore, patients dying with heart failure usually suffer more physical distress than those dying with cancer. Breathlessness, nausea and vomiting are considered by most patients to be worse than pain. The chances of someone being alive one year after an admission to hospital with heart failure are only about 30%.

Causes of blood and fluid accumulation

Several conditions which I have listed above can prevent the heart pumping enough blood round. So is there any mystery to be solved in understanding heart failure? I think there is. We need to know exactly why water and salt are retained in the body in excess, causing either oedema of the legs or of the lungs.

The simplest conceivable situation is easy to understand. Consider the relation between the pressure of blood perfusing a kidney and the rate at which the kidney excretes salt and water. My former colleague Jon Thompson and I removed kidneys from anaesthetised rabbits, put cannulas into the main kidney artery and vein, and perfused the excised kidneys with blood from another (anaesthetised) rabbit. We used a series of three or four different pressures and measured the rate at which urine flowed out and the salt (sodium) concentration of the urine. Our pooled results are shown in Figure 29. The rate of excretion of both salt and water went up exponentially as the pressure of the perfusing blood was raised from 50 to 110 mmHg. Similar results have been obtained in many other animals.

A failing heart may not raise the blood pressure high enough to supply blood to vital organs. Any fall of blood pressure will be detected by the so-called arterial baroreceptors in the chest and neck which I have described elsewhere. Their specialised nerve endings send messages to

233

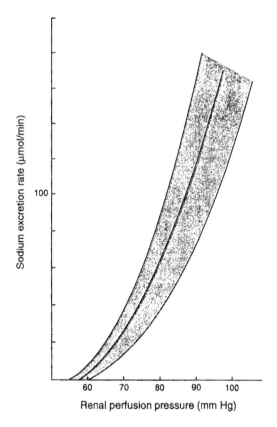

Figure 29 Average results (mean) obtained from 16 excised rabbit kidneys perfused with blood over a range of pressures, showing how the rate of excretion of sodium increases ever more rapidly as the pressure of blood perfusing the kidneys is increased. (Drawn from data of Thompson JMA & Dickinson CJ, *Clin Sci Mol Med* 1976;50:223–236).

the brain, continuously reporting the level of blood pressure. If this is unduly low, the brain brings about constriction of blood vessels throughout the body. Constriction of the arterial blood supply to the kidneys reduces the kidneys' rate of excretion of salt and water. Other influences can also increase the blood volume. Water and salt go together. When water is retained the blood concentration of sodium falls. This leads to increased secretion of mineralocorticoid hormones such as aldosterone, which make the kidneys retain sodium. When sodium is retained in the body, the hypothalamus in the brain detects an increase in osmotic strength of the blood, vasopressin secretion is inhibited and thirst is stimulated. Blood volume and blood pressure both increase.

Treatment of heart failure: Implications for causation

Since all forms of heart failure are associated with excess blood volume and excess interstitial fluid volume – which cause most of the symptoms – 'diuretics' are always needed unless the pumping function of the heart can be greatly improved. Diuretic drugs act on the kidneys in various ways. Most reduce the reabsorption of salt (i.e. sodium) from the glomerular filtrate (p. 146) so that the body loses some of its excess sodium. The brain contains receptors in the hypothalamus (Fig. 7, p. 45) which sense the strength (osmolality) of dissolved substances in the blood passing through it. If the osmolality of the blood has been reduced by diuretic drugs, the hypothalamus signals to the rear part of the pituitary gland to reduce its secretion of the anti-diuretic hormone (vasopressin). This allows the kidneys to excrete more water.

People with heart failure lose most of their symptoms when the excess fluid is removed by the administration of diuretic drugs. Most such drugs promote the excretion of salt (sodium) in the first instance. Water follows.

Some diuretic drugs act in different ways, e.g. specifically acting on chloride rather than sodium excretion. But any drugs which reduce the strength of dissolved substances in the blood will also reduce the amount of water in the body and reduce the symptoms and signs of heart failure.

The work the heart has to do obviously depends on the blood pressure. The higher the blood pressure, the more work for the heart. It is thus nearly always beneficial in people with heart failure to reduce blood pressure, providing that by doing so the blood supply of the brain is not imperilled. In most circumstances drugs antagonising the action of circulating angiotensin (p. 359) lower blood pressure without reducing blood flow to the brain. They are standard therapy for heart failure. Most such drugs are 'angiotensin converting enzyme' (ACE) inhibitors. A few people who develop a dry cough on such drugs can be alternatively treated with 'angiotensin receptor blocking' (ARB) agents.

Beta-blocking drugs

The effects of adrenaline and increased sympathetic nerve stimulation of the heart are to increase heart rate and the strength of cardiac contraction. Common sense suggests that these effects, classified as 'beta-stimulation' must in most circumstances be beneficial and that blocking their effects must be damaging. It certainly can be. Before beta-blocking drugs had been introduced into the treatment of heart failure I personally precipitated a hypertensive middle-aged man into severe heart failure, with pulmonary oedema, by administering a beta-blocking drug in an attempt to lower his blood pressure. It took careful study of the emerging medical literature on the subject to appreciate that my mistake had been to give the beta-blocking drug too suddenly and in too large a dose, without first increasing the patient's dose of diuretic and giving him an ACE-inhibitor drug.

We now know that once excess fluid has been removed from the body with adequate doses of diuretic drugs, and once the ill effects of angiotensin have been eliminated with ACE inhibitors, it is not only safe but nearly always beneficial to give beta-blocking drugs to people with heart failure.[7] It is essential to start with a low dose of the beta-blocking drug and only very gradually to increase it over a month or more.

> I am not convinced that we understand precisely why this treatment helps people with heart failure. For me, this remains a real medical mystery. Do beta-blocking drugs help by preventing damaging rhythm disorders? I have read many reviews, without being entirely convinced by any of the answers suggested so far. In her recent review, Lynne Stevenson[8] mentioned the possibilities that gene expression in heart muscle may be changed by beta-blockade, and that reduction in heart rate may increase the fraction of ventricular volume ejected with each heart beat. The most popular beta-blocking drugs used in heart failure (carvedilol and slow-release metoprolol) have additional actions which include some blocking action on alpha-receptors, with beneficial dilation of arteries. They may also reduce the secretion of renin by the kidneys and thus lower angiotensin concentrations. I suspect that beta-blocking drugs will be found to have many other actions which we have yet to discover.

There has been a good recent review of current treatment options.[9] It is a sad reflection on medical practice in the UK and in many other developed countries that many patients with heart failure are not currently being treated with ACE inhibitor drugs, many are not receiving beta-blockers, and some are not even being given diuretic drugs. Claude Lenfant has made the point most eloquently that many recent clinical research discoveries of these valuable and effective therapeutic and prophylactic advances have been 'lost in translation' to established clinical practice.[10]

Summary

'Heart failure' in standard medical use signifies abnormal expansion of the amount of blood and interstitial fluid, either in the body as a whole (congestive heart failure) or more selectively in the lungs (pulmonary oedema), when the heart is primarily at fault. Poor function of the heart may result in the blood pressure becoming too low, which impairs kidney function and prevents the kidneys excreting the required amounts of water and salt. But sometimes blood pressure may be apparently adequate, but only at the expense of undue nervous and chemical influences on kidney function brought about by the brain and by circulating hormones when the brain detects inadequate heart function.

Treatment of heart failure nearly always requires the administration of a diuretic drug, which increases the rate of excretion of water and salt and prevents them piling up in the body. Drugs which antagonise or prevent the secretion of renin and angiotensin by the kidneys (e.g. the so-called ACE inhibitors) are additionally beneficial. In recent years, evidence has accumulated that both better heart function and improved survival, with fewer symptoms, may accrue from cautious adrenergic beta-blockade by drugs, though at present we do not understand clearly why and how this beneficial result comes about.

22

CLUBBING OF THE FINGERS

Doctors describe 'clubbing' of the fingers as a 'physical sign'. Clubbing is not a disease, but it is a marker for a lot of different diseases. It was first observed and recorded by Hippocrates in the fifth century BC. He noted that in severe lung infections with pus collecting in the chest the finger-nails became curved and the fingers warm, especially at their tips. We now recognise the earliest manifestation of clubbing as increased thickness of the nail bed and of the soft tissues below it. The most objective criterion is that clubbing is present when the depth (i.e. top-to-bottom thickness) of the last segment of the index finger (measurement A in Fig. 30) is the same or greater than the depth of the terminal finger joint (measurement B). The finger pulp is swollen and infiltrated with white blood cells. When clubbing is severe the fingers really look like small clubs. The minute finger-tip blood vessels

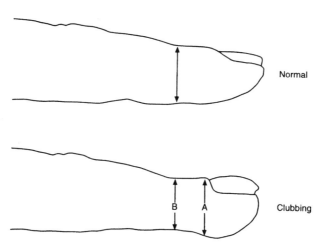

Figure 30 A normal and a typical 'clubbed' index finger, viewed from the side. Clubbing is present when measurement A (the thickness of the finger just proximal to the nail bed fold) is the same or greater than measurement B (the thickness at the distal joint).

(capillaries) are dilated and the number of blood vessels is increased. Most authors have reported that blood flow through the fingers is also increased.

When clubbing is severe it may be associated with changes in the wrist bones. These may become painful and swollen: a condition known as 'hypertrophic osteoarthropathy' (Greek: *hyper* = excessive; *troph* = growth; *osteon* = bone; *arthron* = joint; *path* = suffering). There is new bone formation at the distal ends of long bones, especially the lower arm bones at the wrists, which may be hot and painful, with increased blood flow through new blood vessels.

Association of clubbing with disease

1. Clubbing can (rarely) occur in families as an inherited dominant characteristic and even sporadically without evidence of any gross underlying disease or anatomical abnormality. In most other cases it should be regarded as abnormal and pathological. In many situations it is a sinister physical sign.
2. It is always present in 'blue babies' (with 'cyanotic' heart disease) and also in blue adults. Such people are born with some abnormality of the heart causing unoxygenated blue blood coming from the veins in the body to be pumped straight into the systemic arteries, without passing through the lungs. The shunt is definitely the cause of clubbing in these circumstances because clubbing disappears if the shunt is surgically closed.
3. Clubbing also occurs in some diffuse lung diseases associated with poor oxygenation of the blood, in which there is a right-to-left shunt of blood through underventilated parts of the lungs.
4. Generalised clubbing, of fingers and often toes as well, is characteristic of longstanding subacute bacterial endocarditis (a blood-borne infection of the heart valves). It disappears after successful treatment of the infection.
5. Localised clubbing, affecting only one upper or lower limb has been observed when there has been severe infection in an arterial graft in a large artery supplying that limb. In such cases the localised arterial infection has clearly caused the clubbing. It disappears in those cases in which the infection can be eradicated or the graft replaced.
6. Some longstanding infections of the lungs and chest cavity can cause clubbing without necessarily being associated with low arterial oxygen content and blue blood. Examples are lung abscess, empyema (pus in the chest), cystic fibrosis and bronchiectasis. The

causal relationship here also seems clear, because clubbing has often been noted to disappear after successful treatment of the underlying condition, e.g. draining pus from an empyema.

7. Clubbing has been noted to accompany chronic liver disease and to disappear when cirrhosis has been treated by liver transplantation.[1] The liver disease must therefore have been the underlying cause.

8. Tumours of the lungs and lung linings are also often associated with clubbing. This can occur even if the blood is well oxygenated. Clubbing may disappear if a cancer is successfully removed.

9. Clubbing is well known to occur sometimes in chronic inflammatory diseases of the gut (especially Crohn's disease: Chapter 25).

Previous theories to explain clubbing

The number and apparent diversity of recognised causes or associations of clubbing at first sight make any single hypothesis of pathogenesis untenable. Let me begin by concentrating on the most consistent occurrence of clubbing: in cyanotic congenital heart disease. In this situation large amounts of blue (deoxygenated) venous blood coming to the heart pass directly into the systemic arterial circulation without going through the lungs. This suggests that as blood passes through the lungs of normal people, either a clubbing-producing factor is removed from the blood, or a clubbing-preventing factor is added to the blood. The second possibility seems less likely since there are no obvious secretory glands or tissues in the lungs. Most authors have therefore speculated that normal lungs remove a clubbing-producing factor. But none has yet been generally accepted as a plausible candidate.

A large number of circulating substances have been studied. I have summarised all these in a review.[2] In each case there has been considerable overlap of blood concentration of the suspect material between clubbed and unclubbed patients. None of the previous theories explained why clubbing should occur beyond infected large arteries or arterial grafts, nor its common occurrence in sub-acute bacterial endocarditis. Venous blood, low in oxygen and high in carbon dioxide (the waste gas), will obviously lower the blood oxygen and raise blood carbon dioxide concentrations if it gets into the arteries unchanged. But these gas changes in the blood definitely do not cause clubbing. I have seen many people almost at death's door with longstanding airways obstruction, causing gross cyanosis, without becoming clubbed. Indeed, when clubbing is seen in chronic lung disease and respiratory failure, an associated cancer of the lung can usually be found.

In her review in 1965 Jean Ginsburg wrote: 'It is tempting to speculate on the possibility that a vasoactive substance, produced by tissue metabolism, but normally destroyed during the passage of blood through the pulmonary capillaries, is thus released into the general circulation in amounts sufficient to influence vascular caliber; but it is not proposed to add another unsubstantiated theory to the present confusion ... The problem at present is not the provision of a new theory, but a lack of precise data on biochemical and other changes in patients with clubbing or osteoarthropathy'.

The megakaryocyte/platelet clump hypothesis

Despite Ginsburg's warning, in 1987 John Martin and I proposed an entirely new theory: that particulate matter rather than a soluble factor was the cause of clubbing.[3] This idea was stimulated by recent work on megakaryocyte and platelet physiology. Megakaryocytes (Greek: *mega* = large; *kary* = nut; *cyt* = hollow/cell) are large cells produced in the bone marrow. Each megakaryocyte breaks up into many hundreds of platelets. Platelets are tiny cells with a vital role in blood clotting. (Aspirin protects against coronary thrombosis mainly by reducing the stickiness of platelets.) Megakaryocytes are relatively abundant in venous blood but scarce in arterial blood, whereas platelets are more abundant in arterial than in venous blood. Calculations about the sizes of platelets and megakaryocytes and the relative numbers of each led to the proposition that most platelets are produced in the lungs, in lung capillaries, by physical fragmentation of megakaryocytes.

Normal lung capillaries are narrow. Suspended particulate matter of average diameter greater than 20–50 microns (three to seven times the diameter of a red blood cell) are too big to pass through normal lung capillaries. Consequently, only the denuded nuclei of megakaryocytes are seen in arterial blood, together with clumps of platelets. Megakaryocytes can often be observed apparently stuck in lung capillaries when lungs are examined after death.

A large right-to-left shunt of blood, such as blue babies have, will necessarily let megakaryocytes themselves, large fragments of megakaryocytes, and large platelet clumps straight through into the systemic arterial circulation. This is confirmed by observations that the size distribution of platelets and platelet aggregates, in congenital heart disease with a right-to-left shunt of blood, is exactly what would be expected of the passage of abnormally large particles into the arterial blood. Large particles in flowing blood tend to travel in a central (axial) stream. They will therefore preferentially tend to land up in the tips of the fingers and toes, which is where clubbing occurs.

Growth factors in platelets

Platelets and megakaryocytes contain growth stimulating chemicals, one of which is 'platelet-derived growth factor' (PDGF). Although the three forms of this small polypeptide were first recognised in platelets, they have since been found in many other cells and tissues. PDGF is a general growth promoter of connective tissues. It increases blood vessel permeability. Especially in one of its forms (known as '-BB') it stimulates the growth of new blood vessels and attracts white cells out of the bloodstream. It plays a part in inflammatory reactions. Thus the impaction of a megakaryocyte or a large clump of platelets in a finger-tip might locally release high concentrations of PDGF.

Another powerful blood vessel growth promoter is 'vascular endothelial growth factor' (VEGF), the effects of which could also account for all the pathological changes of clubbing, e.g. increased thickness of the nail bed and pulp, accumulation of excess tissue fluid and increased blood vessel growth. I have discussed arterial growth factors further in Chapter 7.

> Yet another potential similar factor present in platelets is 'transforming growth factor beta-1' (TGFβ1). This material can be detected in higher concentrations of the blood in patients with clubbing than in those without. We do not at present know the relative importance of PDGF, VEGF and TGFβ1. They might all be involved in producing the pathological changes of clubbing.

Conditions explicable by the megakaryocyte/platelet clump hypothesis

The hypothesis obviously accounts for the occurrence of clubbing in the presence of gross right-to-left shunts (category 2, above); but it also accounts well for clubbing in category 3, in which blood travels through distended pulmonary blood vessels. When people with pre-existent clubbing move to live at high altitudes, clubbing has been seen to increase. This can be logically explained because the increased flow of blood through the lungs must involve dilation of the blood vessels of the lungs. This would make it more likely that megakaryocytes and platelet clumps would pass through unchanged. In addition, megakar-yocytes exposed to low oxygen concentrations may increase their production of PDGF. In respect of category 4 above, loose platelet clumps form on heart valves in sub-acute bacterial endocarditis. Platelets are known to clump in a similar way in damaged and ballooned-out arterial walls (aneurysms) and in infected arterial grafts (category 5, above).

Chronic inflammatory conditions of the lungs and pleura

Although clubbing is rare in those chronic lung infections which do not produce pus (e.g. tuberculosis), it is common in lung abscess, empyema, bronchiectasis and cystic fibrosis (category 6, above). In these conditions it is reasonable to assume that in the neighbourhood of the infection there will be dilated blood vessels. In addition, inflammatory conditions of this sort may predispose to platelet aggregates and clots in veins draining the inflamed areas. Such infections might be relevant both to categories 3 and 4, above.

Clubbing in liver disease

At first sight, clubbing in liver disease (category 7, above) is not explicable by the megakaryocyte hypothesis. The diseased liver must be at fault, because clubbing has been observed to improve or disappear after successful liver transplantation, and to reappear if a liver transplant is rejected. But the lung circulation is abnormal in severe liver disease. Patients are sometimes blue and in bygone days have even been wrongly diagnosed as having congenital heart disease with a right-to-left shunt. In some cases of chronic liver disease (cirrhosis) many small abnormal connections between arteries and veins in the lungs have been shown on X-ray or by other means.

Tests of the lung circulation have been made in man by injecting into an arm vein radio-active particles of different sizes (usually technetium-labelled macroaggregates of albumin). Because of their radioactivity these labelled particles can be followed to the lungs by detectors to find whether the particles get through or stick there. In severe liver disease there are abnormally large lung blood vessels which allow particles of 20 to 50 microns diameter to pass through. Even more convincing is a report of the effects of liver transplantation carried out to treat a patient whose liver was damaged by 'biliary cirrhosis', a very serious disease (p. 123). The clubbing previously present disappeared at the same time that the abnormal shunts closed. Particles larger than 20 microns diameter could no longer pass through the lung circulation.

Lung tumours associated with clubbing

Lung cancers are often associated with clubbing (category 8, above). Clubbing has also been observed in tumours of the pleura (the lining membrane of the lungs). It has been observed to disappear after successful treatment, e.g. with radiotherapy or chemotherapy. In these situations, the tumour itself may supply a vascular shunt conveying blood from right to left heart without being filtered through pulmonary capillaries (category 3, above). This could therefore provide at least part of the explanation for clubbing in category 8. In addition, lung tumours may themselves produce a number of growth factors. They may also be associated with larger than normal megakaryocytes and an increased platelet count. The relatively frequent association of hypertrophic osteoarthropathy with lung tumours suggests that factors additional to a local right-to-left shunt may be involved.

Clubbing in other conditions

There is not much information about the lung circulation in other conditions (e.g. category 9, above). The platelet excess often observed in these conditions might have something to do with the clubbing sometimes seen in Crohn's disease (p. 271). I shall discuss later (in Chapter 36) the possible relevance of gut factors to the lung circulation.

To summarise, although the reason for some of the associations remains uncertain, the megakaryocyte/platelet clump hypothesis provides an explanation for most causes of clubbing. It is not disproved by any currently available evidence.

Pathological support for the megakaryocyte/platelet hypothesis

A preliminary report by Stephen Fox and his colleagues[4] gave strong support to the hypothesis. At the time of post mortem (necropsy) examination they looked through the microscope at the nail beds of 24 unclubbed patients and 7 patients who had died with clubbing present. The latter included four cases of lung cancer and one of fibrosing alveolitis, all with unequivocal clubbing, and two cases with mild or early clubbing. Two specimens were taken from each cadaver and stained with specific dyes to show platelet aggregates in nail bed capillaries. All five patients with notable clubbing had numerous tiny aggregated platelet clots (microthrombi) in their nail-bed capillaries; the two

245

with mild or early clubbing had fewer platelet microthrombi. By contrast, in only 4 out of 25 controls were 'very occasional platelet and whole blood microthrombi identified'. Dr Fox has kindly allowed me to mention two of his further (unpublished) observations on nail bed punch specimens taken during life from two patients with clubbing of unknown cause. In both of these numerous platelet microthrombi were identified in nail bed capillaries.

I found these observations, independently confirming exactly what the hypothesis had predicted, immensely exciting. In an ideal world a scientist first identifies a problem, thinks how it might be explained and finally carries out the appropriate observation or experiment himself. Some people deride those who just propose hypotheses and go no further. This is unfair. The failure to pursue a particular line of investigation may certainly be due to laziness, but maybe the necessary techniques or facilities were not available at the time. There have been many successful theoretical predictions in physics which were not immediately testable but which would not have been later examined if the hypothesis or prediction had not been made in the first place.

Objections to the megakaryocyte/platelet clump hypothesis

The strongest potential criticism of our hypothesis is that the large right-to-left shunt present before birth in the 'fetus' (the technical term for a baby as yet unborn) is not accompanied by finger clubbing. (This objection, of course, applies with equal force to all current theories which ascribe clubbing to something carried in the blood and normally inactivated during passage through the lungs). Megakaryocytes are present in near normal numbers in fetal bone marrow in the last months of pregnancy. There are about the same numbers of platelets in the blood of the newborn baby as in the adult, but more megakaryocytes in fetal arterial than in venous umbilical cord blood. Megakaryocytes undoubtedly populate the systemic arterial blood of the fetus. Many must inevitably arrive at the finger tips. Since newborn babies are not normally clubbed, is the hypothesis wrong?

Fetal platelet function

Although they work well as far as blood clotting is concerned, platelets of the fetus and the newborn are far less reactive than platelets of the adult. Platelets in fetal or newborn blood do not clump together normally. There is an 'intrinsically defective release reaction which may reflect immaturity of membrane structure'. They have a 'defect in the release of their dense-body contents, most marked in response to

246

adrenaline'.[5] All these markers of platelet immaturity disappear within a few days of birth. I cannot find any information about the content or release of PDGF or VEGF by platelets of fetuses or of the newborn. But in view of the many measures of immaturity already identified, especially the inability of fetal platelets to release a number of substances when activated, it would be most surprising if PDGF or VEGF function was not also reduced. In evolutionary development this would obviously be desirable, otherwise there could be unrestrained and random growth stimulation at many sites of impaction of fetal megakaryocytes, which are in high concentration in fetal arterial blood.

Hypertrophic osteoarthropathy (HOA)

People with this condition have almost invariably severe clubbing, but we do not know if it has a different cause. HOA is relatively common in people with cancer of the lung, being found in about 10% of cases, though it is less common and much less florid in people with cyanotic congenital heart disease. One difference could be in megakaryocyte function. I have reviewed elsewhere (see note 2) reasons for the slightly different predisposition of various diseases to clubbing and HOA.

Unresolved problems

A good hypothesis should not only be testable and falsifiable: it should spawn further work. One obvious subject needing study is the occurrence of congenital and familial clubbing, in the absence of discoverable pathology. Do such patients have distended pulmonary vessels or multiple small connections between pulmonary arteries and veins, as in liver disease? Is megakaryocyte and platelet physiology normal, especially in respect of PDGF or VEGF production and release? In inflammatory bowel disease with clubbing are similar changes found in the lung blood vessels as have already been shown in severe liver disease accompanied by clubbing?

Clubbing is unusual in longstanding airways obstruction, such as occurs in severe chronic bronchitis and emphysema (Chapter 1). The hypothesis would therefore predict that despite the low oxygen in the blood there would not be significantly enlarged shunt channels. This prediction has not so far been specially looked for. As I have already mentioned, the hypothesis also predicts, in comparison with the situation in adults, that fetal platelets should have reduced PDGF or VEGF content or impaired PDGF release, or that fetal tissue growth factor or receptor function should be impaired. Nothing appears to be known yet about any of these possibilities. None the less, on a personal note, I have been delighted by the striking success of the original hypothesis. It has not so far been disproved. It has provided a plausible explanation for clubbing in the great majority of situations.

Summary

'Clubbing' of the fingers (and toes) is the name given to swelling of the tips of the digits and curvature of the nails. It has been recognised for more than two thousand years as a physical sign which can occur in many different diseases, including pus in the chest and blue (cyanotic) congenital heart disease. Many different explanations have been put forward over the years. According to the most recent and so far cautiously accepted explanation, clubbing may be due to the impaction of megakaryocytes and platelet clumps in the fingers and toes, to which these particles have passed in an axial stream of blood travelling from the heart to the tissues. A pilot necropsy study has confirmed the expected findings in nail beds of people with finger clubbing. It seems likely that at the site of impaction 'platelet-derived growth factor' (PDGF) is released. This material is a general growth promoter. It is known to have effects which include all the pathological changes recognised to occur in clubbed digits. Other platelet-derived factors may also play a part.

In congenital heart diseases with a right-to-left shunt of blood large particles can pass directly from bone marrow to the main arterial circulation without getting broken up in the lungs, as they normally are. In sub-acute bacterial endocarditis and in arterial aneurysms or infected arterial grafts, platelet clumps form locally on heart valves or on the damaged arterial wall. Then they become detached and pass peripherally. This mechanism accounts well for localised clubbing affecting only a single limb.

In those lung diseases in which clubbing is common there may be not only local shunting of blood through abnormal right-to-left blood vessel connections, but also local aggregations of platelets. In some cases there is also altered platelet function. In severe liver disease, clubbing can be accounted for by multiple small artery-to-vein shunts in the lungs.

Clubbing might be expected in the newborn, because blood largely bypasses the lungs during fetal life, but it is not found. The likeliest explanation is that fetal platelet PDGF release is undeveloped or inhibited, as are many other fetal platelet release functions.

Hypertrophic osteoarthropathy (HOA) is a painful disease of the ends of long bones. It is usually associated with severe clubbing. A mild degree of this condition can be found in congenital heart disease with right-to-left shunts, but its special occurrence and severity in certain diseases suggests that some factor additional to a right-to-left shunt of blood may be operating.

23

HEPATITIS: VIRAL DISEASES OF THE LIVER

'Hepatitis' comes from the Greek: *hepar* = liver. The suffix '-itis' has its usual meaning, i.e. 'inflammation of'. Most inflammation of the liver other than that due to alcohol excess is caused by inanimate infectious particles (viruses). These can get into the body from the gut, entering either through the stomach or the small intestine lining. All the blood supplying the gut returns via the liver, before it gets back to the heart and thence to the rest of the body. It is not surprising that many viruses that come in through food or water find a home in the liver. In addition, any break in the skin, e.g. by a needle prick, may directly transmit a few virus particles into a recipient's bloodstream. Drug users transmit viruses to each other when they directly inject into their bloodstreams. Although hepatitis viruses mainly attack the liver, which seems to be particularly vulnerable, many other organs can be infected.

Virus infections of the liver, classified by the letters A, B, C, D, E and G, are major causes of liver disease across the world. Current estimates are that 350 million people are chronically infected with hepatitis B and 150–200 million with hepatitis C. Blood itself and blood products are now routinely screened against hepatitis B and C. Protective vaccination is available against hepatitis B, but viral hepatitis remains a massive public health problem. Acute virus infections cause debility and chronic ill health, but may also lead eventually to liver cancer. In the UK primary liver cancer only accounts for about 2% of all cancers, but it is much commoner in certain parts of the world. For example, there is an annual incidence of 100 cases of liver cancer for every 100,000 men in parts of South Africa and South East Asia. Many cancers will have been caused or triggered by a previous virus infection of the liver.

Any form of liver injury, by virus infections, by liver poisons such as alcohol in excess, or by other poisons such as carbon tetrachloride, can stimulate stellate cells in the liver to produce collagens 1 and 3 and various growth factors. These ultimately cause the deposition of fibrous tissue and the formation of nodules in the liver – changes which are

251

recognised as cirrhosis. Early fibrosis is reversible but eventually the liver structure may become so distorted that normal function cannot be restored. Liver failure may follow, with jaundice and other gross disturbances of the body's internal chemistry.

Liver cell damage by viruses is mainly, perhaps exclusively, mediated by the release from T-lymphocytes of various chemokines – small protein cytokines which are involved in producing or modifying local inflammation. A large number of chemokines (currently about 20) and the chemical receptors with which they react have been identified.[1] They are obvious targets for new drug development, in the hope that damaging inflammation-producing infections can be suppressed or controlled.

Hepatitis A (HA)

The first virus infection of the liver to be recognised (some 50 years ago) was that due to hepatitis A (HA). This virus causes what was at one time called 'catarrhal jaundice', or 'infectious' or 'epidemic' hepatitis. It is commonly encountered in epidemics, e.g. in children's school boarding houses, where bad food handling in the kitchen allows virus particles from the faeces of infected individuals to be transmitted from unwashed hands to uncooked food. Children often suck food and solid objects which have already been licked by other children. Prevention of cross-infection in infant schools is well-nigh impossible. An investigation in Saudi Arabia reported that 3% of pre-school children had antibodies to HA in their blood, but this percentage had risen to 80% in older children and to 93% in adults.[2] Many classy pieces of epidemiology have been reported which have identified a specific source of an outbreak in an institution where many people eat the same food, e.g. the custard on the pudding on a particular day and at a particular meal. Since most pre-school children have not previously encountered the virus and have therefore not developed immunity to it, it is sometimes easy to pinpoint the source of infection, even though the incubation period of HA (the time between ingestion of the virus and the first symptoms of gut disturbance or jaundice) is between 3 and 5 weeks.

After a period of generally feeling unwell and losing appetite, an infected individual may get a low-grade fever. The severity of the disease is very variable. Some infected people will just be off colour for a day or two, others ill for a week or two. Stomach emptying is delayed and many sufferers complain of indigestion for this reason. Others may develop severe jaundice and remain ill for several weeks.

One of my former medical chiefs, Max Rosenheim, had been a

consultant physician in the British Army in Italy during the slow advance up that country by Allied armies in 1944. He told me about an epidemic of what must have been hepatitis A that he had seen at close quarters. A soldier would first report feeling sick and weak, with a slight fever, and complete loss of appetite. A few days later jaundice would appear and the soldier would start to feel better – whereupon (so my chief told me), he would be sent straight back to rejoin his regiment, to continue fighting. Brigadier Rosenheim could recall no adverse effects from this somewhat harsh programme of clinical management. In civilian life also, most patients (my wife was one) recover quickly and their appetite returns. Despite the jaundice they feel much better. Then the jaundice fades and they recover completely, although in about a third of patients jaundice accompanied by itching may last for up to three months.

The virus of hepatitis A is technically a ribose nucleic acid (RNA) virus, which does not immediately become part of the genetic material of the host cells that it infects. But it is able to interfere with protein synthesis in those cells and divert them into making multiple copies of the virus. A human liver infected with HA virus is usually enlarged because of accumulation of white cells from the blood, i.e. there is 'inflammation'. It is often slightly tender on pressure. The swelling may impede the normal flow of yellow bile from the liver into the small intestine. This is the cause of the jaundice. Some liver cells die during the active infection, but their supporting fibrous framework of 'reticulin' (Latin: *reticulum* = a little net) persists and usually allows full regeneration after a few weeks. A halt to further liver cell damage is due to the body making the circulating protein antibodies which combine with and neutralise the virus. Antibodies in the blood give good evidence of previous infection, and also provide protection against further infections with this virus.

Epidemiology of hepatitis A infection

Hepatitis A infection is an important health problem in many parts of the world. It is completely preventable by vaccination and is the commonest vaccine-preventable disease in travellers to developing countries. In developing countries more than 70% of adults have been infected, though infection is rare in infancy. Poor sanitation, especially infection of water supplies, is the major contributor to HA in developing countries. Person-to-person contact is usually responsible for infection in developed countries. Nowadays about 15% of new cases in adults are associated with travel, especially with air travel. New infection of adults is more severe than new infections in children. In developed countries about 70% of adults infected with HA develop jaundice. Almost all recover, thought there have been a few deaths from acute liver failure in patients already debilitated from some other cause.

Hepatitis B (HB)

Hepatitis B virus is a DNA (deoxyribose nucleic acid) virus which can get into the genetic material of host cells and is a much more serious infection than HA. It also differs from HA in that it is spread directly through the bloodstream and never via the gut – hence the old name for HB infection: 'serum hepatitis'. I imagine either that acid digestive juices in the stomach can destroy the virus, or that the HB virus is not excreted in the faeces of an infected person and thus does not enter the food chain. But once a HB virus particle has got into the bloodstream it can multiply in the liver and elsewhere, usually causing jaundice some 60–180 days after exposure. The time delay probably depends on the number of virus particles which have entered the bloodstream. Sexual intercourse is an important cause of infection. Male homosexuals are at high risk. Even microscopic breaks in the skin or in the delicate lining membranes of the sexual organs allow virus to get into the bloodstream. Considerable trauma can be involved in anal intercourse.

The first evidence of infection with HB may be jaundice, which usually clears after a week or two. The virus multiplies inside liver cells and releases into the circulation various 'antigens', i.e. portions of the virus which can be recognised by immunological tests.[3] These appear on the surface of infected cells and can generate circulating antibodies. The first one, which was formerly known as 'Australia antigen', appears in the blood several weeks before there are any symptoms and before the appearance of jaundice. Other antigens appear later, relating to various parts of the virus. These in turn stimulate the production of other circulating antibodies and cell-mediated defensive systems. By analysing the patterns of appearance and the timing of HB virus antigens and their corresponding antibodies it is possible to get an indication of the likely course and severity of the disease.

The multiplication of HB virus particles inside liver cells is not in itself very damaging. The liver damage derives mostly from immune inflammatory responses by the infected host. Liver inflammation, if prolonged, may eventually distort the microscopic liver architecture, causing 'cirrhosis' – a Greek word which initially described the tawny naked-eye appearance of the liver, but which is now simply used to mean 'scarring'. Chronic HB infection can also lead to cancer of the liver, even when it does not produce cirrhosis.

Epidemiology and clinical effects of hepatitis B infection

Most HB infections are followed by a good recovery with no relapse. A few infections progress to fulminant liver failure and death, but the majority (about 85%) of infected people eventually get rid of the virus, usually within 6 months. Some 5–10% of those infected in childhood or adult life, and 100% of those infected from birth, develop persistent (chronic) HB infection. This is a carrier state in which their blood contains infectious virus particles. Some 300 million individuals in the world are in this state and able to infect other people, usually without suffering ill effects themselves. About 4% of UK residents have evidence of previous HB exposure, but only 0.04% (20,000) have chronic infection.

The anti-viral agent 'interferon-α' has been the mainstay of treatment, but more recently other drugs (e.g. lamivudine) have been introduced. These work by blocking virus replication within liver cells. Such drugs are greatly improving the health prospects for people infected with HB virus.

But even with modern drugs, hepatitis B is always a potentially serious disease. Many years ago I was the host examiner in a large London teaching hospital and responsible for organising the clinical examination for the diploma of Membership of the Royal College of Physicians of London (the 'MRCP'). This required the collection of a wide range of patients with different medical diseases, to make it possible for the clinical examiners to test the practical diagnostic and management skills of aspiring young physicians. One of my patients who kindly volunteered to help with the examination – as did almost all my patients – was an elderly man with a severe longstanding neurological disability which had paralysed his legs. He was in hospital for physiotherapy and also to give his devoted wife and carer some rest. During the three days of the examination this man was questioned and examined at length (for about an hour) by a different candidate on each day. My co-examiner and I tried to assess the clinical competence of each candidate at the patient's bedside. As an aside, I should say that although many parts of this traditional examination for the MRCP diploma can be substituted by all manner of multiple choice questions, computer simulations and other ingenious techniques, most physicians still believe that at some stage it is necessary to watch a candidate examine a real rather than a simulated patient. Most examiners will want to find out whether a candidate can achieve good rapport with the allocated patient, record all the relevant parts of the medical history and competently perform the accepted routines of clinical examination.

One important part of a standard clinical (i.e. bedside) examination of a patient with symptoms or signs of a disorder of the nervous system is to test various kinds of sensation, such as light touch, vibration sense, joint position sense – and pain. At the time I am remembering (the late 1960s) many physicians carried in their lapels a few ordinary pins, so that patients could be asked to distinguish between light pressure on the skin with the head of the pin or with its point. It is reasonable to assume that my patient had been tested for pain sensation in this way on the three occasions on which he was examined and that one or more ordinary pins had been used by the examination candidates – as was standard clinical practice at that time. Some two months after the examination was over, after my patient had left the ward and gone home, he was readmitted with a low-grade fever and with jaundice, which later proved to be caused by a very severe hepatitis B virus infection. Since my patient had been given no injections or blood transfusions when in hospital, and since hepatitis B virus is not transmitted through the gut, it seems almost certain that my patient acquired the virus infection while being examined neurologically some two months earlier, presumably by an examination candidate carrying a pin which had already been used to examine someone else whose blood contained particles of the HB virus. I reported this case to the Examinations Board and elsewhere, and am pleased to be able to record that nowadays the dangers of pricking patients with pins is well known. All neurological examination trays in British hospitals are equipped either with sterile needles, or (better) with a box of ordinary pins, each of which can be discarded when it has been used once to test sensation in a patient. But this very worrying case has served ever since to remind me that a minute number of infective virus particles – perhaps only a single particle – can survive on the point of a pin for days or weeks and transmit a potentially serious disease.

Hepatitis C (HC)

This RNA virus was formerly known as 'non-A, non-B', but the infectious agent is now identified.[4] Its mode of transmission (through blood and blood products) is similar to that of HB. It was originally more difficult to identify than HB, although it was at one time the commonest form of hepatitis associated with blood transfusion. Screening of blood to detect HC virus is now routine before blood is used for transfusion into someone else. It is not surprising that HC infection is extremely common amongst intravenous drug users, who often share the same needle.

In its clinical manifestations HC infection resembles HB infection, but HC generally causes a milder disease. Jaundice or cirrhosis may be delayed for decades. A recent comparison between recipients of a blood transfusion contaminated with the HC virus and matched controls receiving HC-negative blood showed no excess death rate during the first ten years,[5] though doubtless the infected patients will do less well in the end than the uninfected ones. Many HC-infected patients have been diagnosed as having so-called 'ME' – chronic fatigue syndrome (Chapter 38). The symptoms and signs of HC infection and chronic fatigue syndrome are very similar and non-specific. Before HC was recognised, many patients chronically infected with HC virus were incorrectly diagnosed as having 'ME' or 'CFS'.

The HC virus may damage parts of the body other than the liver, e.g. the kidneys. But it is difficult to incriminate damage from the HC virus in any one particular organ because the carrier state is so common and because the course of HC infection is so indolent.

HC infection can trigger a form of auto-immune chronic hepatitis, probably because of a chemical similarity between parts of the HC virus and a specific microsomal antigen in liver cells. There is now evidence that white blood cells (monocytes) can also become infected with the HC virus. Some of these infected cells develop into microglial cells in the brain, where they may contribute to some of the CFS/ME-like symptoms complained of by CFS/ME patients, by interfering with nerve cell function and nerve conduction.

Epidemiology of hepatitis C infection

An oft-quoted rule-of-thumb estimate suggests that once HC infection is established it takes 10 years for the changes of chronic hepatitis to develop, a further 10 years for cirrhosis to appear and and other 10 years for liver cancer to develop. Excessive amounts of iron in the body (haemochromatosis: Chapter 26) may contribute to the development of cirrhosis in infected people. Some infected people can mount an effective immune response and clear the virus from the body, but the majority (80%) become carriers even though they may not suffer any symptoms themselves.[6] This is because protective T-cells from the blood migrate into infected tissue and secrete natural anti-virus chemicals which destroy infected cells, thus preventing the virus multiplying. HC-infected carriers are thought to number about 200 million world wide. The estimates are rising steadily. Liver failure due to HC liver damage is the commonest reason for liver transplantation in the USA.

The very mildness and slow development of symptoms of HC infection has contributed to the virus being spread by various common procedures involving breaking the skin, e.g. tattooing, ear piercing, acupuncture, use of shared toothbrushes and razors, and careless dental treatment with inadequately sterilised instruments. Like HB, the HC virus can survive for at least 4 hours – possibly much longer – at room temperature.

Unfortunately it has not yet been possible to make a vaccine to protect against HC. There are several reasons for this, one of which is the number of different virus sub-species and variants. Fortunately, effective drug treatment for HC infection is available, e.g. ribavirin[7] plus modified ('pegylated') interferon. But one recent estimate of the costs of treatment of HC-infected patients with drugs and by liver transplantation is that costs could reach several billion pounds over the next 20 years in the UK. Similarly alarming estimates have been made for the USA.

Other viruses which can damage the liver

Another liver-infecting virus known as hepatitis D (HD) can come in on the coat-tails of HB infection. HD virus seems to use the outside envelope of the hepatitis B virus as its own coat. Double infections with HB and HD are more severe than with HB infection alone. Another virus, hepatitis E (HE), has also been recognised.[8] It has caused sporadic and epidemic hepatitis in many developing countries and is clinically very similar to HA. It can occasionally cause very severe hepatitis. In addition, the recently recognised hepatitis G virus has been found to be associated with slight inflammation of the liver, in the absence of evidence of HB and HC infection.[9] It also reproduces itself (replicates) in lymphoid cells, and slows down the clinical course of human immunodeficiency virus (HIV) infection. Other newly-discovered viruses (the 'SEN' family) can cause post-transfusion hepatitis and may impair the response to treatment of co-existing infections with HC.[10]

Causes

There is no question that the inanimate particles called hepatitis viruses are the immediate cause of liver inflammation and of the many complications that follow. But many mysteries remain. In the first place, why do people react in so many different ways to the same

258

virus? So far we have very few clues about this. In addition there are many problems about the role of auto-immunity in causing disease. This is especially the case for HB infection. Many different parts of that virus seem to be able to stimulate the body to mount defensive antibodies and generate appropriately targeted defensive white cells against them. This also applies, though less strongly, to HC infection.[11] In some diseases – rheumatoid arthritis is an example already discussed in Chapter 9 – the damage produced by defensive mechanisms (e.g. by tumour necrosis factor α) seem to be much worse than the damage brought about by the initiating agent.

One aspect of this is the association being increasingly recognised between chronic virus infections of the liver and autoimmune damage to the kidney filters (chronic glomerulonephritis: p. 365). It is likely that in many situations a vicious circle can be started by an initiating agent such as a hepatitis virus and lead to consequent damage elsewhere:

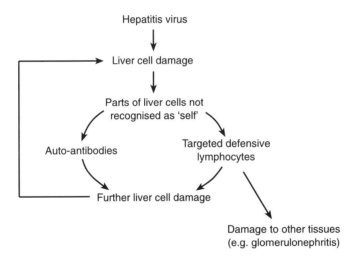

Vaccination has been notably successful in man and in primates in controlling the spread of HB infection, but so far it has not proved possible to vaccinate people or populations to prevent HC infection. Attempts to infect chimpanzees with HC virus have so far failed, but there is some evidence that experimental vaccination may have induced some resistance in infected animals. HC infection amongst intravenous drug users places such a huge economic burden on health services that there is current interest in the possibility that successful vaccination might at least reduce the total quantity of virus and its persistence in infected people, thus reducing the severity of the illness.[12]

Summary

Viruses get into the liver either from the gut (hepatitis A and C) or directly into the bloodstream (hepatitis B and C). Hepatitis A is an RNA virus and only causes a mild and self-curing disease. Hepatitis C is more serious and in the majority of cases reaches a carrier state which allows the infection to be transmitted to other individuals. This may also lead by slow degrees to scarring of the liver (cirrhosis) and eventually also to liver cancer. All virus infections of the liver can be made worse by liver poisons, especially alcohol.

Hepatitis B infection is the most serious of the virus infections of the liver. Although spontaneous recovery quite often occurs, infection can also lead to acute liver failure, to cirrhosis and to liver cancer. Associations have also been recognised between hepatitis B and hepatitis C infections and kidney damage (Chapter 33).

24

IRRITABLE BOWEL SYNDROME

The 'irritable bowel syndrome', often abbreviated to 'IBS', describes an extremely common intermittent disorder of bowel function. It is one of those medical mysteries like 'essential hypertension' (Chapter 31) which is a diagnosis made by excluding other conditions. There is no test which proves the presence of IBS. Fortunately full investigation is neither necessary nor desirable in young people in whom the possibility of serious disease is remote.

Typically the disorder is episodic, with periods of remission to normal function. It may show itself in many different ways. Abdominal pain may occur at the time of passing a stool (defaecation), or it may be associated with some change in bowel regularity. The pain may be severe, though it is more commonly mild. It may be felt anywhere in the abdomen, or even in the back. There is often increased slime (mucus) in the faeces and sometimes gaseous abdominal distension. There may be a feeling after defaecation that the bowel has not emptied properly, a situation given the neat description: 'rectal dissatisfaction' (tenesmus). Some people have sub-classified IBS into abdominal pain + diarrhoea, abdominal pain + constipation, and abdominal pain + alternating diarrhoea and constipation. Chronic painless diarrhoea has been classified with IBS, but some people believe that it is an entirely separate condition.

Epidemiology

The condition is nearly one and a half times commoner in women than in men. It has been reported from every part of the globe, more often in towns and cities than in the country. A recent survey suggested that one in five people in the United Kingdom will be affected by IBS at some stage in their lives, although only about half of them will consult a doctor. The incidence of new cases tends to decline with age. In the UK between 30% and 50% of all referrals by family doctors to hospital specialists are for patients suffering from the condition and $2\frac{1}{2}$ million prescriptions are written each year for IBS. Irritable bowel syndrome can be embarrassing and distressing. Its most disabling manifestation comprises frequent bowel emptying with occasional rectal incontinence. This can make patients frightened even to travel to work. Although most sufferers continue to work normally, IBS is almost the commonest reason for people taking time off work. Very frequent and urgent visits to the toilet are also socially disabling. Curiously, the urge to empty the bowel diminishes at night. Most sufferers from IBS enjoy undisturbed sleep. Diarrhoea interrupting sleep strongly suggests that something more serious is going on, e.g. inflammatory bowel disease – discussed in the next chapter.

Many IBS symptoms, especially pain, can occur in completely different conditions, e.g. endometriosis (Chapter 17). Diverticular disease of the large bowel (diverticulitis) can be confused with IBS. This is perhaps not too surprising because it is even possible that abnormal gut movements in IBS may actually cause the out-pouchings in the large bowel (diverticula) which can become infected. The early symptoms of cancer of the colon, before bleeding has been noted in the faeces, are often much the same as those of IBS. Thus middle-aged patients are commonly at some stage investigated by someone looking up the anus through a hollow tube with a light at the end, or with an instrument in which the image at the end is transmitted to the viewer through closely packed tiny glass rods (a flexible colonoscope). In older patients, in whom cancer is a greater risk, an X-ray of the lower bowel is usually also taken after flushing in a 'barium enema' which contains finely-powdered barium sulphate. This insoluble material is opaque to X-rays.

Cause

There is no general agreement about its cause, though most evidence suggests that the symptoms of IBS are due to defective or incoordinated movements of the gut. No structural abnormalities can usually be discovered by investigation during life, or even at post mortem examination. So the mystery remains. What causes the abnormal gut movements?

Control of gut motility

The gullet, stomach, small and large intestines are not just passive tubes. Rings of coordinated contraction in all these organs slowly propel gut contents from the mouth towards the anus. Figure 31 is a record of pressure changes in a section of human small intestine.

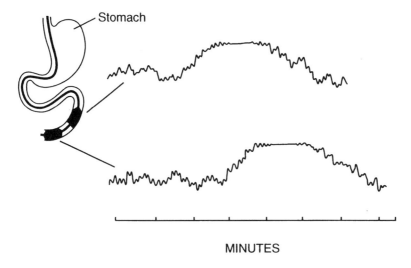

MINUTES

Figure 31 Waves of contraction moving slowly along the upper human small intestine, recorded as pressure changes in two fluid-filled balloons in the jejunum. An upward movement of the record signifies increase of pressure. The time scale is shown below. Contraction waves evidently move along the gut very slowly. The upper trace shows pressure changes in the upper balloon (the one nearest the stomach). The lower trace is from a second balloon a few inches lower down the gut. The maximum pressure comes about a minute later in the lower trace. (From an original record obtained by Michael Atkinson).

Contraction waves come along every minute or so and get alternately weaker and stronger over a 90-minute cycle. Since the human gut is some 30 feet long when stretched out and since the waves of contraction come along quite slowly it may take a day or more for the residues of ingested food to be excreted. Contraction waves are generated by a network of nerves running in the gut wall. These are 'hardwired' into the gut itself. The network, described as a nerve 'plexus' (Latin: braid) can almost be regarded as an independent brain which sends nerve messages up to the head and receives nerve messages in return to control gut movements. Slow moving contraction waves called 'migrating motor complexes' moving in the appropriate normal direction can be seen in lengths of animal colon even when these are isolated and studied outside the body.[1]

Although such coordinated movements can take place in isolated gut, overriding control is normally exerted by the nervous system and by local or circulating chemical factors. Nervous control is transmitted through the so-called autonomic nervous system, which is mostly outside conscious control.

263

The 'autonomic' nervous system (see also Note 6 for Chapter 14)

The autonomic nervous system comprises parts of the brain stem at the back and base of the skull, together with nerve tracts running in the spinal cord. As its name suggests the autonomic nervous system is predominantly outside willed control. Its activities are mostly unconscious, though some of its effects may become obvious in emotional situations, e.g. blushing, or very rapid forceful beating of the heart. Its best known manifestations concern blood pressure control, which I shall discuss further in Chapter 31. The two main components of the autonomic nervous system are the 'sympathetic' nerves (mainly constricting blood vessels and increasing the heart rate and force of contraction) and the 'parasympathetic' nerves (slowing down heart rate and dilating some blood vessels). These two main divisions of the autonomic nervous system have opposite effects on the gut. Excessive activity of sympathetic nerves slows gut movements down and causes constipation, while excessive activity of parasympathetic nerves causes colicky pain and diarrhoea. It also increases gut secretions. Many circulating or locally secreted chemicals (hormones) mimic actions of the autonomic nervous system.

The multiplicity of factors influencing gut motility makes systematic study of IBS very difficult. The control centres in the brain stem are getting vast amounts of information about our internal organs continuously, every second of our lives, day and night. The brain also has information about how much food there is still in the gut, and where it is. It gets this information by means of its connections with the nerve plexus which runs within the whole length of the gut wall.

Possible role of infection in causing IBS

Irritable bowel syndrome often begins as persistent diarrhoea months after an attack of infective gastroenteritis. All of us have experienced attacks of infective diarrhoea, just lasting a few days. Such symptoms are usually attributed, correctly, to 'food poisoning'. Most such attacks clear up on their own, so doctors seldom investigate them by sending a stool specimen to the lab. A low-grade gut infection with some as yet unidentified disease-producing organism might be the trigger which starts off IBS. Such an infection might involve a virus, bacterium or protozoon.

Viruses are minute complex chemical structures which can only survive and replicate inside the cells of the body. They are usually parasites: that is, their replication and activity is damaging to the cells they infect. The human bowel contains about 1200 different viruses, but most of these are harmless to human beings. Many viruses are so-called 'phages' which destroy potentially harmful bacteria. Several common viruses disturb bowel function, especially in their early invasive stages, e.g. rotavirus, astrovirus and Norwalk virus.

Bacteria are larger but can still only be seen with a microscope. They are single-cell organisms which in most cases have some ability to survive and multiply outside body cells. Many different bacteria can infect the bowel (e.g. *Salmonella* species are common causes of so-called 'food poisoning' as well as of typhoid fever). *Vibrio cholerae* causes the serious tropical disease cholera.

Protozooa are single-cell organisms, larger than bacteria, with a definite nucleus. *Giardia lamblia* is a protozoon which is a common cause of mild but tiresome diarrhoea. It is usually acquired by drinking infected water. *Entamoeba histolytica* is another example of a protozoon which causes diarrhoea and much more severe inflammation of the bowel. Infection of the bowel by fungi has been looked for in IBS but not found. When 'thrush' (the fungus infection candidiasis) involves the anus there has usually been some loss of normal immunological function, e.g. because of AIDS (p. 37). But unless one of these infections persists in the bowel wall – for which there is no evidence in IBS – it is not clear why the symptoms should continue.

One suggestion has been that there might be a disturbed balance between different bacteria within the colon itself. There have been reports that antibiotics given to women before gynaecological operations such as hysterectomy may trigger IBS. Many different bacteria can be found in the colon, including harmless and protective ones (e.g. some of the lactobacilli) and harmful ones such as certain 'entero-pathogenic' (gut-harming) strains of *Escherichia coli*. Current estimates are that there are 300–400 different species of bacteria living together in the large bowel and that there are some 500 million living bacteria present in each ounce of intestinal contents. Some physicians get IBS patients to swallow cultures of certain harmless bacteria (e.g. *Lactobacillus plantarum*) in the hope that 'good' bacteria will drive out harmful ones. Eating live yoghurt is often recommended. But in view of the enormous variety of different bacteria present such an approach seems a bit naive. The large bowel possesses a property called 'colonisation resistance', largely the result of immunological defence mechanisms. This protects against damaging bacteria taking hold, but makes it more difficult to change the microbial environment or indeed to restore it after the inappropriate use of antibiotics.

Possible role of malabsorption

Another possibility is that sufferers don't absorb certain sugars properly (e.g. fructose, lactose and sorbitol). In some cases this could be due to relative lack of a digestive enzyme (e.g. of lactase, which is necessary to split lactose into its two separate sugar components before it can be absorbed). Accumulation of undigested sugars might perhaps lead to undue fermentation in the colon and local irritability of the bowel wall. But careful comparisons of IBS patients with normal people have not revealed any failure of absorptive function in IBS. None the less, patients sometimes report that eating sugary things produces symptoms or makes existing symptoms worse.

Food allergy or intolerance

IBS may overlap in its symptoms with the syndrome of intolerance to gluten, a protein found in wheat. Gluten intolerance of severe degree causes 'coeliac disease', in which the lining cells of the small intestine become atrophic and do not absorb fats properly. This condition is often associated with diarrhoea. Avoiding dietary gluten relieves the symptoms of coeliac disease. Some patients who don't have the gut changes which characterise coeliac disease have reported improvement in their IBS symptoms by avoiding wheat gluten.

Diarrhoea in children is well known to be sometimes associated with intolerance to cows' milk. It is less well known that chronic constipation in children can also be due to cows' milk. It is not known whether cows' milk could occasionally play a part in producing the symptoms of IBS in adults. The possibility might repay further investigation.

Nervous and psychological factors

Many investigators, perhaps most, believe that psychological factors are important.[2] Sufferers from IBS have more often experienced severe anxiety or depression in the past than people without IBS. Hypnosis or self-hypnosis has benefited some patients. Sufferers often complain of undue fatigue. Symptoms sometimes overlap with those of the chronic fatigue syndrome (Chapter 38). Patients with IBS seem to have a reduced pain threshold to distension of their gut by balloons. An interesting observation is that IBS sufferers spend more time in the phase of sleep associated with dreaming and rapid-eye-movements than comparable people without IBS. This would fit in with the idea that sufferers have a built-in (intrinsic) alteration in central nervous system function.[3]

Emotions can have profound effects on gut function because the nerve networks in the walls of the gut are connected to the brain. When we experience an attack of diarrhoea in a frightening situation the brain has sent messages to the large bowel via the autonomic nervous system. Isolated rear gunners in bombers during the 1939–45 war were well known to be troubled by rectal incontinence. Certain local chemicals which are neurotransmitters (p. 203) can modify and sensitise the connections between brain and bowel. Serotonin is one such substance, antagonists of which are being investigated for treatment of IBS.[4] One trouble is that such treatment reduces bowel motility. It risks converting uncomfortable diarrhoea into equally troublesome constipation.

Many investigations have been made of gut movements in IBS. They have been notably inconsistent, though the rate of transit of food through the gut has usually been found to be increased.

If sufferers from undue anxiety or stress are more likely than normal people to complain of IBS symptoms, does this mean that the cause lies in the brain? Not necessarily. Maybe a primary disorder in the gut itself is sending nerve messages to the brain which result in feelings of anxiety. Furthermore lots of people have IBS without any evidence of psychological disorder. Many investigators are not convinced that IBS is a manifestation of an inner psychological disturbance, even though irritable bowel disorder is one of those conditions in which there may be a good response to so-called 'placebos', treatments masquerading as active drugs when they are not. Perhaps the cause should not be regarded as psychological, but rather as representing some defect in the way the brain processes information coming from sensory nerves running from the bowel to the brain, somehow leading to uncoordinated muscle movements of the gut wall.

Apart from serotonin, many other chemicals influence gut movements and might be released from nerve endings in the gut walls (e.g. acetylcholine and 'vaso-active intestinal peptide' (VIP). Undoubtedly IBS symptoms are made worse by the so-called 'affective' psychological disorders – those involving emotional disturbance. But they are probably not *caused* by them because IBS symptoms usually appear before the psychiatric ones. Severe IBS symptoms might, obviously, so disturb someone's life that the symptoms themselves might initiate an affective disorder. (This is one of the many situations in medicine and psychiatry where a 'chicken or egg' problem arises.) So far there is no universal agreement about either the cause or the best treatment of IBS, though drugs which relax the specialised muscle tissue in the bowel wall can help a bit (e.g. peppermint oil, mebeverine or alverine). Diarrhoea can be treated by various drugs reducing gut movements (e.g. loperamide or codeine). Constipation may be improved by a high fibre diet, though this is disputed. If certain foods seem to be triggers, they should obviously be avoided.

I am very suspicious of psychological explanations for bodily symptoms. As a general physician ('internist') I have seen many people complaining of apparently inexplicable symptoms such as abdominal pain, indigestion, bowel disturbance, loss of appetite, loss of weight, low-grade fever, chronic fatigue and dizzy attacks, in whom a physical cause eventually became apparent. When I was a junior doctor working long hours I started to get episodes of cramping central abdominal pain which I thought (at first) were probably due to stress and anxiety. They were immediately cured after I passed a round worm (*Ascaris lumbricoides*) in my faeces and gave myself appropriate eradicatory treatment. This reminds me of a maxim that I have found surprisingly useful: a patient willing to accept a psychological explanation for bodily symptoms is probably suffering from a physical disorder; conversely, one who rejects the possibility of a psychological cause probably has one. This may sound nonsensical but any experienced physician can think of examples.

My best guess is that most otherwise normal people who have an episode of the irritable bowel syndrome have acquired it from what they have been eating. Food may be contaminated with infectious material. One thinks of the frequent salmonella scares. It seems likely that an infecting bowel bacterium, one of the *E. coli* variants, for example, could achieve an uneasy half-symbiotic/half-parasitic relationship with its host, causing IBS symptoms whenever it gained the upper hand. I am also intrigued by the potential rivalry between 'good' and 'bad' bacteria in the gut. There is, of course, every reason to expect that someone's emotional state can aggravate, modify or suppress an irritable bowel syndrome caused in the first instance by food intolerance or allergy. Man shares many genes in common with lower animals and plants. Foreign proteins are often the triggers for allergic reactions. So there are good theoretical reasons for supposing that vegetable products could well act as low grade 'allergens' (substances able to provoke an allergic reaction). People in developed countries eat such an enormous variety of different foods that it may be very difficult for an affected individual to identify one specific dietary item as a precipitant of IBS symptoms. Tinned foods in particular contain many different chemicals as preservatives, artificial flavouring or colouring. True food allergy is rare. Careful studies suggest that it may affect 1.4% of the adult population and between

5% and 7% of children.[5] But IBS might yet be brought about by a low grade allergic reaction only affecting gut movements, without causing gut inflammation.

The symptoms of IBS can be so severe that some victims have been prepared to have an abdominal operation to allow a full-thickness specimen of their bowel wall to be examined. Preliminary results have been fascinating.[6] They suggest that although the superficial layers of the gut wall always look normal under the microscope, the deeper layers may contain infiltrating lymphocytes, suggesting that chronic inflammation of the bowel wall might underlie IBS. If these results are confirmed they could provide a focus for further research. But whatever the main cause of irritable bowel syndrome eventually proves to be, its discoverer will earn a great debt of gratitude from the many sufferers from this common condition.

Summary

Irritable bowel syndrome is a common condition of unknown cause which can cause abdominal pain and bowel disturbance. There is often increased slime in the stool and sometimes gaseous abdominal distension. There may be a feeling after defaecation that the bowel has not emptied properly. Irritable bowel syndrome has been sub-classified into abdominal pain + diarrhoea, pain + constipation, and pain with alternating diarrhoea and constipation. Although there seems to be disturbed gut motility, numerous investigations have been notably inconsistent – though there is some new evidence for an underlying chronic inflammatory process. Perhaps something in ingested food, possibly a low-grade bacterial infection, might be its cause.

The symptoms of IBS may be augmented by psychological disturbance; but psychological disturbance may also arise from the bowel symptoms themselves. It is often difficult for the physician, let alone the patient, to sort the problem out.

25

ULCERATIVE COLITIS AND CROHN'S DISEASE

I am discussing these two conditions together, because it can be difficult and sometimes impossible to distinguish between them. Ulcerative colitis (UC) is almost exclusively a disease of the lower part of the bowel (the colon and rectum) – the so-called 'large bowel'.[1] The colon is a wide tube running in a loop from the lower right abdomen upwards, across and down to the lower left abdomen. It terminates in the wider rectum. Ulcerative 'col(on)itis' means that there is inflammation of the colon causing ulceration, although the disease invariably begins in the rectum. Food residues are mainly liquid when they enter the colon. The colon absorbs water and dries up the food residues, which are eventually passed into the rectum and out through the anus.

Crohn's disease (CD), named after the man who first recognised and described it, used to be called 'regional ileitis.' Typically the lower part of the small bowel (the ileum) is inflamed.[2] 'Crohn's disease' is now the preferred name because the disease can affect parts of the gut other than the ileum (Fig. 32) and because its cause is still unknown. It shares many features with ulcerative colitis though there are some differences. In both diseases there is inflammation of the wall of the bowel, but inflammation in UC only affects the large bowel (rectum and colon), and is largely confined to the superficial (mucosal) layer of the bowel wall. In CD inflammatory changes extend throughout the entire thickness of the bowel wall. Ulcerative colitis can be cured by surgical removal of the colon, but cutting out bits of gut affected by Crohn's disease, though it may relieve symptoms for a year or two, seldom leads to permanent cure. The disease recurs in new sites, almost invariably at the junction of the two gut ends (the 'anastomosis'). With each operation to remove some of the small intestine its absorptive capacity is reduced. Widespread Crohn's disease can threaten life simply through failure to absorb enough food. In days before permanent artificial feeding had become a practical proposition I once had the devastating experience of helplessly watching one of my patients, a young man with extensive Crohn's disease and multiple surgical resections, slowly and inexorably starve to death.

271

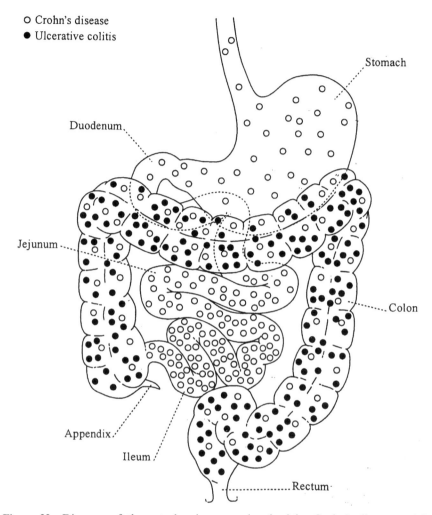

○ Crohn's disease
● Ulcerative colitis

Stomach

Duodenum

Jejunum

Colon

Appendix

Ileum

Rectum

Figure 32 Diagram of the gut showing parts involved by Crohn's disease and by ulcerative colitis. Crohn's disease can affect any part of the gut, though predominantly the ileum; ulcerative colitis exclusively involves the large bowel.

In both conditions there are all the changes of inflammation (p. 83). The bowel lining may ulcerate, leading to bleeding. Pain may occur anywhere in either condition, but is commonly felt in the central lower abdomen in UC. In Crohn's disease pain is often felt in the lower abdomen on the right side, where it may mimic grumbling appendicitis. In UC there is often bright red blood in the faeces. In CD the bleeding tends to be of lesser degree, but may be enough to produce iron deficiency anaemia. In addition, the involvement of the ileum in Crohn's disease can interfere with the absorption of vitamin B_{12}. This can lead to a different type of anaemia. Under the microscope all the changes of inflammation may be seen in both conditions, though in Crohn's disease there may also be tiny pale granules (granulomata) in the bowel wall. These look like the 'tubercles' characteristic of tuberculosis.

The effects of smoking are interesting. Cigarette smoking is a definite precipitating factor for CD, whereas smoking seems to be protective against UC. This may be because nicotine stimulates nicotinic acetylcholine receptors in cells lining the bowel wall. Activation of these receptors probably increases the production of protective mucus by the lining of the colon. In addition, nicotine may inhibit Th2-lymphocyte activity, which predominates in UC. Nicotine has even been used therapeutically in ulcerative colitis.

Despite these and other differences, it is often difficult to distinguish between CD and UC because parts of the colon may be affected by Crohn's lesions, with typical granulomata. This can give rise to symptoms identical with those of UC, a situation described as 'Crohn's colitis'. When only the colon is affected by inflammatory changes, classification is impossible in some 15% of cases. But when manifestations of disease do *not* first appear in the rectum, the condition can be confidently identified as Crohn's colitis.

Steroids are the most effective drugs for inducing remission in either condition, but their use is limited by side effects which include muscle and bone weakness, high blood pressure, diabetes and obesity of the trunk. In UC, steroid therapy can be given by enemas. This leads to less absorption into the body, with consequently fewer side effects. It is doubtful whether the newer steroids (e.g. budesonide) are superior to standard steroids such as prednisone. They are certainly much more expensive.

The early symptoms of ulcerative colitis are similar to those of the 'irritable bowel syndrome' (IBS), discussed in the last chapter. There is often lower abdominal pain with frequent loose stools or diarrhoea. But in IBS, by definition, there is no inflammation present in the wall of the bowel and there is no ulceration. In both UC and CD there is loss of the normal thin lining layer of cells, the bowel 'epithelium'. (This word has an interesting Greek derivation, from *epi* = above/upon and *thele* = nipple. It was chosen to emphasise the thinness of the lining layer of cells, resembling the thin skin overlying the nipple.)

Epidemiology

The prevalence of ulcerative colitis in Europe and USA is about 150 per 100,000 population. UC is not an uncommon disease. The number of newly diagnosed cases is about 10 per 100,000 population annually. Crohn's disease is slightly less common and its prevalence is about 100 in every 100,000. White races are more often affected than black. Ulcerative colitis is commoner in Jews than in non-Jews. Young adults (aged 15–40) are the most common victims of both diseases, which are typically diagnosed some 10 months after the first symptoms appear.

Genetics

Anyone with a first degree relative with UC or CD has at least a 10% risk of developing ulcerative colitis. The risk is higher for those who have relatives with CD than for those with relatives with UC. Identical twin pairs are only about 10% concordant for UC but someone who has an identical twin with Crohn's disease has about a 45% chance of also getting that disease. In non-identical twins the risk is only a few percent. Clearly in both diseases environmental and genetic factors are both important. Most surveys suggest that several genes determine susceptibility to both CD and UC. Some genes are common to both conditions.

> There are genes on chromosomes 16 and 12 which appear to determine whether someone will develop IBD or not. A gene called NOD2 on chromosome 16 is strongly associated with susceptibility to Crohn's disease but not with susceptibility to ulcerative colitis. Someone inheriting this gene from one parent is about 3 times more likely to develop Crohn's disease than people without the gene, and someone inheriting the disease gene from both parents has about 20 times the risk. But environmental trigger factors are at least as important as genetic predisposition, probably more so.

Cause

Identifying the cause of human diseases often advances quickly when there is an example of the same condition in animals. Spontaneous inflammatory bowel disease in animals is very rare. The ideal animal model has not yet been found, though the surgically-created 'ileal pouch disease' has many features in common with IBD. It certainly suggests that bacteria or their toxins play a big part in the inflamma-

274

tory process. Longstanding inflammatory changes in the gut wall of animals can be induced by a large variety of external damaging agents.

Many people with ulcerative colitis believe that their disease is caused, or at least exacerbated, by psychological stress. Some doctors share the same opinion. Indeed, one celebrated and charismatic English physician used to claim that he could always cure UC by sufficiently forceful psychological intervention. His claims have not withstood the test of time; but there is no doubt that psychological stress can substantially affect immune responses and modify the distressing symptoms of the disease. Animals also may respond adversely to psychological stress. For example, certain primates (cotton-top tamarins) develop spontaneous colitis only if they are held in long-term captivity.

The way that ulcerative colitis starts in the rectum makes one think that perhaps an infecting organism gains access to the large bowel from the anal orifice, from which it spreads upwards. I have found no reports linking previous anal intercourse or anal trauma with the onset of ulcerative colitis, but I imagine that this rather obvious possibility must have been carefully examined in the past. In early cases of UC there may be a clear line of demarcation between the lower inflamed bowel wall and the upper unaffected part. (This finding normally suggests that a trial of local medical rather than surgical treatment should be the first step.) It remains a complete mystery why whatever causes UC never ascends the gut above the colon. Is this because of the inborn structural difference between colon and lower small intestine (ileum)? Or is the difference chemical or bacteriological?

Many chronic (i.e. long-standing) diseases such as multiple sclerosis and rheumatoid arthritis (Chapters 3 and 9) have a strong association with certain groups of human leucocyte antigens (HLA: p. 474). A strong HLA association suggests that the condition may be one of the so-called 'infective/immune' groups of diseases, in which an external infecting agent so closely resembles some human tissue or organ that the circulating antibodies and defensive lymphocytes which the body produces to combat the infection react in a damaging way against its own tissues or organs. HLA associations have been sought in IBD, but have not yet been convincingly identified.

Does infection initiate IBD?

I have already described in the last chapter the complex microbial environment of the gut, especially the enormous numbers and variety of bacteria normally present in the large bowel. The sudden way in which IBD often begins suggests that it may be started by an intercurrent infection, or by some damaging dietary or microbial product. But neither in Crohn's disease nor in ulcerative colitis is there consistent evidence of any specific infecting organism. The parts of the gut wall involved by either disease become more permeable to bacterial toxins and even to living bacteria (so-called 'translocation'), but whether this is cause or effect is unclear. In Crohn's disease it may reflect an impaired acute inflammatory response.

There is recent interest in the possible protective effect of bananas, which may prevent bacteria attaching to the intestinal wall. The synthetic drug sulfasalazine has antibiotic activity and is useful in treatment of both diseases, but probably works more as a suppressor of the inflammatory reaction rather than something which kills an infecting organism. Its active principle (5-aminosalicylic acid) is an aspirin-like drug.

A few years ago an attempt was made to implicate the measles virus in causing Crohn's disease. This relationship was not established and tests for measles virus in CD tissues drew a blank. However, the original suggestion had also raised the possibility that measles vaccination, especially the use of the measles, mumps and rubella (MMR) vaccine might predispose to Crohn's disease. Careful studies have found no evidence for this.

By unfortunate chance there seems to be a slight but significant association between Crohn's disease and autism. The latter is a common and distressing behavioural disorder in children, which first shows itself at about the same age that children are given the MMR vaccine. A statistically unjustified report was published in *The Lancet* (a leading English medical journal) suggesting that the MMR vaccine might also cause autism. This made many parents in the UK and elsewhere so anxious about having their children protected by the MMR vaccine that there is now a serious risk of a major measles epidemic in the UK, despite the suggested association having since received no reliable support. Somehow distrust of the MMR vaccine strikes a responsive chord in the minds of many otherwise intelligent people who seem to snatch at any chance to discredit decent science in favour of poorly supported ideas.

Some people enjoy constructing their own pseudo-scientific theories using crazy logic. I once had admitted under my care an elderly professional man who was reckoned by his family and friends to be highly intelligent. I found him unconscious and almost at point of death from a massive series of fits associated with gross neck stiffness and all the signs of an acute meningitis or severe bleeding into the brain. His relatives told me that his doctor (in Harley Street) had injected him intravenously with ozone. Ozone is an intensely poisonous and irritant

276

gas which is a form of oxygen (chemically O_3), and which is a powerful oxidant (oxygen supplier). The apparent logic behind this treatment was as follows: swimming baths are treated with ozone to get rid of harmful contaminants and to destroy infecting organisms; my patient suffered from psoriasis (a usually mild, harmless but disfiguring skin disease); since swimming baths are cleansed of harmful agents by bubbling ozone through the water supply, my patient's skin disease might be improved or cured by the same treatment. My patient's doctor had bought an expensive but commercially available electrical generator which enriched oxygen (from a cylinder) and generated ozone at preset concentrations. I had this machine in my office for a few days and satisfied myself that it did indeed generate ozone. The smell was unmistakeable! My patient's doctor had connected this machine to an oxygen cylinder in his office and collected some 20 cubic centimetres of ozone-enriched oxygen into a syringe. He then injected the gaseous contents directly into an arm vein of his patient. The patient immediately started to shake violently and then became unrousable. An ambulance was summoned and he was admitted to St Bartholomew's Hospital under my care. When I saw him, he was febrile. His neck was stiff and rigid. He showed all the signs characteristic of a severe pyogenic meningitis. His blood, and the fluid surrounding his brain, showed a vast excess of inflammation-associated white cells (neutrophil polymorphs). All these effects might have been expected by the known biological effects of ozone. My patient slowly improved over the succeeding week and survived. He was lucky. It was a close call.

Possible intercurrent infections and IBD

An interesting pointer to the possible role of infection causing ulcerative colitis is the well-established observation that people who have had their appendix removed early in life are less likely than other people to get UC. Because of the dangers of an inflamed appendix bursting and because the certain diagnosis of acute appendicitis is difficult, surgeons often remove normal appendices to be on the safe side. As a junior doctor (a 'house surgeon') I removed several normal appendices myself. Although it may appear that preceding inflammation of the appendix protects against UC, removal of a normal appendix has not yet been shown to confer any protective effect. Perhaps people who are for some reason less predisposed than others to get UC may also be less likely to get acute appendicitis. Epidemiological observations can be difficult to interpret!

The suddenness of onset in many cases of IBD might be explained by the affected individual meeting for the first time a particular chemical antigen. This might have been a component of a new infecting organism. It could equally well have been an unusual article of diet. In either case the antigen might have acted as a trigger which set off a chain of immune reactions which then became self-sustaining. We do not know what the responsible antigen might be, though many possible candidates have been suggested.

Cyclosporin, an immunosuppressive drug, improves symptoms in Crohn's disease by inhibiting the production by specialised T-lymphocytes of damaging cytokines such as IL-2 and IL-6. Its effectiveness strongly suggests that there has been a harmful activation of the immune system. Considerable improvement has been obtained in Crohn's disease (e.g. in closing gut-to-skin fistulas) by giving antibodies which neutralise the damaging cytokine TNFα. This is present in large amounts in and around inflammatory cells in the gut wall. Infliximab is one such antibody, developed from a human-mouse chimera. The improvement brought about by giving antibodies to TNFα has been compared with that obtainable by the same treatment in rheumatoid arthritis. But as in that condition, antibodies tend to develop to the antibody. Its benefits are therefore limited. By analogy with rheumatoid arthritis anti-TNFα antibody probably needs to be given together with low-dose methotrexate.

Trials are in progress to evaluate antibodies to yet another cytokine, IL-12.

Another drug which has had some recent success in treating Crohn's disease is thalidomide (previously discussed in another connection on p. 78). It is an immunosuppressive drug which reduces the production of tumour necrosis factor-α. Interleukin-1 (IL-1) is another cytokine which has also been strongly associated with damaging inflammatory reactions in IBD. Yet another promising approach to the management of Crohn's disease is to antagonise so-called 'adhesion molecules' on the surface of lymphocytes which help them stick to the inner lining of small blood vessels. An antagonist to integrin α_4 (natalizumab) has been reported to reduce inflammation in Crohn's disease.[3] This is the same drug which has been used with some success in controlling relapses in multiple sclerosis.

Clearly many different inflammation-producing cytokines are involved in CD. By analogy with asthma, the transcription factor NFκB is a potentially attractive target for inhibitory therapy because it controls synthesis of so many cytokines. Several trials are under way.

There is much genetic diversity in the way in which different people react to damaging cytokines. This may account for differing individual susceptibilities to CD or UC. Despite considerable success in controlling symptoms, no anti-cytokine therapy has so far produced improvement which continues after treatment has stopped. Several groups of investigators have tried to identify a genetic factor which predisposes to inflammatory bowel disease. One which has been suggested is a defect in a gene responsible for repairing damaged DNA.

Minor degrees of predisposition to IBD have been noted for certain articles of diet and for some common intercurrent infections. The associations are too weak to suggest that they are important causes of either disease, though the consumption of margarine was rather strongly associated with ulcerative colitis in a Japanese study.[4] The problem about this sort of study is statistical. If the consumption of a large number of individual items of food is related to their apparent associations with inflammatory bowel disease it is inevitable that some relationships will be discovered which seem to be more than chance occurrences. At best such studies can only be used as pilots for larger surveys which concentrate on the association of interest.

Crohn's disease is often associated with what seem to be immunological complications in organs outside the gut, e.g. inflammation of joints, eyes and skin. These observations raise the possibility that the disease is triggered by infection with a ubiquitous bacterium to which only certain unfortunate individuals are susceptible. The genetic element in susceptibility to Crohn's disease might be of this nature. Susceptibility might lie in defective function of the lining cell layers of the gut, or in the nature of the immunological response to damaging material entering the gut wall.

Because the granulomata seen in the intestinal wall in Crohn's disease resemble those seen in tuberculosis, search has often been made in microscope sections of bowel wall for tubercle bacilli, but none has been seen or successfully cultured. There are close resemblances between some segments of DNA detected in Crohn's disease tissue and DNA extracted from a paratuberculosis bacterium related to the tubercle bacillus itself. One such organism is the paratuberculosis mycobacterium which causes Johne's disease, an inflammatory granulomatous condition of the gut in ruminants. This is an exciting observation; but unfortunately the same genetic material has been found in normal people and in other conditions. As I mentioned earlier, infection of susceptible people with the measles virus has also been suggested as a cause of CD but strenuous attempts to prove a link have failed. This is an area which cries out for resolution between research groups holding conflicting views.

Perhaps the putative organism needs to infect a susceptible person to cause disease but is harmless to most people. This is no means an uncommon situation. For example, most of the adult population of the UK have been exposed to, and infected by, the Epstein-Barr virus in childhood, without suffering any serious disease. But when susceptible young adults get infected with the virus they can get glandular fever or even a lymphoma, as I mentioned in Chapter 9.

Although currently used anti-tuberculosis drugs are ineffective in CD, some success has recently been achieved with drugs which have shown to be effective against the paratuberculosis bacterium. If I had to bet at present I would put my money on the cause of Crohn's disease, and possibly of ulcerative colitis as well, being an acquired infection with a paratuberculosis organism.

Could the blood supply of the gut be important?

I have a personal reason for wondering whether the blood supply of the gut might be of some importance, perhaps by making the gut more vulnerable to infection. Some 25 years ago I made the diagnosis of Crohn's disease in a young woman. Some years later I was consulted by her sister, who was complaining of rather vague abdominal pain associated with eating. Blood tests had provided no evidence of inflammation such as is usually seen in Crohn's disease. The 'ESR' was normal. When I examined her abdomen I heard a regular rushing noise over the upper abdomen in time with each beat of the heart. Our Professor of Surgery was also impressed by this. He arranged an angiogram of the superior mesenteric artery (an X-ray taken after arterial injection of contrast material). This showed very severe narrowing of the main artery which supplied all the small intestine and quite a lot of the large intestine too. While further tests were awaited the woman developed what appeared to be acute appendicitis. The excised appendix showed under the microscope typical changes of Crohn's disease. My surgical professorial colleague and I had official complaints lodged against both of us by the family, for failing to make the diagnosis of Crohn's disease earlier.

At that time I had no knowledge that Crohn's could be associated with premature atheromatous disease making the large arteries narrow; but there has since been some suggestive evidence of the association. This experience made me wonder at the time, and since, whether a poor blood supply might make the bowel wall less resistant than normal to bacterial or virus invasion. This could be relevant if Crohn's disease is started by an infection. Second infections with *Mycobacterium tuberculosis* (the bacterium which causes human TB) usually appear in the apices of the lungs – the upper parts, where blood supply is poor. In days before streptomycin and other specific antibiotics became available, bed rest was the cornerstone of anti-TB treatment. It is now thought to work by improving the blood supply to the upper parts of the lungs.

Another reason for speculating that the gut's blood supply may be important is the almost invariable recurrence of Crohn's disease at the site of the join (anastomosis) when a segment of small intestine has been cut out. It seems likely that at this region the blood supply could have been damaged by the previous surgery.

Responses to therapy in inflammatory bowel diseases

There are differences in the response to therapy in Crohn's disease and ulcerative colitis. Dietary control and certain antibiotics (notably metronidazole) are helpful in CD but not in UC. Aminosalicylates such as sulphsalazine are useful in UC but rather less so in Crohn's. Apart from steroids – which help anyway by increasing mucus synthesis – other immunosuppressants such as azathioprine, methotrexate, cyclosporin and mycophenolate may be useful but carry risks of their own. The merits and dangers of each new immunosuppressant drug has to be assessed in careful clinical trials against the gold standards which azathioprine and methotrexate provide. I have already mentioned the use of cytokine-neutralising drugs. As in many other fields, the rate of discovery of new drugs vastly exceeds the rate at which each can be critically evaluated against the others.

Psychological factors, anxiety and depression, are sometimes invoked as potential causes of inflammatory bowel disease. Psychotherapy has been tried, particularly in UC, though with little success. Anyone who has seen, as I have, many patients with ulcerative colitis transformed psychologically by surgical removal of their diseased large bowel will find it difficult to believe that psychological disturbance is an important cause of the condition. Patients are anxious, but this is only to be expected for such a disabling and unpleasant condition.

Summary

Ulcerative colitis (UC) and Crohn's disease (CD) are both relatively common inflammatory conditions of the gut. UC affects only the colon, but CD can involve not only the lower small intestine (the ileum), but also other parts of the gut, including the colon. Both conditions cause substantial constitutional symptoms as well as diarrhoea and abdominal pain. UC can be permanently cured by removal of the colon. Removal of the whole small intestine for CD is not feasible because of its essential absorptive function. Both conditions can be improved, though not cured, by immunosuppressive therapy. Removal of affected parts of the small intestine may relieve Crohn's disease symptoms temporarily, but the disease seems always to come back somewhere else.

It is difficult to summarise a host of different views about the cause of Crohn's disease and ulcerative colitis, but a reasonable synthesis might be along the following lines: first the gut wall is attacked either by an infecting organism or by an external toxin; this leads to increased permeability of the gut wall to many other damaging materials; if the patient has the appropriate genetic susceptibility to cytokines (inflammation mediators) the inflammation becomes self-perpetuating. Immune reactions may then affect other tissues outside the gut. This especially applies in Crohn's disease.

Crohn's disease and ulcerative colitis share many attributes but are distinctly different diseases. They almost certainly have different triggers which set off the diseases even though they share many attributes, especially reactions to damaging cytokines.

26

HAEMOCHROMATOSIS: DISORDERS INVOLVING IRON

Haemochromatosis (Greek: *haima* = blood; *chroma* = colour; suffix -osis = too much of) is the name of a disease or a group of diseases caused by having too much iron in the body. This can give the skin a rather unhealthy-looking greyish or sunburnt appearance. The body may contain ten or more times its normal amount of iron, with damaging effects in many organs, notably the liver, heart, pancreas, testes and joints. Haemochromatosis is one of the most common inherited liver diseases in the United Kingdom. It has often been classified as the commonest well-recognised human genetic disorder.[1] A genetic predisposition to the disease is present in about one in every 250 people in most populations. It is ten times as common as cystic fibrosis.

Most medical mysteries involve a mixture of genetic and environmental factors. This particularly applies to haemochromatosis, but the disease is unusual because of the overwhelming importance of genetic factors. These mainly determine who gets the disease, and in how severe a form.

Iron is one of the most stable of all the elements in the universe and is not subject to radioactive decay. It comprises much of the solid mass of stars and planets. So it is not too surprising that living creatures have made use of its unique chemical properties. Iron can take two forms, the highly reactive 'ferrous' form and the chemically stable 'ferric' form. Students of chemistry are familiar with the pale green colour of the chemically reactive (divalent) ferrous compounds, and the orange/brown colour of the stable (trivalent) ferric compounds. All iron left exposed to the air eventually turns into the fully oxidised ferric compounds which we recognise as rust.

Energy to maintain life comes principally from that released when foodstuffs are combined with oxygen gas (i.e. oxidised). Oxygen is a rather insoluble gas. Circulating blood could not carry round the large amounts of oxygen that the body needs (250 cubic centimetres each minute for an adult at rest) simply dissolved in the blood. Instead the body makes use of the chemical properties of iron, carrying round oxygen in combination with the red iron-containing protein, haemoglobin. This is the main constituent of the red cells of the blood. Haemoglobin has a bright red colour when it is fully oxygenated. It is dark bluish/purple when it has given up its combined oxygen. When someone loses blood from an injury, dark blue blood almost immediately turns bright red, by taking up oxygen from the surrounding air. These two states of haemoglobin (red and bluish) can be thought of as containing 'ferric' and 'ferrous' iron respectively.

Iron also makes up part of the oxygen-carrying muscle protein 'myoglobin' and of many other chemical catalysts (enzymes) and cytochromes. The latter are chemicals involved in a chain of chemical reactions by which oxygen – an intensely poisonous gas – is tamed and controlled within the body. This then allows foodstuffs to be oxidised to produce a controlled supply of energy without the body going up in flames.

Iron in the body

Despite its overwhelming importance in the body's internal chemical reactions, collectively described as metabolism, the total amount of iron in the human body is small, only 3 to 4 grams (one tenth of an ounce). Most iron is contained in the protein haemoglobin, in the red cells of the blood. Most adults absorb 1–2 milligrams of iron daily from their diet. About the same amount is lost each day from the gut and from skin scales. Men only need 0.8 mg of iron each day to meet their needs. Iron deficiency is not a problem for men unless they are losing blood from the gut. But women in the reproductive age group need more (at least 2.2 mg daily), because they lose menstrual blood each month. Pregnant women, who are passing on iron to their fetuses, also need more. The officially recommended minimal dietary iron intake is 10 mg/day.

Lack of enough iron prevents the body making enough haemoglobin. Symptoms (e.g. weakness and breathlessness) ensue because of anaemia, when the circulating blood cannot carry round enough oxygen for the tissues to work properly. Normal growth is inhibited. Worldwide, two billion people are currently suffering from iron deficiency anaemia.

The body has no way of controlling the excretion of iron. To prevent either iron deficiency or iron overload, systems have evolved to regulate iron absorption. Absorption needs to increase when body iron is deficient and decrease when the body is overloaded with iron. Regulation takes place in the gut.

Absorption of iron mainly takes place in the duodenum, the first part of the small intestine. Most iron in food is in the unreactive ferric form. To allow its absorption through the intestinal wall it has to be reduced to the ferrous form by digestive enzymes working in the acid medium which stomach secretions provide. A protein known as 'divalent metal transporter-1' (DMT-1) is located on the surface of absorbing cells lining the duodenum. It plays a part in the binding and transport of iron (and of other important divalent metals such as copper, manganese and zinc) from the gut into duodenal cells. Inside the cells lining the duodenum, ferrous iron combines with protein to make 'ferritin' (a specialised iron-storage protein), some of which is stored in the lining cells. Some is transferred into the plasma (the fluid part of the blood) and some is lost when cells lining the gut slough off at the end of their life. The delicate balance between iron absorption and iron loss mainly depends on the function of the cells lining the duodenum.

Iron balance in the body is also complicated because the haemoglobin-containing red cells of the blood only survive for about 120 days. Decaying red cells release about 20 milligrams of iron every day. This iron has to be recycled within the body so that new red cells can be filled with newly made haemoglobin.

Several regulatory mechanisms control iron absorption. If iron-containing food in the diet is increased, iron uptake in the duodenum is automatically slowed down. Another system seems to be able to sense the total amount of iron in the body, possibly by the degree to which the iron-carrying protein in the blood ('transferrin') is saturated with iron. When the blood is only partly saturated with iron, absorption is increased. When it is fully saturated, absorption is decreased. In addition the body seems to be able to sense the requirements for iron of newly made red blood cells. Iron absorption is greatly increased after someone has lost blood and the rate of red blood cell production by the bone marrow is increased. Iron absorption is also increased in some kinds of anaemia. The detailed regulatory mechanisms have not yet been completely unravelled.

It is curious that in some anaemic states (notably thalassaemia[2]) iron absorption from the gut is increased, making iron overload and consequent iron toxicity a big clinical problem. Yet in other anaemic conditions (e.g. sickle-cell disease and auto-immune haemolysis) iron absorption is not much increased. Why the body should react differently to different kinds of anaemia is a mystery. Iron absorption seems to depend on the maturity of the red blood cells. Mature red cells which are destroyed in peripheral tissues such as liver and spleen do not stimulate increased absorption of iron from the gut.

Ill-effects of too much iron in the body

In haemochromatosis the concentration of iron in the blood plasma is greater than can be held harmlessly combined with the carrier-protein transferrin and with other less well known proteins in a combination known collectively as 'nontransferrin-bound iron'. Iron plays an important part in immune reactions and in the body's defence mechanisms against infection. But free iron is damaging to most body tissues. When deposited in many organs it can cause cell death and consequent scarring. This occurs notably in the liver, the pancreas and the heart and results (respectively) in cirrhosis, diabetes and heart failure. Cirrhosis may also lead on to liver cancer. Impotence may be caused by iron deposition and fibrosis in the testes and can also result from the associated diabetes. The pituitary gland may be damaged. Fatigue is a frequent symptom. Iron excess may be deposited in certain parts of the mid-brain, causing a type of weakness and tremor similar to that seen in Parkinson's disease (Chapter 28). Osteoarthritis, especially of the hands, knees and hips, is present in 20–50% of cases. The second and third knuckles (metacarpophalangeal joints) are particularly affected. The recently-noted statistical association between osteoarthritis of the hands and coronary artery disease might be linked with iron overload.

Another feature of haemochromatosis is excessive liability to bacterial infections of many kinds. Susceptibility to tuberculosis is greatly increased. On the other hand, some infecting organisms have critical requirements for iron to survive and multiply e.g. *Yersinia enterocolitica*. The ability of some bacteria to extract iron from the environment is an important factor determining how virulent and damaging they are.

Cirrhosis of the liver has many causes other than haemochromatosis, e.g. alcohol, and virus hepatitis B and C (see Chapter 23). A good case has been made to incriminate haemochromatosis rather than alcoholic excess as the prime cause of Beethoven's cirrhosis and abdominal pains.[3]

A less serious type of iron overload is seen in over-transfusion and in some types of increased red cell destruction. In these situations the iron released from dying red cells is taken up by scavenger cells (macrophages) and does little damage.

A certain diagnosis of haemochromatosis can be made by biopsy of the liver, but blood measurements of ferritin concentration or transferrin saturation may provide enough information to avoid the need for liver biopsy, particularly when analysis of a suspected individual reveals a genetic predisposition to the disease.

There is a strong suspicion that excess iron in the body is not only associated with but probably causes premature arterial disease.[4] Iron is sometimes infused intravenously for the treatment of severely iron-deficient patients and has sometimes been thought to have accelerated arterial disease. There is some evidence that iron excess can damage the endothelium, the inner lining of blood vessels. The lower prevalence of arterial disease in women compared with men has even been partly attributed to women's lower levels of body iron. The link between iron and arterial disease remains tantalisingly unproven. It has been observed that the iron-depleting drug desferrioxamine may reduce the extent of so-called 'reperfusion injury', when blood flows back to heart muscle previously damaged by arterial obstruction. Clinical trials are going on at present to determine whether the deliberate removal of iron could provide a cost-effective protection against arterial disease. There is a nice epidemiological study waiting to be done to find whether regular male blood donors suffer less arterial disease than men who do not donate their blood – though comparisons will be difficult because the conscientiousness of donors might well be linked with other confounding factors such as dietary preferences.

Fortunately all the ill effects of excess iron can be prevented by removing the excess from the body, providing that scarring and fibrosis of organs have not already developed. When the disease is recognised in time, the usual clinical practice is first to remove one pint of blood weekly. (One pint of blood contains about 200 mg of iron.) Once transferrin saturation or plasma ferritin concentration have gone down to normal levels, undue iron accumulation and cirrhosis of the liver can be prevented just by removing a pint of blood a few times each year.

It is also possible to remove excess iron by 'chelation': the administration of a chemical which combines strongly with free iron in the body and converts it to a harmless soluble form which is excreted in the urine. There is some current interest in a compound of this type known as EGCG, which is contained in green tea. But since bleeding is so effective and so safe I cannot imagine that such treatment has much of a future.

Cause: Genetics

People with haemochromatosis absorb two or three times as much iron from the gut as do normal people. The diagnosis is usually suspected in men when the transferrin in the blood is more than 50% saturated with iron. Although haemochromatosis is an inborn, genetic condition, its inheritance is extraordinarily complicated. Furthermore, the 'penetrance' of haemochromatosis genes is very variable. People with apparently highly unfavourable genetic makeup may show little evidence of disease.[5]

The most important genetic link in haemochromatosis is with the human leucocyte antigen (HLA) system on chromosome 6 (HLA-A3), and also when a related sugar-containing protein product (a glycoprotein called 'HFE') is altered by a mutation designated as C282Y.[6] This mutation is extremely common and found on one or both chromosomes in about 10% of individuals of North European extraction. Inheriting the C282Y mutation from only one parent has no effect on health or life expectancy, but inheriting it from both parents predisposes to clinically significant haemochromatosis. Some 80–90% of people with haemochromatosis are in this situation. Children who inherit the mutation from only one parent may also get the disease if other disadvantageous mutations on chromosome 6 (e.g. H63D) are also present.

The high prevalence today of the C282Y mutation, since its first appearance – probably in a Viking ancestor some 70 generations ago – suggests that it must have conferred substantial survival advantages, though we do not know what they were. The most likely and obvious possibility is that the haemochromatosis gene may have prevented iron deficiency anaemia in those young women who inherited it, by increasing the amount of iron they absorbed from their food. Iron-deficiency anaemia would have reduced the energy of affected women, perhaps even affected survival when food was in short supply. Thus women protected by this haemochromatosis mutation may have had a survival advantage over women without it. I imagine that the different geographical prevalence of the HLA-A3 gene in different parts of the world (e.g. 100% in Australia, but only 60% in Italy) probably reflects the patterns of previous migration of Europeans, as well as the availability of iron in local foods. The C282Y mutation is common in northern Europe, but less common in Greece and Italy.

The other genetic influence of iron excess on disease is the carrier protein DMT-1, which can interact with the mutated HFE gene product in haemochromatosis. We still do not understand how the HFE gene product affects the intestinal uptake of iron. In addition, other factors such as the recently identified compound 'ferroportin' (an intestinal protein which is also an iron-carrier) and a transferrin receptor protein (TFR2)[7] have to be taken into account. The genetics of the rarer forms of haemochromatosis comprise a very fast-moving research field at

288

present. When all these newly discovered factors can be identified and quantified we may eventually understand why some people with a genetic predisposition to haemochromatosis develop the full-blown disease whereas others remain well throughout life.

There has been a useful recent short review of the function of HFE protein and the genetics of haemochromatosis.[8]

Screening for haemochromatosis

Since haemochromatosis is a completely treatable disease if recognised in time, it might seem that a good case could be made for comprehensive population screening and prophylactic removal of blood. The subject has been hotly debated.[9] In many genetic diseases, especially haemochromatosis, the 'phenotype' (that is, the clinical signs and symptoms of a particular genetic make-up) doesn't consistently reflect the 'genotype' (the underlying genetic make-up itself). People with two copies of the C282Y mutation (one from each parent) do not always suffer from iron overload. And a few people get heritable iron overload, of unknown cause, without having inherited the C282Y mutation from either parent. Many mysteries remain to be solved.

Summary

Haemochromatosis describes a disease which results from the body containing too much iron. Iron excess is deposited in many organs, causing liver cirrhosis and diabetes mellitus. There are also adverse effects on the heart, the ductless glands, the testes, the joints and (in very rare cases) the basal ganglia of the brain.

The cause of the disease is excessive absorption of iron from the diet. This usually has a genetic cause, associated with a mutation in a gene on chromosome 6. This mutation is extremely common and when the defective gene is inherited from both parents haemochromatosis ensues in many cases. The precise relation between the abnormal gene and its effects on iron absorption are not fully understood. The merits and cost–benefits of screening populations for haemochromatosis remain hotly debated. It seems certain that many interacting genetic influences still await identification. These may in the end explain how people with apparently similar genetic constitutions can behave so differently.

27

FOLIC ACID AND NEURAL TUBE DEFECTS

The body's need for vitamins

Vitamins are simple chemicals in our diet, found mainly in vegetables and fruit but also in certain animal organs. Small amounts are essential for life and health, because they cannot be synthesised within the body. Deficiencies of some vitamins cause well-recognised diseases, e.g.:

B_1: beri-beri;
B_6: pellagra;
B_{12}: pernicious anaemia;
C: scurvy;
D: rickets and osteomalacia.

Folic acid is not a natural compound; but when it enters the body it is converted to the natural vitamin (tetrahydrofolate), which is required for all cell divisions and cell renewals. Adequate amounts are specially necessary in pregnancy. Folate is a member of the 'vitamin B_2 complex' family. In the past it has been known as vitamin B_{10} or B_{11}. Its name came from Latin (*folium* = leaf) because it is found particularly in green vegetables.

No named disease has so far been linked with folate deficiency, though in adults lack of folate may cause neuropsychiatric disorders which resemble the neurological complications of vitamin B_{12} deficiency.[1] These may be relieved, even 'spectacularly', by the administration of folic acid 5–10 mg daily.[2] A subnormal concentration of folate in the blood appears to increase the risk of premature atheromatous arterial disease, probably through the association of low folate concentrations with increased blood concentrations of the amino-acid homocysteine. This is recognised as an important causal link to arterial disease. Figure 33 illustrates in outline one of the chemical interrelationships which keeps the concentration of homocysteine low. The vitamin B_{12}-requiring enzyme (catalyst) methionine synthetase links folate supply with homocysteine metabolism. Lack of a supply of

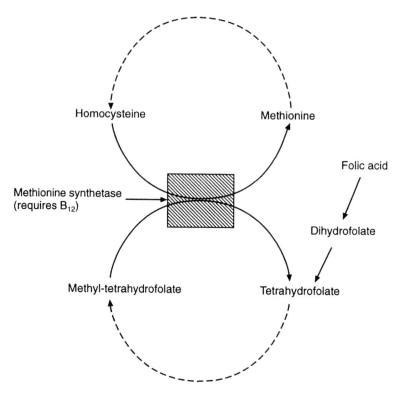

Figure 33 Diagram of one of the main chemical pathways which interrelate the chemical (metabolic) pathways by which the body keeps the concentration of homocysteine low by converting it into methionine. This is only possible if there is an adequate supply of folate and also of vitamin B_{12} (necessary for the action of methionine synthetase).

folate causes a build-up of homocysteine because its conversion into methionine is impaired. There are other chemical reactions involving the B-vitamin pyridoxine (vitamin B_6) as well as folate, which act to prevent a harmful rise in the blood concentration of homocysteine.

Tetrahydrofolate is necessary for many chemical reactions, particularly those involved with the synthesis of the building blocks of DNA. Folate deficiency interferes with the formation of blood cells. It can also damage the inner lining (endothelium) of blood vessels.

Folic acid-like drugs are used in the therapy of some malignant diseases. Thus folic acid could theoretically antagonise and potentially interfere with anti-cancer drugs like methotrexate which may themselves work in part by interfering with folic acid metabolism, but there has been little to suggest that this is a significant or serious problem. Although folic acid has in the past been sometimes thought to accelerate malignant changes, the opposite is more likely to be the case. Folic acid has been found to protect against some cancers in animals.[3] In pregnancy there is some evidence that folic acid administration reduces the risk of premature births. It may also reduce or prevent other disorders of development such as cleft palate and certain brain tumours in children. But the most important effect of folic acid is the protection it gives against neural tube defects.

Folate protects against nervous system maldevelopment and disease

The spinal cord is a slim (about $\frac{1}{2}$ inch diameter) cord of nerve cells and nerve fibres, running from the back of the brain to the middle of the back. It is normally protected from injury by being enclosed by bony arches protruding from each of the vertebral bodies which make up the spine. During development the two sides of each vertebral arch close, thus forming the 'neural tube' which protects the delicate spinal cord within it. But sometimes development is incomplete. The vertebral arches do not close properly. This may allow the spinal cord coverings, or the delicate cord itself, to protrude out of the lower back, a condition described as a myelocele (Greek: *myelo* = marrow; *kele* = hernia). Many different severities of this condition can occur. All run the risk of damage to the spinal cord. This can cause a lifelong stiff paralysis of both legs (spastic paraplegia) or worse defects.

In the huge multi-centre British Medical Research Council trial a daily supplement of 4 mg folic acid by mouth, before and during pregnancy, reduced by two thirds the risk of a woman having an affected baby.[4] The risk is even substantially reduced for a woman taking a supplement of only one tenth of this (0.4 mg folic acid daily throughout pregnancy), compared with one taking no supplements. Other vitamins make no significant difference. We do not know for sure whether all mothers-to-be need extra folic acid before and during pregnancy. Concentrations of folate in red cells of the blood have been found to be less in women who have had children with neural tube defects than in a matched control group with normal children. Folate levels were lowest in women who had three or four affected offspring.

One important factor predisposing to neural tube defects may be an inherited disorder of folate metabolism causing a fault in body chemistry which has the same effect as that seen in actual folate deficiency. This could explain why many mothers of neural tube defective children can have blood folate levels well within the accepted normal range. The concept of a metabolic block has received further support from a comparison of dietary intake and folate levels between mothers of normal children and mothers of children with neural tube defects.[5] There may be an increased rate of folate breakdown in the body in pregnancy and a consequent extra need for folate. Another possible factor preventing a developing embryo getting enough folate is a blockage of the chemical receptors for folate because of the development of auto-antibodies. These have been found in a significant proportion of mothers who have borne neural-tube defective children.

Clearly all women should take folic acid supplements before and during pregnancy. Under most circumstances 0.4 mg daily is probably enough, but more than this (i.e. 4 or 5 mg daily) may be better, to overcome one of the possible metabolic blocks.

The possible bad effects of folic acid

The blood disease called 'pernicious anaemia' (PA) was recognised around 1900. It is now known to be due to a failure to absorb enough vitamin B_{12} from the diet, usually because of stomach disease. This is commonly 'atrophic gastritis', in which stomach lining cells have been damaged by an auto-antibody (p. 68). The description 'pernicious' was given because, in addition to anaemia, patients developed unpleasant and ultimately fatal neurological complications (see below). In the 1930s, folic acid was found usually to correct or prevent the anaemia of vitamin B_{12} deficiency when taken by mouth. Unfortunately it was later found not to prevent the neurological complications. This was particularly unfortunate because although folic acid is active by mouth, vitamin B_{12} is not. It has to be given by injection.

We now recognise that giving folic acid to a patient with B_{12} deficiency can mask underlying disease and allow neurological deterioration. This should not happen if doctors are properly educated to check (by a simple blood test) for vitamin B_{12} deficiency in any person complaining of leg weakness, unsteadiness of gait, or of feelings of numbness or 'pins and needles' in the legs. Anaemia should not be regarded as a necessary accompanying sign of the neurological disorder.

Is folic acid a neurological poison for people with B_{12} deficiency?

Normal individuals have never been harmed by taking extra folic acid, even in a dose as large as 20 mg daily. But folic acid has a bad reputation in pernicious anaemia because of the suspicion that it is actually harmful when vitamin B_{12} is deficient. In days before B_{12} treatment was introduced, PA patients who did not die of anaemia often

294

succumbed to the unpleasant neurological condition known as 'subacute combined degeneration of the spinal cord'. The speed of neurological deterioration was extremely variable.

Unfortunately there were some reports of rapid neurological deterioration in people given folic acid as sole therapy for some types of anaemia. Such experiences led to a widely-quoted editorial in 1947 in *The New England Journal of Medicine* (the world's most influential medical journal) warning that an 'explosive onset' of neurological symptoms had been seen in many cases of pernicious anaemia treated with folic acid alone. The editorial stated that 'whereas although subacute combined system disease may start acutely, it does so rarely'.

Sometimes strong clinical impressions unsupported by rigorous statistical analysis become accepted truth. As a student I was taught that folic acid damaged people with B_{12} deficiency. This view is still widely accepted today. But it is always worth questioning accepted truth. The issue is important because of its relevance to food fortification. So I made a library search of clinical studies of pernicious anaemia published before 1930, before the introduction of either folic acid or B_{12}. These revealed that neurological deterioration was often quite as rapid and severe in otherwise untreated patients not given folic acid as in those given the vitamin, once it became available in the 1940s.

In situations like this, animal evidence can be helpful. Large fruit-eating bats can be made deficient in vitamin B_{12} by manipulating their diet, whereupon they develop serious neurological deterioration and eventually die. There has been some evidence – indeed the only animal evidence we have (apart from a very small dog study) – that giving folic acid to vitamin B_{12}-deficient fruit bats hastens neurological deterioration. I examined the evidence carefully and was unconvinced, for reasons which I published in a review.[6] The big question remains: does folic acid cause or accelerate neurological damage to humans with B_{12} deficiency? There has never been a controlled, let alone a double-blind, comparison between the rate of neurological deterioration in pernicious anaemia with and without folic acid.

Theoretically, folic acid could act in various ways.[7] The most obvious is that it might reduce plasma B_{12} concentrations and hence accelerate neurological damage. There is no good evidence for this. Folic acid might have a direct effect on vitamin B_{12} metabolism, but no evidence has been found for this either. The relation between vitamin B_{12} and folic acid is complex. The cause of the neurological disturbances in vitamin B_{12} deficiency is not yet known. It may involve some as yet unidentified vitamin B_{12}-dependent enzyme. The speed of progression of neurological symptoms and signs in untreated pernicious anaemia is extremely variable. It can be rapid, with notable deterioration occurring over a few weeks. In the many published reports from 1947 onwards on folic acid being given to people with pernicious anaemia, I could find no evidence that the speed of neurological deterioration had been any faster than in untreated cases. In all the reports, serious neurological deterioration in pernicious anaemia patients treated with folic acid as sole therapy took between 6 weeks and 24 months to develop.

Subacute combined degeneration of the spinal cord is an alarming and unpleasant condition. It is not surprising that a doctor watching a patient over a few months become incoordinated, spastic, and unable to walk might describe the deterioration as 'explosive', perhaps not appreciating how rapidly progressive the untreated condition can be. Since giving B_{12} produces a complete cure of PA, whereas folic acid does not, it is now impossible – ethically – to compare the rates of neurological deterioration in untreated PA with PA treated with folic acid alone. But the proposition I arrived at by research in the library – that folic acid even in full dose (e.g. 4 or 5 mg daily) will neither cause nor accelerate neurological deterioration in pernicious anaemia – is not refuted by any solid published evidence. Nor is it reliably contradicted by the only available animal evidence. I conclude that folic acid is intrinsically safe.

The case for food fortification with folic acid

Folic acid can be added to flour for making bread and pasta. It does not deteriorate during baking. Fortification of flour would ensure that most women would have enough folic acid in their bodies to protect against having a damaged spastic child. Many pregnancies, even as many as 50%, are unplanned and unexpected. Not all parents are both responsible and fully informed about the importance of folic acid supplements. Thus a very strong case can be made for fortifying flour with folic acid,[8] especially since the need for the vitamin is greatest in the first few weeks of a pregnancy. However, bread in shops is eaten by everyone. Some elderly people with pernicious anaemia will undoubtedly have their anaemic symptoms suppressed by folic acid, even by a small dose. How serious is this risk?

The pros and cons of food fortification

Having reviewed the evidence I suggest that the risk of doctors failing to diagnose pernicious anaemia early enough is now negligible. All doctors recognise the need for checking blood B_{12} concentrations in anyone with unexplained neurological symptoms or signs. The test is simple and cheap. The hypothetical side effects of flour fortification with folic acid have to be balanced against the certain benefit of preventing neural tube defects in unplanned pregnancies. I suggest that the case for universal fortification of bread and other cereals is thus very strong. The American Center for Disease Control Working Group recently calculated that if one third of a milligram of folic acid was added to each 100 grams of cereal grain, only 5% of the population would receive more than 1 mg daily of folic acid. This modest dose, which should prevent between 25 and 50% of neural tube defects, might be enough to prevent patients with vitamin B_{12} deficiency from becoming anaemic. But surely it will soon seem absurd that doctors need to see their patients become anaemic before they can make the diagnosis of vitamin B_{12} deficiency. As I have mentioned earlier, folic acid deficiency is suspected of causing mental deterioration, serious neurological symptoms and developmental abnormalities. It is therefore likely that some elderly people will be spared neuropsychiatric and other disorders if their usual diet contains extra folic acid. I have already mentioned that folic acid supplements lower the level of homocysteine and thus may also protect against arterial disease.

The possibility of inadvertently improving anaemia with big doses of folic acid in someone with vitamin B_{12} deficiency during pregnancy is small, because pernicious anaemia usually arises after the menopause. Furthermore, vitamin B_{12} deficient women are often, though not always, sterile. Inadvertent folic acid administration may occur when multivitamin preparations are given and continued despite the appearance of neurological symptoms. Doctors need to bear this possibility in mind because many people take extra vitamins without consulting their doctors. Some anti-epilepsy drugs can cause an anaemia which gets better with folic acid. So if an epileptic individual was in an early stage of developing pernicious anaemia and received added folic acid, the neurological symptoms of B_{12} deficiency might be masked. This seems only a theoretical risk. Anti-epileptic drugs are prescribed by doctors, who should be aware of this possible problem. They should therefore check the plasma vitamin B_{12} concentration in all suspicious cases.

As long as doctors are properly educated to have blood vitamin B_{12} concentration measured on everyone presenting with pins and needles or other odd sensations in the legs, unsteadiness, or unexplained limb weakness, no harm will ensue, though the situation will need careful monitoring. Most doctors are anyway aware that vitamin B_{12}

deficiency is a common cause of odd neurological symptoms in people over 35, and that there is a high prevalence of borderline or actual vitamin B_{12} deficiency in the elderly. Neuropsychiatric symptoms have been observed in nearly a third of people with subnormal B_{12} levels, even though many were not anaemic. It seems to me that to withhold folate fortification of food because patients with pernicious anaemia may then not become ill enough for doctors to make the diagnosis promptly is absurd. It is as absurd as would be stopping the routine administration of iron tablets to pregnant women, for fear that the occasional case of polyposis coli[9] might be overlooked. Even as long ago as 1951, probably as a result of improved general nutrition, patients with pernicious anaemia were beginning to present themselves more often than before with neurological rather than anaemic symptoms.

How to proceed?

Although I believe that the current prejudice against universal folic acid fortification of food is based on anecdotal and scientifically invalid evidence, and that the benefits outweigh the risks, a compromise of some sort may be needed. I hope that universal folic acid fortification of cereal grain may soon come about in the UK. Careful observation and recording of possible ill effects in the elderly should be combined with recording of what I anticipate will be beneficial effects: protection against neuropsychiatric, arterial and malignant disease. I have been an examiner in general medicine in many medical schools in Great Britain and abroad and can testify that most clinical students know that the neurological signs and symptoms of vitamin B_{12} deficiency may occur without anaemia.

We still do not know exactly how folic acid works, nor do we know why lack of vitamin B_{12} damages the nervous system. When these mysteries are solved it may become easier for everyone to accept the desirability of folic acid fortification of flour and to overcome the widespread natural prejudice against food fortification, even with a natural vitamin.

Summary

If an expectant mother takes a modest supplement of folic acid (one of the B_2-complex vitamins) before and during pregnancy she will prevent at least two thirds of the expected number of neural tube defects in her child. Folic acid also protects against a number of neuropsychiatric conditions in the elderly and may give some protection against coronary arterial disease.

Unfortunately it does not prevent the neurological complications of vitamin B_{12} deficiency, although it does prevent and correct the anaemia. Although folic acid is believed by some people to aggravate or even cause the serious neurological complications of vitamin B_{12} deficiency this fear is probably unfounded. The case for universal fortification of cereal grain with folic acid now appears to be extremely strong.

28

PARKINSON'S DISEASE

This illness was first recognised as an entity nearly 200 years ago by James Parkinson, an East London physician who practised in Hoxton, only a mile from the Institute in which I work. He described the disease since known by his name as a 'shaking palsy' (paralysis agitans). It is the second commonest of the so-called neurodegenerative diseases, after Alzheimer's disease.

Parkinson's disease (PD) has an insidious onset, usually after age 40, though it may begin earlier. Fifteen per cent of people develop their first symptoms before the age of 45. One famous victim of early-onset PD was the Arsenal and Liverpool footballer, Ray Kennedy, who tragically developed his first symptoms at the age of 33, while still playing for Swansea City – as described by Andrew Lees in his book *Ray of Hope* (Penguin Publications: London). However, the typical age of onset of the disease is 55.

The first symptom is commonly repetitive shaking of an arm or hand, at 4–6 shakes/second. Intentional (willed) movements are slow, weak and stiff. As the disease progresses other muscles become affected by tremor, weakness and rigidity. Tremor is present at rest, decreased by action and disappears in sleep. It is increased by emotion or stress. I remember watching an unfortunate bass walking forward on the opera house stage to deliver Sarastro's aria which opens the second act of *Magic Flute*. It is one of the most sublime solemn pieces of music Mozart ever wrote. The singer had to control the emotional effect of the moment by grasping one of his shaking hands with the other hand, to stop the 'pill-rolling' movements of the affected hand. With much difficulty he successfully finished the aria, whereupon the tremor disappeared.

Coordination and control of muscles become impaired by PD. Walking is difficult. 'Festination' (uncontrolled hurrying) is characteristic. It tends to occur when a patient already leaning forward, loses his balance and has to run forward with tiny steps to prevent himself falling over. The late Fuller Albright, who was at the time the world's greatest authority on metabolic bone diseases, had the misfortune to suffer from Parkinson's disease. He was often observed having difficul-

301

ties in the hospital canteen holding a tray steady and moving to his table without spilling his lunch. Once he had started festinating he often could not stop. Obstinately, but helplessly, he collided into walls while his horrified colleagues watched. On a lighter note, the late London society surgeon Dickson Wright once greatly impressed a porter in his consulting rooms by ushering out a Parkinson's disease sufferer who had been carried up immobile to rooms on the third floor. The patient started to hobble back to the lift, lost his balance, and festinated at high speed all the way down the stairs and into his waiting Rolls Royce. 'He's not a surgeon: he's a ruddy magician,' was the porter's verdict.

Parkinson's disease has to be distinguished from another condition, 'benign essential tremor' in which a Parkinson-like tremor is present throughout life, but with none of the other accompaniments of PD. A well-known English professor of medicine suffered from benign essential tremor. When he was performing a lumbar puncture – a procedure involving inserting a needle in the back – one of his patients is reputed to have complained that he felt like a tree being attacked by a woodpecker. But if the professor's tremor had been due to Parkinson's disease, it would have stopped during the willed movements involved in performing a lumbar puncture.

In most cases PD is slowly progressive and may be associated with depression, constipation and a gradual slowing down of all willed movements. Blood pressure is lower than would be expected for the age. Elderly people with Parkinson's disease become demented rather more often than people of the same age without the disease. Dementia, sometimes with hallucinations, is increasingly recognised as a symptom of PD in the elderly.[1] In the past, in the absence of effective treatment, most patients had a much shortened life expectancy, dying prematurely from bronchopneumonia and other conditions associated with immobility. Drug treatment has improved the situation but Parkinson's disease still significantly shortens life as well as causing disability.

Under the microscope the brains of Parkinson's disease sufferers in all cases show substantial loss of the 400,000 deeply pigmented dopamine-containing nerve cells in the substantia nigra of the mid-brain (Fig. 34). This paired layer of cells runs from the upper border of the pons in the brain stem to the level of the hypothalamus. Dopamine, chemically related to adrenaline and noradrenaline, is one of the numerous but specific chemical neurotransmitters which enable nerve cells to communicate with one another. Recognisable symptoms begin to appear when some 80% or more dopamine-containing nerve cells have been lost from the substantia nigra.

302

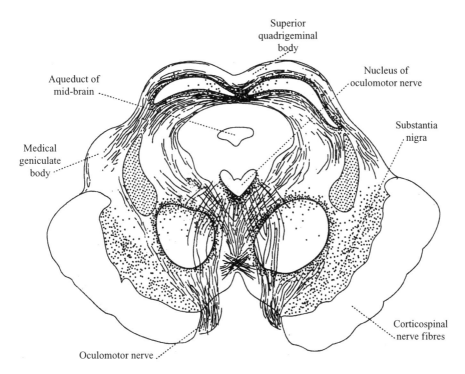

Figure 34 Diagram of the appearance of the human mid-brain cut across transversely. This part of the mid-brain contains the 3rd (oculomotor) nerve nucleus, giving rise to nerves which supply the eye muscles. Large tracts of nerve fibres (corticospinal nerve fibres) pass from the cerebral cortex to the brain stem and spinal cord, to control skeletal muscle movements. The pigmented nerve cells comprising the substantia nigra lie between these motor nerve fibres and parts of the brain concerned with coordinated muscle movements.

Current estimates suggest there is usually a period of about 5 years between the time at which dopamine-containing neurones begin to be lost to the time of appearance of the first clinical manifestation of the disease. The loss of dopamine function is partly compensated for by an increased turnover and secretion rate of dopamine by the remaining neurones, together with an increased sensitivity of the chemical receptors with which dopamine combines to transmit its message from one cell to another.

In addition to the loss of dopamine-containing nerve cells, there is also loss of noradrenaline-containing cells in the brain stem, with consequently decreased activity of the sympathetic nervous system. This often results in poor postural maintenance of blood pressure as well as a below average blood pressure during the day.

Degenerating nerve cells contain various abnormal minute particles, collectively described as cellular inclusions or 'inclusion bodies'. In the case of Parkinson's disease these are typically 'Lewy bodies' – spherical particles, 15–20 thousandths of a millimetre in diameter, made up of protein remnants of thin fibres (microfibrils) and the proteins α-synuclein and ubiquitin. Lewy bodies can be stained with the red dye eosin.[2] Other filamentous inclusions called 'Lewy neurites' have the same protein composition as Lewy bodies. When they are first formed, each Lewy body contains only about 25 molecules of α-synuclein. These are thought to be directly damaging to neurones. A current theory suggests that the much larger mature Lewy bodies containing aggregates of α-synuclein and ubiquitin represent the reactions of affected cells – perhaps one might almost say 'infected' cells – which have incorporated the damaging protein aggregates.

Damage to neurones in Parkinson's disease is now being increasingly attributed to misfolding of cell proteins, thus bringing it into the same stable as motor neurone disease and Alzheimer's disease, which are discussed elsewhere, in Chapters 42 and 19 respectively.

Epidemiology and genetics

There are no great geographical differences in the prevalence of PD across the United Kingdom nor indeed across the world. This makes it likely – though not certain – that the disease has existed in all populations throughout history, even though neither in Shakespeare's plays nor in the Bible is there any clear reference to tremors or shakes in the elderly. The apparently lower prevalence of PD amongst Asians and African black people might be explained by a lower rate of diagnosis. Prevalence has remained stable in the last 30 years and is about 150 for every 100,000 people, with a slight excess of men over women.[3] Amongst people of 70 and older its prevalence rises to at least 1 in 200. Over the age of 80 some 10% of the population is affected. Clearly, age is the single most important risk factor. In North America more than a million people have the disease. An epidemiologist has reckoned that by the year 2040 Parkinson's disease with dementia and motor neurone disease (Chapter 42) will together become the second most common causes of death.

There is curiously quite a strong *negative* association of PD with smoking. A smoker of either sex is less likely to get PD than a non-smoker of the same age. Smoking appears to be protective, although we do not know why. Some physicians have even advised their non-smoking patients to take up the habit. Patients with PD are also less likely to get cancer of the lung from smoking than are normal people.

There may also be a protective effect of caffeine (from coffee), though it is uncertain whether caffeine is itself protective or whether habitual coffee drinkers benefit from not drinking something else which is damaging.

When one member of an identical twin pair has the disease, it rarely also affects the other, unless the first twin has early-onset disease. This observation speaks strongly against an important inherited (genetic) influence in most sporadic cases. However, some definite rare genetic associations have been recognised. Someone with a parent or sibling with the disease has almost twice the expected risk of developing the disease themselves.

A rare mutation in a gene on chromosome 4, controlling the expression of a protein found in nerve tissue (α-synuclein) and in Lewy bodies has been found to be closely related to PD in some families. Members of families inheriting a single extra copy of the α-synuclein gene have been observed to develop an autosomal dominant, but an otherwise entirely typical form of the disease. Another genetic association of PD, on chromosome 6, is with the protein 'parkin'. This association has been reported in Japanese and some other families. Parkin appears to play a vital part in the survival of dopamine-producing neurones. Recently a modified parkin protein has been found to interact with α-synuclein.[4] Several other rare conditions manifesting dominant inheritance of PD-like symptoms have also been recognised.[5] But these exceptions serve to emphasise that by far the greater number of people in the UK or North America suffering from PD do *not* have the disease amongst their immediate family members.

Another confounding problem is that some hereditary diseases carried by autosomal dominant genes may show only small degrees of so-called 'penetrance', i.e. these individuals have a recognised genetic fault which is known in other people to be associated with Parkinson's disease, but they show no signs of the disease. This situation makes unravelling the heredity of PD extremely difficult.

Cause

The most striking association of a specific infection with Parkinson's disease was revealed by the occurrence of 'encephalitis lethargica', a disease which reached worldwide epidemic proportions for about a decade after 1917. The illness ran a course similar to that seen in known virus causes of acute brain inflammation (encephalitis), such as that associated with the mumps virus. But encephalitis lethargica left some of its victims suffering from what was called 'post-encephalitic Parkinsonism', with degenerative changes in the substantia nigra of the brain. These looked exactly the same as those seen in the brains of modern-day sufferers from PD. Many of the victims of post-encephalitic Parkinsonism who survived the acute illness were left in a nearly comatose state. The dramatic animating effects of drug treatment with dopamine or dopamine-generating drugs were described by Oliver Sacks in his book *Awakenings*, which was later made into a successful film.

The cause of the encephalitis lethargica epidemic was never established at the time. No virus has ever been grown from or identified in the brains of victims. Encephalitis lethargica has sometimes been linked with and attributed to the world influenza epidemic which occurred at about the same time, suggesting that the influenza virus could have caused the encephalitis epidemic. This is wrong. The influenza epidemic of 1918 came *after* the encephalitis lethargica epidemic. Furthermore, post-encephalitic Parkinsonism has not followed any recent influenza epidemic. Recent work (from Great Ormond St Childrens' Hospital and from Queen Mary, University of London) now strongly suggests that encephalitis lethargica is caused by a neurotoxin produced by a particularly virulent streptococcal bacterial infection. In the last few years a significant number of children and young people who have had a recent sore throat have been observed to get Parkinsonism-type symptoms and neurological disability.

It might seem strange that a specific infectious disease – or perhaps a specific bacterial toxin – could have picked out selectively a particular group of mid-brain neurones. But the well-studied virus disease acute poliomyelitis – which disabled Franklin D Roosevelt in his prime – is an example of a specific virus disease which selectively targets and destroys a particular group of nerve cells in the brain stem and spinal cord, leaving most others intact. (The affected neurones are those which send fibres to activate the skeletal voluntary muscles.)

Although there has been some suggestive evidence that a rural way of life may predispose to PD, there is no definite evidence that modern pesticides (for example) are potential causative factors. The uniform prevalence across the world speaks against rare specific causal factors. One intriguing potential cause is the infectious bacterial agent associated with and frequently causing peptic ulcer: *Helicobacter pylori*.[6] This infection is common and occurs worldwide. Surveys have suggested a link between infection with this agent and the prevalence of PD. This needs further investigation because of the possibility that control of *H. pylori* infection could reduce the incidence or severity of PD.

One might anticipate that intense investigation of 'Lewy bodies' (the characteristic signature of Parkinson's disease left inside nerve and glial cells in affected parts of the brain) would provide a clue to the cause of PD. But so far their significance remains obscure. Lewy bodies may be inactive particles of non-functional debris, perhaps toxic protein remnants, which nerve cells have been unable to extrude or dispose of. Alternatively their presence might signify that the synthesis of neurofibrils in the axons of nerve cells is impaired so that they cannot join up properly to make functional nerve fibres. Small numbers of Lewy bodies are sometimes seen in a few other degenerative diseases. They can also be found in the brain cells of some elderly people without manifest Parkinson's disease.

It is curious that spontaneous Parkinson's disease has not been recognised in animals, nor can the human disease be transmitted to animals. Non-human primates are totally resistant to Parkinson's disease even when affected human brain tissue is surgically implanted into animal brains. The toxic material MPTP (see below) which causes PD in man can also produce a similar disease in primates. This primate model is under intense scientific scrutiny. But so far no consistently damaging natural material has been identified. The most likely reason for primates' apparent immunity to spontaneous PD is that animals do not live long enough to get the disease. For this reason alone it seems to me most unlikely that experiments on animals are going to find the cause of Parkinson's disease in man.

Apart from difficulties with the genetic differences between human and non-human primates, primate studies will be far too cumbersome, slow and expensive to allow rapid progress in identifying toxic factors in the environment and genetic susceptibility factors in individuals. Perhaps we need to devise ways of growing dopamine-containing nerve cells in test-tube culture so that very slow potential damage from environmental agents can be examined. Such agents might account for differing susceptibility between individuals for nerve damage brought about by a host of different environmental agents.

Stem cells in the brain

It is generally assumed that nerve cells in the adult brain remain there during life, though their interconnections may wax and wane according to the prevailing level of electrical activity. This may not be exactly true. There is some evidence that primitive 'stem' cells are present in many parts of the brain and that they can transform into mature neurones. The quicker and better recovery after brain injury in young people compared with older ones may be due to stem cells in the young being able to turn more readily into fully functional neurones. Recently some recovery of function in Parkinson's disease has been achieved by grafting multi-potent stem cells into damaged regions of the brain, where they may be able to synthesise dopamine and alleviate the neurological defect.

Clues from treatment

Because there was known to be a deficiency of dopamine-containing cells in PD, the dopamine precursor drug levodopa soon became the cornerstone of treatment. It is a so-called 'first-line' drug, but is often combined with an inhibitory drug to reduce side effects. Selegiline, which prolongs dopamine action at nerve junctions, has had some success, though one of my patients reacted very strongly against the drug and had to stop using it. Many other related drugs have been used. Recently physicians have begun to go back to starting treatment with a single drug despite the worry about induced tolerance. The therapeutic pendulum has swung back. There is now less tendency to blame the early use of levodopa for causing later drug tolerance. Many neurologists now recommend levodopa use throughout the illness. There is no good evidence that levodopa is actually toxic to nerve cells, though it has been blamed for causing dyskinesia (Greek: *dys* = bad; *kinesis* = movement), i.e. abnormal writhing movements. A recent study suggested that ropinirole, which stimulates dopamine receptors, causes less dyskinesia than levodopa itself.[7] The vomiting-inducing drug apomorphine has been found to be effective in relieving episodes of sudden deterioration in PD, but is not used as long-term treatment.

Surgical removal of certain parts of the brain (e.g. 'pallidotomy') has helped dyskinesia in many patients, though it has been a disaster for others. The rationale behind the treatment is that in PD certain parts of the brain are overactive and cause excessive release of a neurotransmitter called GABA, which inhibits dopamine-containing neurones. At present it seems that of the heroic (i.e. brain-invasive) treatments available, stimulation of the subthalamic nucleus by previously implanted electrodes has given the best results and has spectacularly improved motor function in some patients. Another approach has been to implant normal fetal neurones or stem cells to produce dopamine in parts of the brain where dopamine-producing neurones have been lost. But I find it difficult to believe that heroic treatments such as these are going to find an established place in the management of Parkinson's disease.

The MPTP story

About 15 years ago some drug addicts in California were trying to synthesise a substitute for heroin. They experimented with a contaminant called MPTP and many developed all the symptoms and signs of Parkinson's disease, sometimes within only 2 weeks of exposure. MPTP is converted in the body to another compound which selectively destroys vulnerable nerve cells in the mid-brain. It generates highly reactive chemical fragments (free radicals) and interferes with the generation of energy from food by mitochondria (p. 464). Some victims of MPTP poisoning showed the same relentless progression associated with spontaneous sporadic Parkinson's disease, even though they took no more of the chemical. These observations obviously raise the possibility that sporadic PD might be caused by a single episode of poisoning of the brain which triggers off progressive loss of dopamine-containing brain cells. But the uniform distribution of sporadic cases of the disease across the world makes this possibility rather unlikely. So far researchers have not been able to incriminate any plausible causal material resembling MPTP. Studies of primates given MPTP may eventually throw up some genetic susceptibility clues, because non-human primates share so many genes with man.

> The MPTP story triggered off a worldwide search for other drugs and naturally-occurring substances which might account for sporadic PD. Recently there has been interest in two natural so-called neurotrophic factors (GNNF and BDNF) which stimulate nerve growth. These have been found to ameliorate Parkinson-type symptoms in MPTP-treated primates, suggesting that deficiency of some neurotrophic factors might play a causal role in PD.
>
> Finally, by analogy with other age-related degenerative neurological diseases (Alzheimer's and motor neurone disease) the possibility needs to be considered that protein misfolding in nerve cells might result both in defects in nerve transmission function as well as in the formation of ubiquitin and protein-containing Lewy bodies.[8] Almost certainly Parkinson's disease is not a single entity with a single specific immediate or genetic cause, but rather a group of diseases with similar symptoms but disparate causes.

Summary

Parkinson's disease (PD) is the second commonest neurodegenerative disease. It is strongly age-related and usually strikes in middle-age, most typically at 55. It may begin either as tremor, usually in a single upper limb, or as weakness and unsteadiness in walking. Later there is typically slow relentless spread gradually involving the rest of the body. Disease symptoms may continue throughout life usually leaving intelligence and thinking powers intact. But PD is now increasingly recognised sometimes to lead to abnormal behaviour and frank dementia in its later stages.

The immediate cause of PD is the loss of a group of pigmented nerve cells in the mid-brain (the substantia nigra). These cells contain large amounts of the neurotransmitter dopamine. Symptoms appear when more that 80% of the cells have been lost. This slow process takes about 5 years. The symptoms can usually be alleviated for many years by giving dopamine or other drugs which are chemically similar to dopamine or which increase its concentration in nerve cells.

There is growing recognition of an important hereditary element which may comprise genetic susceptibility to many widely distributed toxic agents. Although the synthetic nerve toxin MPTP can produce an illness indistinguishable from PD there is no evidence that sporadic PD is due to poisoning either with MPTP or with any other known specific toxic agent.

29

PAGET'S DISEASE OF BONE

Sir James Paget was a famous surgeon and teacher at St Bartholomew's Hospital in London. In 1877 he described a disease of bone called 'osteitis deformans' but more often known simply as 'Paget's disease'. (One should add 'of bone' since Paget's name is associated with other quite different diseases.) The condition is a curious mix of bone softening and bone overgrowth. It affects most often the lower bones of the spine (the lower lumbar vertebrae and sacrum), the skull and the pelvis, though long bones may also be involved. In about 10% of cases only a single bone or even part of a bone is involved. The disease seldom appears before the age of 40. Thereafter the incidence of new cases steadily increases in frequency. Men are more often affected than women. The first symptom may be pain in the affected bone or bones. If the main lower leg bone (the tibia) is affected, the bone first softens and bends forwards. If the thigh bone (the femur) is involved, it bows outwards. Later the bones thicken, harden and re-ossify in their new shape, which may look 'as though they have been bent by the hands of a giant'. Bones are affected apparently at random and usually asymmetrically, hence the 'deforming' label attached to the disease. One or more bones of the pelvis are commonly involved. The skull is often affected. When men usually wore hats, an early symptom of Paget's disease was the need for a larger size of hat. Bony overgrowth in the skull may compress the auditory nerve on one or both sides, leading to deafness.

The sufferer from extensive Paget's disease has a short squat figure. The shoulders are bent and the enlarged head hangs forward. The gait is waddling and the sufferer commonly uses a stick. Though muscles are not much affected the bony deformities can make balanced walking difficult, as Figure 35 shows. Paget's disease may affect only a single bone, e.g. one vertebral body in the spine, or one lower leg bone. Figsure 36 shows Paget's disease affecting a single bone in the lower arm (the radius). Figure 37 is an X-ray of the involved bone. In such cases the diagnosis may be made by accident, or perhaps when a routine X-ray is taken. I have seen Paget's disease of the collar bone (clavicle) on one side unexpectedly revealed in a routine chest X-ray.

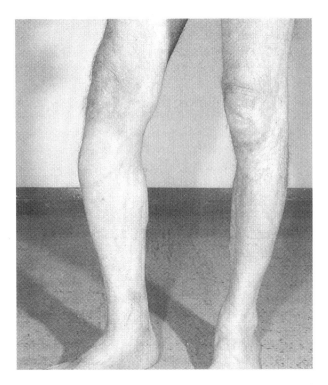

Figure 35 Bowing forwards of the main bone in the right leg (the tibia) in a man with Paget's disease. (Photograph courtesy of John Kanis.)

Under a microscope the bone structure in Paget's disease is grossly disturbed. It has been likened to an irregular mosaic of cement lines. The pattern is due to numerous successive phases of bone absorption and bone regeneration. There is an excess of bone-dissolving cells ('osteoclasts') (Greek: *osteon* = bone; *clast* = destruction) but also uncoordinated activity of bone-forming cells (osteoblasts) (*blast* = bud,germ). Although the affected bones are thickened, enlarged and distorted, they are porous and not as strong as their gross appearance suggests. Although affected bones very occasionally develop a rare malignant tumour (an osteosarcoma), Paget's disease generally runs a benign course. Lesions develop slowly and the disease seldom shortens life.

Epidemiology

In unselected post mortem examinations Paget's disease has been recognised in 3–4% of cases. X-ray population surveys in the USA

312

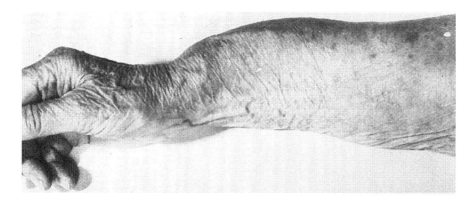

Figure 36 Bowing forwards of the main bone in the lower arm (the radius) in a patient with Paget's disease. (Photograph courtesy of John Kanis.)

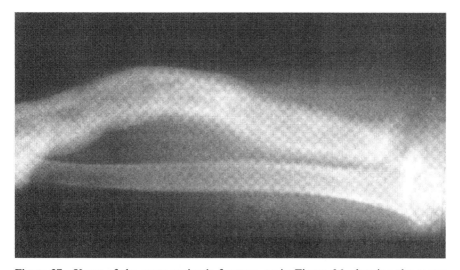

Figure 37 X-ray of the same patient's forearm, as in Figure 36, showing the coarse enlargement of the radius bone, with increased length and deformity. The adjacent (normal) thin ulnar bone is not affected. In this conventional type of X-ray picture bone appears white and soft tissues and background are dark. (X-ray courtesy of John Kanis.)

and northern Europe suggest a higher prevalence, up to 6% of the adult population. The disease is common in Europe, the USA and Australia; but it is uncommon in China, Japan, Scandinavia, the Middle East and Africa. Its prevalence in South America and Mediterranean countries is midway between these. Within the UK the disease

313

is more prevalent in northern than southern parts. All these observations ought to give a clue as to the probable cause. Is this an infection spread in confined spaces? Or is its occurrence favoured by low external temperatures? Most of the commonly involved bones (skull, vertebrae, pelvis and thigh) have a good blood supply, which is increased in Paget's disease. (One clinical sign suggesting that a particular bone is involved in Paget's disease is an increase in the temperature of the skin over the bone concerned.)

Cause

Most experts at present attribute Paget's disease to a virus infection which gets into bones of a predisposed individual and activates osteoclasts. Electron microscopy of osteoclasts in Paget's disease shows that many have abnormal particles ('inclusion bodies') inside cells, or even inside the cell nuclei. These are not found in normal osteoclasts, but might be viral or bacterial products. Possible viruses include the paramyxoviridae, especially measles (MV), respiratory syncytial virus (RSV) and canine distemper virus (CDV). Simian virus 5 and para-influenza virus type 3 have also been implicated. Various identifiable portions of viruses (e.g. antigens of MV and RSV) have been demonstrated in inclusion bodies inside cells, though not – so far – whole viruses.

There are difficulties in accepting the virus hypothesis. The virus components and inclusion bodies in osteoclasts certainly suggest that viruses could be the cause of Paget's disease. But they might just be opportunistic travellers. A recent reviewer[1] pionted out: (1) that there is little evidence of different blood concentrations of antibodies to MV, RSV, CDV or para-influenza viruses when Paget patients are compared with normal subjects; (2) not all osteoclasts in Paget's disease contain the (presumed) viral inclusions; (3) similar inclusions have been observed in some rare conditions, e.g. non-pagetic giant cell tumours, osteopetrosis, pycnodysostosis and familial expansile osteolysis: thus the inclusions would have to alter osteoclast function differently in non-Paget disorders; (5) no infectious agent has yet been extracted from pagetic tissue; (6) the paramyxoviridae are ubiquitous whereas there are striking geographical differences in Paget's prevalence.

Paget's disease seems to be unique to man. Why is this? Necropsy and radiological surveys from Europe estimate a 3% prevalence for the population over 40 and 5% for the population over 55. It is extraordinary that there is no animal model for such a common human disorder. Paget's is a disease of the elderly: perhaps animals don't live long enough to get it? Is there some exclusively human habit of diet, posture or social behaviour which predisposes to the disease? The enormous variations in prevalence in different parts of the world and different ethnic groups point to an environmental cause. People in Europe, North America and Australasia are more affected than those in the third world. Paget's disease often runs in families; but truly genetic influences are not strong. It is somewhat comical that one group of investigators has reported that chromosomes 18 and 6 seem particularly important in some pagetic pedigrees,[2] whereas another group of scientists have suggested that genes on chromosomes 2, 5 and 10 are specially significant in another pedigree![3] Only five examples of Paget's disease in identical twins have been recorded. It is almost impossible to rule out the influence of shared family environments such as diet in causing familial aggregation of cases. Might it not be sensible for the time being to forget genetics in today's search for a cause for Paget's disease?

Why should the disease pick out certain bones preferentially, e.g. the long leg bones, pelvis, spine and skull? It is said that the right side of the body is more often affected than the left. If so, why? Since bone destruction seems to start Paget's disease off, it seems relevant to ask what external agents might start off bone weakening by stimulating the osteoclasts, the specialised cells which actively dissolve or destroy bone.

Osteoclast stimulation by bacteria: An alternative hypothesis to explain Paget's disease

Suppose viruses are irrelevant. Suppose they are simply picked up by pagetic osteoclasts and do not make those cells grow larger and more active. Is there any other extrinsic source of material known to stimulate osteoclasts strongly and which could enter bone via the bloodstream? (The natural history of Paget's disease seems best explained by the initiating agent arriving in the blood and settling at random in bones.) Many well-known bacteria are able to destroy bone, though bone abscesses (collections of pus) are not seen in Paget's disease. But many less virulent non-oxygen-requiring ('anaerobic') bacteria can destroy bone. In particular, a bacterium called *Actinobacillus actinomycetemcomitans* (AA) has potent bone-resorbing activity. It causes local infection of tooth sockets (periodontitis) especially in children.[4] Antibodies to this organism and to many other mouth bacteria can be detected in the blood of people with periodontitis.[5] The antibodies produced may have a protective role.

315

Since circulating antibodies to several anaerobic mouth bacteria can often be found in normal people, the organisms responsible must presumably get into the bloodstream. I have speculated[6] that AA (for example) might get into bone and lodge there, perhaps in thick bone tissue in which oxygen tension might be relatively low. The frequency of involvement of long bones is proportional to their volume. If AA get into bone and are taken into osteoclasts – which share most properties of scavenger cells (phagocytes) and probably derive from a common precursor – they would not be expected to cause inflammation.

Bacteria were looked for in affected bones in Paget's disease nearly a century ago and intermittently since, without success. But AA is a small fastidious non-motile bacillus (a particular type of bacterium) which is slow-growing and difficult to study. It might persist only in a single small focus within each affected bone and might have been overlooked. For example, *Tropheryma whipplei* (causing Whipple's disease, a serious condition initially affecting the intestinal wall) and *Helicobacter pylori* (causing peptic ulcers) were overlooked for decades. AA bacteria can grow and even multiply inside cultured human cells.[7] If symbiosis (Greek: 'living together') between AA bacteria and osteoclasts became established within bone, the infected osteoclasts might be spared immunological destruction, as are human cells infected by *Tropheryma whipplei*.

When growing in test-tube cultures, outside the body, AA bacteria produce several powerful osteoclast-stimulating chemicals. Some of these can be readily washed off the surface of AA bacteria in culture. Is it possible that material from a small focus of AA infection could diffuse within bone, stimulating and changing osteoclast function in the surrounding region? The rate of progression of Paget's disease can be followed using serial X-rays. From its origin in a long bone the disease process moves along very slowly, at a rate of between $\frac{1}{4}$ to $\frac{3}{4}$ of an inch per year (Fig. 38).[8] Such a slow rate of progression would be entirely compatible with the very slow diffusion of osteoclast-stimulating material through bone matrix (see Table 1, p. 75).

An advancing front of Paget's disease created by the very slow diffusion of large protein molecules seems to me a more credible explanation than the advance of an incredibly slow infection down a long bone. The way in which the advance of Paget's disease may peter out half-way along the length of a long bone also suggests the progressive weakening of a chemical osteoclastic stimulus. By knowing the rate of progression of the changes of Paget's disease in a long bone it is possible to work out roughly when the disease began in that bone. The data 'suggest that Paget's disease may be a disease of teenagers and

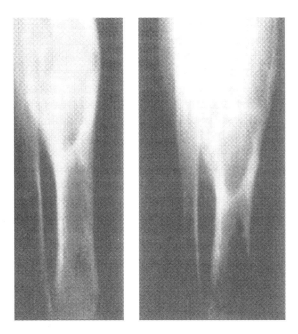

Figure 38 Two X-rays of the same main bone of the lower leg (the tibia), taken at different stages of the disease. The knee joint (not shown) lies above the upper part of the X-rays, and the ankle joint (also not visible) lies below the lower part of the X-rays. The upper part of the tibia is swollen and distorted by Paget's disease. Half-way down the bone a V-shaped line of demarcation separates active disease above, where the bone density is diminished, and normal bone below. The X-ray on the right was taken 3 years after that on the left. It shows how very slowly the disease progresses. The advancing front of disease has moved only about one inch down the leg. (X-rays by courtesy of John Kanis.)

young adults', but one which can take many years to cause symptoms or gross deformities.

Humans with severe periodontitis have increased circulating antibodies to AA bacteria. Simple brushing of the teeth is well known to send bacteria into the bloodstream. Scaling and root planing in people with periodontitis has been observed to increase AA antibody concentrations over a 6–12 month time scale. Is it possible that conservative dentistry, in which people in developed countries take pride, might sometimes spread AA and other potential osteoclast-stimulating organisms from the mouth into the bloodstream and thence into bones? This hypothesis could be tested by examining old embedded pagetic bone sections by the modern technique of immunocytochemistry. If marker antigens of AA or of other pathogenic oral bacteria were found in or close to osteoclasts, or if antibodies to one or more of them were found in high titre in Paget's disease, further investigation of the possible role of bacterial infection would be worthwhile. Unfortunately I have not yet located an academic department of pathology which holds a stock of old embedded sections of Paget's diseased bones and which has sufficient interest to make a pilot study.

My clinical impression is that gross deformities of the Paget's disease type have become much rarer than they were when I was first a medical student. If my hypothesis is correct, this could be due not only to current treatment of Paget patients with biphosphonates, which induce osteoclast apoptosis (p. 97), but also perhaps to the widespread use of broad-spectrum antibiotics to which all mouth anaerobic bacteria are to some extent sensitive.

There are rather few epidemiological data about dental problems in Paget patients, even though dentists often make the initial diagnosis of Paget's disease. In any case, distal bone foci are probably established years before the disease starts to produce symptoms and signs. In 1995 the result of a questionnaire sent to 292 Paget patients about the possible complications of their disease was published.[9] The patients rated the state of their mouth and teeth as unhealthier than that of matched controls. Paget's patients more often reported pain on opening the mouth. The very rare condition of juvenile Paget's disease (idiopathic hyperphosphatasia) is associated with premature loss of teeth.

Invoking mouth bacteria as the cause of Paget's disease helps to account for the unique affliction of man. Most animals' teeth are widely spaced and a roughage diet is protective. Only sheep have periodontitis comparable to ours. AA antibodies have been reported in diseased sheep, though other species of mouth bacteria predominate. Sheep have been kept for up to 15 years, as pets or for antibody production. They sometimes even need false teeth, so it might be worth looking out for Paget lesions in elderly sheep with bad teeth. I have spoken to vets about this, but so far have drawn a blank. This is probably because my hypothesis is wrong; but it would be amusing if it proved to be correct.

Jokes are unfortunately rare in science. In his 1969 monograph on Paget's disease[10] Hugh Barry wrote: 'One feels that when the secret is given up it may be so obvious that it is right there under our noses.' It would be ironic if the cause of Paget's disease eventually proved to lie exactly there!

Summary

Paget's disease of bone is a deforming condition affecting mainly large bones in a random fashion. There is first stimulation and proliferation of bone-destroying cells (osteoclasts). These cause bone softening, usually with bending and distortion. Later bone-forming cells (osteoblasts) take over and proliferate. New bone is laid down, often leaving bizarrely deformed long bones and a curious mosaic pattern when bone sections are examined under the microscope.

Pagetic osteoclast cells usually contain foreign particles (inclusion bodies), some of which might be viruses. However, the viruses apparently associated with these osteoclasts could be opportunistic rather than causative. Some mouth bacteria can destroy bone. One (*Actinobacillus actinomycetemcomitans*) can grow and even multiply inside cultured human cells, producing potent osteoclast-stimulating materials. An (as yet) untested hypothesis is that a small focus in a bone of this bacterium, or of one of the other periodontitis-causing bacteria, might gradually spread its chemical influence to activate osteoclasts, the first stage in Paget's disease. The focus in each bone might be small and easily overlooked, as other intracellular bacteria have been in the past.

30

OSTEOPOROSIS

The hardness of bone comes from it having mineral crystals strongly bound to a protein skeleton. The mineral elements are calcium and phosphorus, combined in the form of microscopic hexagonal plate crystals called hydroxyapatite.[1] The body contains over two pounds weight (one kilogram) of calcium, almost all of which is in bone. An average normal daily diet contains one gram of calcium and a slightly smaller weight of phosphorus. Phosphorus is present in abundance in almost all foods and there is always enough for life and health. But there is often not enough calcium, especially because the human gut is only able to absorb some 20–30% of the calcium in food.

The protein component of bone (collagen) makes up 90% of the bone 'matrix' (Latin: 'breeding animal'). Collagen itself has a strong structure comprising chains of proteins coiled round each other like a rope. The molecular structure of hydroxyapatite crystals fits exactly with the protein molecules of collagen. This allows the two components to bind together to make rigid bone. On the basis of its strength to weight ratio, bone is one of the strongest materials known. When it is first formed, bone matrix comprises a network of interconnected struts (trabeculae) of collagen laid down along lines of mechanical stress. Initially, trabeculae are soft and bendable. Strength and rigidity come later when hydroxyapatite crystals combine with the molecular template provided by collagen.

Once puberty is past and the long bones stop growing in length, the total mass of bone in the body slowly increases until at age 25–35 it makes up about 17% of body weight. For example, the skeleton of a 6 foot man of average build would weigh about 27 lb (12 kg). From its peak in the third decade total bone mass slowly and steadily declines with age, though people who take regular strenuous exercise can slow the process down or even temporarily reverse it.

The word 'osteoporosis' (OP), derives from Greek: *osteon* = bone and *poros* = a pore. The description is accurate. Osteoporotic bones are not filled to their fullest possible extent by interconnected struts. There are too many empty spaces (Fig. 39). This makes the bones unduly fragile. Minor injuries can cause fractures. An unexpected

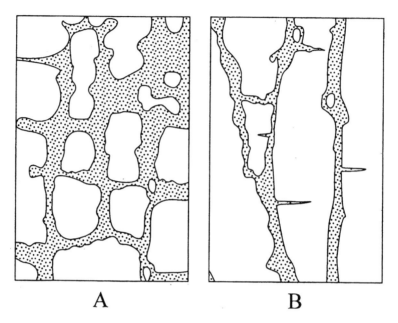

Figure 39 Diagram of the microscopic structure of a normal bone (A) and an osteoporotic bone (B).

fracture of a long bone is usually the first symptom of osteoporosis, though progressive loss of height or an episode of low back pain may suggest that there is weakness of the spine (the vertebral column). Osteoporotic bones do not bend when they are unduly stressed. They break. A severely osteoporotic bone is best likened to an egg shell – rigid to a limited extent but fragile and brittle. The progressive loss of height in people with osteoporosis is due to successive episodes of partial collapse of individual vertebral bones. Each episode usually causes local back pain which lasts for a few weeks. Sometimes crush fractures of the spine are visible on X-rays even though the individual has not complained of back pain. Although the characteristic first symptom of osteoporosis is a bone fracture resulting from minor trauma which would not break a normal bone, human osteoporosis is an infinitely graded disorder. In this respect it resembles other common conditions such as high blood pressure, diabetes and heart failure.

If a previously active adult retires to bed, the muscles become weak and bones porotic with almost frightening speed. Mild weakening of bone structure is sometimes called 'osteopenia' (Greek: *penia* = poverty) but neither for this nor for osteoporosis is there a generally accepted precise definition. Many different measurements of many different bones have been made. Many different criteria for the diagnosis of osteoporosis have been proposed. The best measure of OP is probably the 'bone mineral density' (BMD) at some particular site. This usually requires a special X-ray technique which depends on the fact that the calcium of bone mineral partly blocks penetration by X-rays. The density of any bone in the body can be measured by an X-ray absorptiometer, though there are other more elaborate techniques. Unfortunately BMD measurements are also affected by minor degrees of vitamin D deficiency, causing overactivity of the parathyroid glands and another type of bone weakening (see below).

Total bone mass is greater on average in males than females at all ages. Bone mass rises steadily during childhood and puberty to a plateau which is maintained until the late 30s, after which it declines in both sexes at a rate of about 1% per annum, more rapidly in women in the decade after the menopause. Osteoporotic fractures occur mainly in the elderly. Falls in young people cause bruising but rather rarely break bones. The most serious common fracture in the elderly is of the hip. This means a fracture at the upper part (head) of the main bone of the thigh (the femur). The most accurate predictor of a later fracture of the hip is – as one might expect – a previous measurement showing reduced bone density of the head of the femur. BMD measurements can also be made of the spine, ribs, pelvis, arm, wrist and fingers. Not too surprisingly BMD measurements at the hip correlate better with the risk of a later hip fracture than BMD measurements at any other site[2] even though in the same individual reduction of bone density at any one site correlates reasonably well with reduction of bone density at other sites.

Nomenclature: Osteomalacia

There is an important distinction to make between osteoporosis and 'osteomalacia' (OM). The latter term also comes from Greek: *malako* = soft. The name is accurately descriptive. The bones are too soft and not rigid enough. They don't often break, but they can bend or be compressed. There is plenty of collagen matrix. It is the failure to incorporate enough calcium-containing hydroxyapatite mineral into the bone matrix which characterises osteomalacia. This can be due to low calcium concentrations in blood and body fluids or to low concentrations of phosphate. The arithmetic product of calcium and phosphate concentrations $[Ca] \times [PO_4]$ determines the probability of crystals of hydroxyapatite being deposited. Osteomalacia is usually due to vitamin D deficiency, but some genetic and acquired kidney conditions with low phosphate concentrations may have effects similar to those due to lack of vitamin D.

Osteomalacia affects other tissues than bone. It is often associated with weakness of the upper leg muscles. The initiating event in contraction of any muscle is the entry of calcium into muscle cells. Without going deeply into mechanisms it is easy to understand why a disease characterised by insufficient calcium in bone might also be associated with muscle weakness. In severe cases of osteomalacia the patient waddles rather than walks upright. He or she cannot keep the pelvis level when standing on one leg, or climb out of a chair without using the arms to push the body up.

Osteomalacia can occur in children, when it is known as rickets. The soft leg bones become bowed because of the force of gravity on the heavy body above them. Rickets is seldom seen nowadays in the UK because our diet is better that it used to be and contains plenty of calcium and vitamin D, mainly from milk products.

Epidemiology

Examination of old English skeletons from the Middle Ages suggests that osteoporosis was less prevalent then than it is now in the UK. The (plausible) reason is that in past centuries people took more exercise and regularly lifted heavier burdens than we do today. The same explanation may also account for the relative freedom of modern-day Africans from the relentless age-related increase in hip fractures which is seen in developed countries – about a 1–3% incidence per year in most parts of the world.[3] A few drugs increase the risks of hip fractures, e.g. some tranquillising drugs (benzodiazepines), anti-epileptic and anti-cancer drugs, steroids, heparin and lithium. Caffeine from coffee – but not from tea – has also been incriminated. The difference between the two caffeine sources may be that tea contains more fluoride than coffee, and fluoride increases mineral deposition in bone. Smoking is associated with an increased risk of hip fractures, though we do not know why.

Gravity makes an important contribution to bone health. Lifting heavy weights stresses bones in the arms, spine, pelvis and legs and stimulates the synthesis of bone matrix. Travellers in space are well known to suffer rapidly progressive OP unless they regularly stress their bones by deliberate isometric exercises which increase muscle tension without necessarily moving joints. Simply going to bed for more than a few days starts osteoporosis off. Loss of bone matrix means that there is not enough collagen protein to hold on to the hydroxyapatite mineral which is lost. This results inevitably in an increase in calcium concentration in the urine. Most calcium salts (e.g. phosphate or carbonate) don't dissolve well in water. The urine may become supersaturated with calcium, so that stones made up of calcium carbonate, phosphate or oxalate can form in the kidneys or in the bladder. There may even be a damaging increase in the concentration of calcium in the blood. These are problems with any sudden reduction in bone mass. Loss of bone mass can occur, for example, in overactivity of the thyroid gland (thyrotoxicosis: see Chapter 6) in which body proteins are broken down faster than normal. I have seen stones containing calcium forming in the kidneys of a patient who had suffered extensive fractures of the pelvis and legs. These had forced a previously active young man to stay in bed for many weeks, with consequent loss of bone mass.

Social costs of osteoporosis

Osteoporosis places an enormous burden on health services. Most of this cost in the UK derives from 70,000 hip fractures annually, mostly in women. Men also get osteoporotic fractures, but on average about 10 years later in life than women. The annual costs of medical treatment of OP, related social services and necessary surgical operations amount to about one billion pounds sterling. In addition there are other burdens arising from osteoporotic fractures at the wrist (so-called Colles' fractures) and at several other sites, including spine, ankles, hands and feet. Wrist fractures typically occur from the age of 55 onwards, spinal fractures from age 65 and hip fractures from age 75. Minor trauma can break bones almost anywhere in people with OP. Often the first indication that someone has a serious problem with osteoporosis is that they fall onto an outstretched hand and get a wrist fracture. Another indication of osteoporosis is spontaneous collapse of the body of a vertebral bone of the spine, causing loss of height. One fifth of women who have suffered a vertebral fracture get another one within a year.

Cause

A major mystery, to me, is why muscle movements and stresses strengthen rather than weaken bone. Since crystallisation of many simple chemicals from a supersaturated solution is impaired by keeping the solution stirred, one might think that crystallisation and deposition of calcium in bone would be helped by rest. In the case of bone this is not so: rather the reverse. The more stress that is placed on bone, the stronger it gets, and vice versa. I imagine that stress must stimulate protein matrix synthesis, but we do not yet know how this action is exerted.

One factor increasing the risk of OP and of an osteoporotic fracture includes an early onset of the menopause in women. In adults of both sexes chronic liver disease, alcoholism, food malabsorption, smoking, thyrotoxicosis, rheumatoid arthritis, Cushing's syndrome (steroid overproduction), uncontrolled diabetes mellitus, and sex hormone deficiency can all contribute to OP. All of these can interfere with protein synthesis and hence reduce the mass of bone matrix. All have been shown to be associated with reduced BMD. Women taking hormone replacement therapy after their menopause get significant protection from osteoporotic fractures. There is a strong association of OP with the iron overload disease haemochromatosis, described in Chapter 26. OP in this case is probably due to the associated sex hormone deficiency. Another association of OP – recently recognised – is increased concentrations of homocysteine in the body. This material increases when folate is deficient (see Chapter 27). Trials are now in progress to find whether folic acid supplements might help to prevent osteoporosis.

My intention in writing this book has been to discuss the causes of diseases rather than treatments, but the effectiveness of several treatments for osteoporosis may throw light on its cause.[4] Treatment may strengthen bone by increasing the total amount of bone matrix or by preventing bone matrix loss. Hormone replacement therapy with oestrogens, for post-menopausal women, reduces the natural rate of reabsorption of bone matrix. It is curious that raloxifene, which antagonises some actions of oestrogens and might be expected to make OP worse, improves bone mass by a different and protective action on bone. Certain biphosphonates (e.g. alendronate, risendronate, and clodronate) combine with hydroxyapatite in bone and inhibit bone reabsorption. Since the fault in OP lies in the bone matrix rather than in bone mineral, it is not to be expected that calcium and vitamin D should help OP much. But since elderly people often have some degree of dietary deficiency of both these factors, with some consequential osteomalacia, it is not too surprising that both have been found to help elderly people with osteoporosis. They are widely used prophylactically.

Genetics

Osteoporosis is overwhelmingly (65–80%) an inherited disease even though many environmental factors can make the disease worse. By a technique of what is called 'linkage analysis' some 20 genes (associated with chromosomes 17, 12, 4, 6, 2, 5, 7 and 3) have been identified. All may contribute to the inheritance of osteoporosis. OP is thus classed as a 'polygenic' disease. It has clearly no single genetic cause. Any idea that a single specific treatment will one day be devised seems hopelessly optimistic.

The severely disabling disease 'osteogenesis imperfecta' is caused by a mutation in the gene which governs the synthesis of the protein collagen. This makes bones unusually fragile. Unfortunate children with this condition repeatedly break their bones from minimal trauma. The disease can be regarded as a particularly severe form of osteoporosis, caused by a specific defect in the protein matrix of bone.

The recently discovered protein 'osteoprotegerin' (so-called because it was thought to have a protective function for bone) probably prevents OP, but its ligand (the receptor chemical with which it combines) can cause OP when present in excess. The production of the ligand by certain bacteria, especially those causing infections of tooth sockets (periodontitis), is thought to be one of the main factors causing local bone destruction. Its role, if any, in age-related osteoporosis is uncertain, but the genetics and epidemiology of osteoprotegerin and its ligand will undoubtedly be closely studied in the future. I discussed the possible role of bacterial infection causing Paget's disease of bone in the last chapter.

It is interesting that mice which have overexpressed genes coding for osteoprotegerin have *osteopetrosis* – excessively hard and rigid bone. Conversely, deficiency of osteoprotegerin ligand leads to osteoporosis. Another mutation leading to increased bone density has also been identified: a mutation in a gene on chromosome 11 which codes for a lipoprotein receptor.[5] This has aroused interest by opening up the possibility of supplying the protein product of this gene, in the hope of stimulating osteoporotic individuals to increase their bone density.

Treatments and prophylaxis for weak bones

There is a clear distinction between OP and OM, and between the treatments appropriate for each. Physical exercise and good protein nutrition help prevent OP, whereas prevention of OM depends on achieving high enough concentrations of calcium and phosphate in the blood, to promote adequate mineral deposition of hydroxyapatite. Because vitamin D plays a role in the absorption of calcium from the gut, vitamin D intake is as important as adequate amounts of calcium. Vitamin D in food comes in the form of a precursor, a cholesterol compound which is acted on by ultraviolet light in the skin to form cholecalciferol (vitamin D_3). The liver and the kidneys convert this to its active metabolite 'calcitriol' (1,25 dihydroxycholecalciferol) at a rate which depends on the prevailing concentrations of calcium, phosphate and parathyroid hormone (see below) in the blood. The interconnected metabolic feedback paths are extremely complicated, but it is failure of this vitamin D conversion which causes OM in both longstanding liver and kidney diseases.

As I have already emphasised, OP is the main cause of hip fractures. Elderly folk often cannot afford to eat enough protein. They may also lack adequate vitamin D in their diet. But OM is neither the main nor a common cause of abnormally fragile bones. Since ultraviolet light is necessary for the synthesis of vitamin D in the skin, fully clothed people, those with dark skin, or those living indoors all the time are specially liable to get vitamin D deficiency and hence OM. I have seen gross OM in several Indian women living in London and eating a diet deficient in both calcium and vitamin D. Strict vegetarians (vegans) and Asians are specially likely to suffer in this way. I have also seen a well grown and well nourished 25-year old English woman, a food faddist, who had contrived to give herself gross OM. This was obvious as soon as she waddled into my consulting room. When she was eventually, with difficulty, persuaded (by my colleague Peter Kopelman) to take a modest vitamin D supplement, she quickly got better.

Many people in the UK are intensely suspicious of Government-sponsored or Government-recommended food supplements, even of essential vitamins. This is an important aspect of the vocal, sometimes hysterical and even physically destructive anti-scientific activities of influential groups of people in the UK. They find acquiescent allies in campaigning journalists.

Secondary hormone effects of a low calcium state

Four parathyroid glands, two on each side, lie in the neck at the sides and partly behind the thyroid gland (Fig. 9, p. 62). They are ductless glands, like the thyroid itself, but they secrete into the blood hormones known collectively and simply as 'parathormone' (Greek: *para* = at the side of). Parathormone has an important role in stimulating the absorption of calcium. If dietary calcium is deficient parathormone secretion is increased. Parathormone acts on bone and on the kidneys. It increases bone turnover of calcium and also absorption of calcium from the gut. If the body contains calcium in excess, parathormone secretion is shut down. Normally the entire surface of bone in the adult body is renewed every 2 years, but this rate doubles when the

328

parathyroid glands are overactive, in the condition known as 'hyper-parathyroidism'.

The administration of parathormone (which has to be given by intermittent injections) increases the rate of synthesis of bone matrix. At present parathormone, or one of its components, appears to be gaining favour as a treatment for osteoporosis, even though large doses in animals have provoked the production of malignant bone tumours (osteosarcomas). Strontium compounds are cheaper, and are useful stimulants of bone growth.

Before progressive deficiency of vitamin D has had time to bring about the bone changes of osteomalacia, the reduction of available calcium will have already stimulated the parathyroid glands to secrete more parathormone. This situation is known as 'secondary hyperpar-athyroidism' to distinguish it from the primary disease when there is oversecretion of parathormone by an abnormal gland or by a normal gland acting abnormally. Some degree of secondary hyperparathyr-oidism is common with minor degrees of vitamin D deficiency and also when there is chronic failure of kidney function.[6] Oversecretion of parathormone may make accurate estimation of bone mineral density difficult.

Because of the difficulties in assessing individual needs for calcium and vitamin D, the usual practice of most physicians is to give elderly patients, especially those with previous bone fractures, a vitamin D supplement together with plenty of calcium by mouth, to ensure that no significant element of osteomalacia contributes to the bone weakness of osteoporosis.[7]

Summary

Osteoporosis (OP) is an extremely common condition which becomes more and more significant at ages above 55–60, especially in women after the menopause. As its name suggests, it is characterised by holes or pores in the structure of bone. There is an inadequate number of bony struts (trabeculae). The intrinsic defect lies in the protein matrix of bone, which provides a template for crystals of calcium and phosphate mineral (hydroxyapatite) to bind strongly with it. The closely bound protein + mineral compound creates the great strength of normal bone.

Bone is normally in a state of flux, being slowly removed and resynthesised throughout life. The rate of synthesis of bone matrix is increased by movement and stress, whereas disuse and lack of stress speeds up the normal rate of bone destruction. Poor nutrition and many chronic diseases are associated with OP. Steroid drugs, which are widely used, are well known to cause osteoporosis. Many other drugs can have a similar effect.

Spontaneous bone fractures, or fractures after minimal trauma, are often the presenting feature of osteoporosis. Fractures of the large bones, especially the hip, are of enormous economic importance. They make a major contribution to ill health. The pain associated with bone fractures has a serious impact on the ability of old people to enjoy their later years.

Another condition, osteomalacia (OM), also weakens bones, but here the fault lies in the mineral rather than in the protein content of bone. Deficiency of calcium and also of vitamin D both predispose to OM, which is relatively easy to treat effectively. OM may be associated with (secondary) hyperparathyroidism – increased secretion of parathormone by the four small parathyroid glands in the neck. This complication may also give rise to other symptoms.

31

HIGH BLOOD PRESSURE: 'ESSENTIAL HYPERTENSION'

I have found this chapter the most difficult to write. My main life's work in medical research has been trying to identify the cause of so-called 'essential' hypertension. During my search I have come to hold strong opinions which most fellow scientists in the field do not share. I have probably failed to be fair to rival views. So readers of this chapter must keep an open mind and realise that a bigot is trying to persuade them of his own interpretations. But let me start with a few facts.

Anatomy of the circulation

The simplest way to think about the circulation is that blood goes round the body in a figure-of-eight racetrack. The smaller loop is the lung ('pulmonary') circulation, the larger comprises the rest of the body (the 'systemic' circulation). Although the heart lies at the crossing of the two blood circuits, and the two sides of the heart contract and pump at the same time, there is normally no connection between them in the heart itself (Fig. 40).

The aorta is the main and largest artery in the body. In the adult it is an inch or more in diameter (3 cm) where it leaves the heart. Blood is pumped from the aorta to all the body tissues – brain, gut, and muscles – through a set of large arteries. These branch repeatedly in all the organs they supply, finishing in a network of very small blood vessels (capillaries) which take nutrients to the tissues and remove waste products from them. Capillaries are tubes only about two-thousandths of an inch (8–20 microns) in diameter. They are too small to see with the naked eye and their internal diameter is only slightly larger than that of the red cells of the blood.

Blood is collected from the tissues by veins. The two largest veins (the venae cavae) convey blood into the right side of the heart. The larger veins contain flap valves which allow blood to flow only one

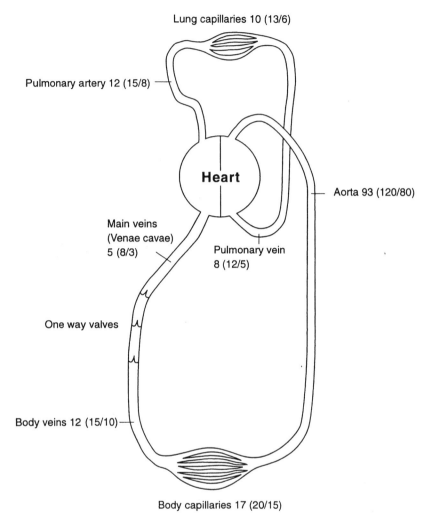

Lung capillaries 10 (13/6)

Pulmonary artery 12 (15/8)

Heart

Aorta 93 (120/80)

Main veins
(Venae cavae)
5 (8/3)

Pulmonary vein
8 (12/5)

One way valves

Body veins 12 (15/10)

Body capillaries 17 (20/15)

Figure 40 Diagram of the two main parts of the circulation, with the typical pressures at each point in a supine subject, in mmHg. The mean pressure is followed by typical values for pressure oscillations, in brackets, also in mmHg.

way, towards the heart. It was by study of these valves in human arm veins some 350 years ago that William Harvey realised that blood had to go round in a circuit. It did not simply oscillate with each heart beat, as people had previously believed.

From the right side of the heart blood is pumped through the pulmonary artery into the two lungs. The air we breathe in and out comes into contact with a fine network of very small blood vessels, the pulmonary capillaries. These surround the tiny air sacs of the lungs (the alveoli). After going through the lungs, blood is collected into the left 'atrium' (Latin: entrance hall) of the heart. Then it enters the main pumping chamber of the heart, the left 'ventricle' (Latin: *ventriculus* = little stomach), and starts its journey round again. At its fastest it takes about 20 seconds for a complete circuit, and maybe only half that during strenuous exercise. But it could take a minute or two for a single blood cell to go round the circuit if it happened to be going a long distance and through a tissue with only a small blood supply (e.g. the bones of the feet).

An adult body contains about 9 pints (5 litres) of blood. More than 90% of this is in the main (systemic) circulation, in the veins and arteries. A small amount is in the capillaries. The left side of the heart (the left atrium and left ventricle) does most of the work because it pumps blood up to a high pressure. The right side only has to pump blood through the lungs, which normally present very little resistance to flow.

Pressures of blood in different parts of the circuit

All parts of the systemic circulation contain blood at a higher pressure than that in the corresponding parts of the pulmonary circulation. Stephen Hales (an English clergyman) directly measured systemic arterial blood pressure in a horse in 1733. He restrained the animal and tied a long tube into an artery. Blood rushed up the tube to reach a height of about 6 feet.

Physicists measure pressure in international standard (SI: Système Internationale) units such as kiloPascals (kPa). But for more than a century doctors have measured pressure in arteries by comparing it with the pressure generated by a vertical column of mercury. This metal, 13 times heavier than blood, is fluid at room temperature and more convenient than using a column of blood. Indeed, Stephen Hales himself made use of a mercury manometer to measure fluid pressures in plants. The 'sphygmomanometer' is used to measure indirectly the pressure in the main arm artery. (The name is derived from Greek: *sphygmos* = pulse; *manos* = rare, thin; *metron* = measure.) A high air pressure is applied to a cuff around the upper arm, then the pressure is gently lowered until the pulse returns to the wrist or until a pulsating rushing noise can be heard by a stethoscope pressed against the main artery below the cuff. At this point the peak or 'systolic' (Greek: *systolo* = contraction) pressure can be read off a graduated column of mercury or from some other pressure-measuring device, since it will be the same as the air pressure in the cuff.

Ironically, doctors and hospitals are now abandoning the mercury pressure measurer because mercury gives off a poisonous vapour even at room temperature. In a glass manometer this is harmless, but mercury manometers get abandoned and broken. The mercury trickles into flooring and crevices so that the level of mercury vapour in the air of hospitals and laboratories can become a real health hazard. The European Union is in process of banning this use of mercury. But so well established is the 'millimetres of mercury' unit for blood pressure measurement, and so many mercury manometers remain in use all over the world, that it will be decades before standard SI units of pressure (kiloPascals: kPa) take over. It will be longer still before all mercury manometers are phased out. But so long as people remain familiar with the unique physical properties of mercury they will probably continue to find it easier to relate arterial blood pressure to the pressure exerted by a mercury column rather than train themselves to think and talk about kiloPascals.

In a normal adult the systolic blood pressure is equivalent to a pressure exerted by a column of mercury just under 5 inches (120 millimetres) high. The measurement is abbreviated to 'mmHg' because 'Hg' is the chemical symbol for mercury (itself an abbreviation of the expressive Latin: *hydrargyrus* = water-silver). This pressure corresponds to about 16.5 kPa. That is only about one sixth the normal pressure exerted by the atmosphere around us and only about one tenth the pressure in an average mains water tap.

When the heart's left ventricle relaxes after discharging its contents into the arteries the pressure falls to a trough level, the 'diastolic' (Greek: *diastole* = dilation) pressure. This is around 80 mm Hg, or 11 kPa. It is detected because of the disappearance of the pulse sound heard via the stethoscope over an arm artery as the cuff pressure in the upper arm is gradually lowered. Doctors conventionally write down the two pressures in shorthand as, for example, '120/80'. Because of the triangular shape of the pressure curve, the diastolic pressure is closer than the systolic pressure to the true average arterial pressure. The best estimate of mean pressure is given by adding one third of the pulse pressure (the difference between systolic and diastolic pressures) to the diastolic pressure. For a blood pressure of 120/80 the mean pressure will be roughly

$$80 + \frac{(120 - 80)}{3} = 93\,\text{mmHg}.$$

In the fine capillaries of the body the pressure is much lower, 15–20 mmHg on average. In the veins the pressure is lower still. It is often possible to see pulsation in the large veins of the neck of someone lying flat because the pressure there oscillates just above and below atmospheric pressure. The directors of television plays have to keep a close watch on the sides of the neck of supposed dead people, in case pulsation in superficial veins gives the game away.

The right atrium collects the blood from the great veins and pumps it into the right ventricle, in which the average pressure is raised to about 10–15 mmHg. This is normally high enough to send blood through the low resistance path of the lungs.

Systemic hypertension

'Hypertension' is a hybrid word (Greek: *hyper* = over, above; Latin: *tens* = stretch). Unless otherwise specified, the term always refers to the systemic circulation and to pressure in the large systemic arteries. Many surveys of whole populations have shown a frequency distribution of blood pressures, at rest, which look like Figure 41. With increasing age of a population the average pressure increases, and there is a wider spread of pressures between individuals. In addition the frequency distribution curves become progressively skewed towards the right in older age groups. Figure 41 shows that there is no clear dividing line at any age between high and low pressures. People with pressures consistently maintained above about 140/90 are described as 'hypertensive'. If this definition is used, about 4% of young adults in most developed countries are hypertensive. The proportion rises with age. By the age of 60 the definition includes about half the population, and by the age of 75 about 65%. The great majority of people in their seventies have a systolic pressure considerably greater than 140 mmHg. Despite the apparent normality of raised blood pressure in the older members of the community, hypertension is not a harmless variation at any age. On average people's life-span is inversely proportional to their blood pressure. People with blood pressures of 160/100 are much more likely than those with pressures of 120/80 mmHg to get arterial complications such as heart or kidney disease and strokes in later life. They will die younger. At the extreme end, a man whose blood pressure is at, say, 300/180 (which is about the highest pressure ever seen) is likely to die soon, within a month or two, probably from a brain haemorrhage, unless he is treated by blood-pressure-lowering drugs.

I am only talking about sustained hypertension. When a normal

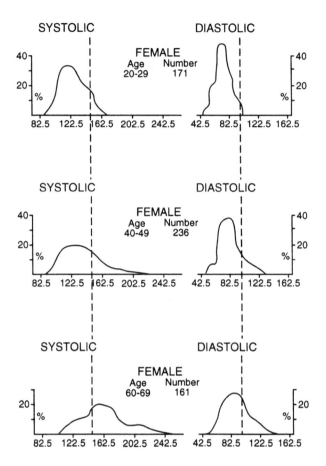

Figure 41 Frequency distribution of systolic and diastolic blood pressure in three groups of women, aged 20–29, 40–49 and 60–69. The curves were drawn by joining the percentage numbers of all cases in each individual group of people within a 10 mmHg range of blood pressure: e.g. 82.5–92.4 and 92.5–102.4 mmHg. The interrupted vertical lines mark off groups of women with blood pressures of 160/100 or more, i.e. definitely 'hypertensive'. Note that more women over 60 have systolic blood pressures greater than 160 mmHg than have systolic pressures less than 160 mmHg. (Drawn from individual data in a population study by Hamilton M et al., Clin Sci 1954;13:20).

person engages in strenuous exercise, especially so-called isometric exercise like lifting heavy weights, the blood pressure in the main arteries goes up a lot, partly because hard muscles squeeze soft blood vessels. When the exercise stops, blood pressure goes back to normal. In established hypertension, on the other hand, blood pressure is consistently above normal even at rest.

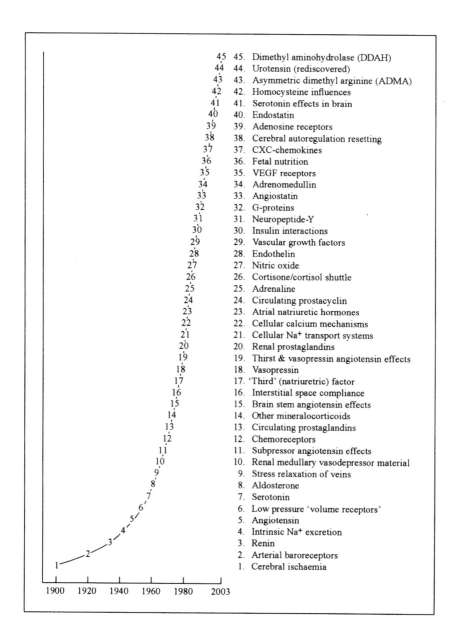

45. Dimethyl aminohydrolase (DDAH)
44. Urotensin (rediscovered)
43. Asymmetric dimethyl arginine (ADMA)
42. Homocysteine influences
41. Serotonin effects in brain
40. Endostatin
39. Adenosine receptors
38. Cerebral autoregulation resetting
37. CXC-chemokines
36. Fetal nutrition
35. VEGF receptors
34. Adrenomedullin
33. Angiostatin
32. G-proteins
31. Neuropeptide-Y
30. Insulin interactions
29. Vascular growth factors
28. Endothelin
27. Nitric oxide
26. Cortisone/cortisol shuttle
25. Adrenaline
24. Circulating prostacyclin
23. Atrial natriuretic hormones
22. Cellular calcium mechanisms
21. Cellular Na^+ transport systems
20. Renal prostaglandins
19. Thirst & vasopressin angiotensin effects
18. Vasopressin
17. 'Third' (natriuretic) factor
16. Interstitial space compliance
15. Brain stem angiotensin effects
14. Other mineralocorticoids
13. Circulating prostaglandins
12. Chemoreceptors
11. Subpressor angiotensin effects
10. Renal medullary vasodepressor material
9. Stress relaxation of veins
8. Aldosterone
7. Serotonin
6. Low pressure 'volume receptors'
5. Angiotensin
4. Intrinsic Na^+ excretion
3. Renin
2. Arterial baroreceptors
1. Cerebral ischaemia

Figure 42 Historical perspective of some of the main mechanisms and systems involved in blood pressure regulation, plotted against the approximate year of their discovery.

337

Causes

There are many recognised specific causes of sustained hypertension. Figure 42 shows the large number of potential influences on blood pressure regulation already identified during the last century. It seems highly likely that many more will be described in the years to come. But we must start somewhere.

Kidney disease is the best understood and will be discussed in the next chapter. Since kidney disease can cause hypertension and hypertension can damage the kidneys we have the ingredients for a vicious circle. But the kidneys appear normal in young people with essential hypertension. None the less, many people believe that subtle changes in the way the kidneys operate can raise the blood pressure even though the kidneys look normal under the microscope. Nothing totally disproves this theory. There is continuing interest in the possibility of hypertension being due to excessive production of blood-pressure-raising 'steroid' chemicals from the adrenal glands, especially aldosterone. Some people have estimated that between 5% and 10% of people with apparently 'essential' hypertension (see below) could be suffering from a subtle excess of aldosterone.

Despite this, for reasons which will become clear, I found it intellectually more satisfying to propose and study a cause for essential hypertension which gives a primary role neither to the kidneys nor to the adrenal glands. Hypertension appearing towards the end of pregnancy is described in Chapter 35. Several causes of human hypertension due to a mutation in a single gene have been identified, but they are very rare. All such causes, together with recognised kidney disorders, account for only some 10–20% of cases of established hypertension. The cause of the rest is unknown. Such people are described as having 'essential hypertension'. This antiquated term has stuck but all it means is 'high blood pressure of unknown cause'. An essential hypertensive individual is defined as one whose blood pressure lies in the upper range of the normal distribution curve of Figure 41 – above the (arbitrary) level of, say, 140/90 – and in whom no specific cause can be found.

Is there a real problem about the cause of essential hypertension?

Sir George Pickering, a former Regius Professor of Medicine at Oxford, challenged the idea that there might be a specific cause for essential hypertension. He regarded it as simply a quantitative deviation from the norm and therefore thought that there was no point in looking for a specific single cause.

I shall illustrate the weakness of his argument by an analogy. Suppose that in the country of Erewhon the sphygmomanometer has not been invented, but that somehow doctors there have invented an instrument which when placed on the chest wall measures the resistance to blood flow in the coronary arteries of the heart. (Don't ask me how the machine works.) Erewhonian doctors call the measurement 'CVR'. Although they don't know exactly what they are measuring, their population surveys reveal skewed bell-shaped frequency/distribution curves of CVR looking just like those for blood pressure (Fig. 41). One of their Regius professors says that there is no point in looking for 'the' cause of high CVR, because it is just 'a quantitative deviation from the norm', even though Erewhonians have noticed that people with high values for CVR die young. But then one of their pathologists correlates measurements of CVR in life with observations made after death. He notes that people with high CVR have lumps of white material (atheroma) partly blocking the coronary arteries, whereas those with low CVR don't. Here is a highly specific condition, the severity of which is normally distributed in the adult community.

Instead of trying to find an all-or-none cause for essential hypertension let us consider that its cause might be both *well-defined* and *infinitely graded*. Random arterial obstruction by atheroma could obviously be described in this way.

High blood pressure and the nervous system

I have written many articles and two monographs (26 years apart) suggesting that the brain initiates most cases of apparently 'essential' hypertension.[1] The word 'neurogenic' in the titles of these books implies that the hypertension is created by the nervous system. Many laymen, and some doctors, regard essential hypertension as a psychosomatic disease. In the USA particularly, the high prevalence of hypertension in black people has been ascribed to suppressed hostility. Fear, anger and mental stress are well known to raise blood pressure transiently. But there is no good evidence that emotions, however strong, cause established essential hypertension. Psychological testing has failed to identify hypertensives in a population of young people who had no prior knowledge of their blood pressure. The strongest rebuttal came from the large trial organised by the British Medical Research Council.[2] Twelve thousand people filled in a well-validated questionnaire before their blood pressures were known. Later analysis failed to find any link between high blood pressure and psychological factors.

Although in the last 100 years huge advances have been made in many other fields, the cause of essential hypertension remains elusive. There seem to be too many contenders rather than too few, as Figure 42 shows. For fun, I calculated the exponential equation relating time (x: in years since 1900) to the number of factors (y) recognised at various times to influence blood pressure:

$$y = 1 + 0.05(x - 1900) + 0.06(0.05x - 95)^4$$

Curves like this suggest that there are certainly lots of presently unknown mechanisms influencing blood pressure which have yet to be discovered. If the curve continues for another 100 years, we might expect another 500 new discoveries. This may sound ridiculous: but just wait!

The influence of breathing on blood pressure

The concentration and effective partial pressure of carbon dioxide (the waste gas produced by food combustion in the body) is closely regulated by the brain, by its control of breathing. Holding the breath raises carbon dioxide concentration; overbreathing reduces it. Increased concentrations of carbon dioxide gas directly dilate blood vessels, but this effect is antagonised by increased sympathetic nervous activity. Curiously it has recently been found that the hormone insulin (deficiency of which causes diabetes) has actions which parallel those of carbon dioxide. Insulin itself is a vasodilator material, i.e. when infused into an artery supplying an organ or tissue it increases the local blood flow (by increasing the rate of production of nitric oxide (p. 140)). But it also acts directly on the brain to increase sympathetic nervous activity. This constricts blood vessels. As in the case of carbon dioxide, the two mechanisms cancel each other out. Insulin has almost no net effect on blood pressure when it is infused or injected. However, there is much interest in the possibility that changes either in insulin secretion or in the chemical receptors with which insulin combines might play a subtle part in causing high blood pressure, especially when high blood pressure co-exists with obesity.

Alcohol in many circumstances raises blood pressure, possibly through an action on the brain; but people with essential hypertension can be lifelong teetotallers.

Genetics

Heredity is certainly an important factor. By comparing identical and non-identical twins it is possible to calculate to what extent someone's

340

blood pressure is determined by heredity and how much by external environmental factors. The answer is about half and half. The genetic influence on blood pressure is 'polygenic', i.e. the result of the interaction of several genes. A large number of genes, each affecting one or more of the important blood pressure control factors shown in Figure 42 might play a part.

A recent scan of the whole human genome has located several parts of the DNA 'library' contained in the human chromosomes which themselves contain genes that influence adult blood pressure. But it has not succeeded in identifying a single all-important chromosome segment or gene which on its own determines whether someone will or will not get essential hypertension.

There has been some suggestive evidence in man that the lower an individual's birth weight the higher his or her blood pressure as a adult will be. These observations originally derived from ancient public health records of birth weights. They have created a lot of interest. Animal experiments manipulating the diets of female rats give some support to the idea that poor maternal nutrition during pregnancy and a consequent lower than average weight of the fetus can raise blood pressure in the adult. Unfortunately, in man there are many possible confounding factors, especially the mother's blood pressure inheritance. A recent survey of a large number of published human observations suggests that on average a new born baby weighing 2 lb (1 kg) less than average will have a blood pressure as a young adult $\frac{1}{2}$ mm Hg higher than average.[3] Such very small differences cannot account for more than about one per cent of the variations in blood pressure between adults. So a low birth weight cannot be looked upon as an important or significant cause of human adult 'essential' hypertension.

Genes influence the degree to which an individual's habitual intake of salt affects blood pressure. In susceptible people, the more salt they eat the higher their pressure. I shall return to this theme in the next chapter.

Negative feedback systems

A major problem in hypertension research is the large number of mechanisms stabilising blood pressure over time. Most of these utilise a 'negative feedback' principle. Blood pressure in the aorta and in the main arteries of the neck is continuously monitored by tiny sensors in the walls of large arteries. Although these specialised nerve endings detect stretch, in effect they sample blood pressure. Hence they are known as 'baroreceptors' (Greek: *baro* = pressure). Specialised 'sympathetic' nerves (part of the autonomic nervous system (p. 481) go from the brain stem to many veins and arteries in the body, making them constrict so that the blood in the circulation is gripped more tightly. Other sympathetic nerves increase the force and rate of beating of the heart.

If the blood pressure falls for any reason, e.g. standing up, or losing blood, the brain detects the fall through its nerve connections. Control centres in the brain stem get second-by-second information about the blood pressure in the large neck arteries and also about the adequacy of filling of the veins from which blood flows to fill the heart. All this information is transmitted by specialised nerve endings in the walls of these vessels and in the walls of the heart itself. The information is in the form of bursts of electrical impulses, conveyed by nerves running up each side of the neck. The rate of discharge of nerve impulses increases when the pressure (and hence the stretch of the vessel wall) is increased.

The kidneys provide another example of a blood pressure stabilising system working by negative feedback. If blood pressure rises, the kidneys excrete more salt and water. This reduces the amount of blood in the circulation and blood pressure goes down. If blood pressure falls, the kidneys hold on to fluid, thirst is increased, the volume of blood rises and pressure is restored. I shall discuss this example of negative feedback in the next chapter.

There are several other stabilising systems. All have one characteristic in common: they stabilise blood pressure over short periods of time but not over long ones. They reset their range of operation. In the context of essential hypertension, it is as if the control system says: 'OK – somebody – I don't know who – wants my blood pressure to go up from 120/80 to 170/120 and to stay at that level. As he insists on this I will have to permanently change my operating system. In future I will keep my blood pressure at 170/120, come what may.' So even if this hypertensive individual loses a pint or two of blood through an accident, blood pressure will be back almost to 170/120 in a few minutes. Retention of fluid will expand blood volume again in less than 24 hours, so that the brain will no longer need to send extra nerve impulses out to make arteries constrict.

To solve the mystery of essential hypertension, we need first to identify the basic master control system. Then we might be able to find why it is misbehaving.

Young inbred hypertensive rats can have their blood pressure kept low for many weeks or months by appropriate drug treatment. When treatment is stopped blood pressure may remain down. This does not seem to happen in man. In one big trial by the British Medical Research Council a large number of hypertensive people were treated for 6 years continuously with blood-pressure-lowering drugs. When treatment was stopped, to find out whether it was still needed, the blood pressure climbed quickly back to its original level 6 years before.[4] Evidently, therefore, people with essential hypertension have undergone some change which prevents the blood pressure being reset back to normal levels, even though pressure has been kept down for months or even years.

Where is the master controller?

This is where I get autobiographical and heretical. In 1958/9 I was a Research Fellow in the Middlesex Hospital Medical School in London. I attended the post mortem room there and looked at the main arteries supplying blood to the brain in nearly 100 people who had died in hospital and who were being examined to find the cause of their death. I had the idea that maybe the cause of essential hypertension lay in the brain, which raised blood pressure when it wasn't getting enough blood. But I must first explain the historical background.

More than a hundred years ago Harvey Cushing, a famous American neurosurgeon, observed that when the arterial blood supply to the head of a dog was restricted its blood pressure went up. This phenomenon is now known as the 'Cushing response'. Drawing on these observations, and on experiments of his own in the 1920s, Ernest Starling, the greatest English physiologist since William Harvey, suggested that essential hypertension might be due to 'gross lesions in the arterial trunks (which) might diminish the average pressure in the arteries of the brain...This condition is well known.' Two observations then came along to put this idea back on the shelf. First, fast-reacting baroreceptor nerve endings were discovered in the walls of the main arteries supplying the brain. When blood pressure in these arteries goes down, the change is detected by the baroreceptors and a signal is sent up to the brain. The brain then puts the blood pressure up again by a reflex action through the sympathetic nervous system. This discovery appeared to remove the need to invoke a contribution to the Cushing response by the brain itself. Secondly, in the 1940s Seymour Kety devised a clever indirect method of measuring total cerebral blood flow (CBF) in awake man. CBF was found to be substantially normal in essential hypertension.

More recent work has shown that total brain blood flow is in fact slightly reduced in essential hypertension, on average. But even if it had been found to be absolutely normal, I never felt that it was logical to argue that hypertensive individuals had nothing wrong with the blood supply to their brains. Could it not be that the rise in blood pressure was the response needed to keep CBF normal? Hypertension could then be regarded as an appropriate response to increased resistance to the flow of blood through the brain.

A simple first test of this hypothesis seemed to be to examine the large arteries supplying the brain (the internal carotids and the vertebrals), both in the neck and within the skull. The main arteries arise within the chest close to the heart, pass upwards along or within the neck bones, through the base of the skull and enter the brain as illustrated in Figure 20 (p. 139). Drew Thomson and I thought that disease of these large arteries might provide enough added resistance to make a rise of blood pressure necessary to maintain adequate blood flow to the brain.

Figure 43A shows X-rays of one fairly normal left internal carotid and vertebral artery in a woman of 43 whose blood pressure had been almost normal during life. Figure 43B is from a woman of 59 with severe hypertension whose right internal carotid and (especially) vertebral artery was irregularly and grossly narrowed. In each case post mortem artery spasm was first fully relaxed with ammonia. Then warm radio-opaque gelatin solution was pumped into each artery (tied off at its ends) and held at a pressure of 140 mm Hg until the gelatin had set. X-rays were taken at the same standard X-ray tube distance in each case.

Clearly there was very gross narrowing of both arteries in the hypertensive woman. The central channel (the 'lumen') of the vertebral artery, which supplied the hindbrain, was reduced almost to pinhole size. The internal carotid artery was larger but also considerably narrowed. Inspection of the arteries concerned showed that the narrowing was due to patchy deposits of 'atheroma', a hard cheesy material mostly made up of cholesterol. It is obvious that extensive disease like this must have greatly increased the resistance to blood flow to the brain during life.

The technical difficulties of this type of study can easily be imagined. But since Drew Thomson and I were only interested in the resistance to the flow of blood through these arteries we decided for our whole series of nearly 100 cadavers just to measure the rate at which water could be forced through the neck arteries from their origin in the chest to their termination inside the skull. This avoided any need to dissect the neck. We used a standard pressure of 140 mmHg, after relaxing post mortem spasm with ammonia.

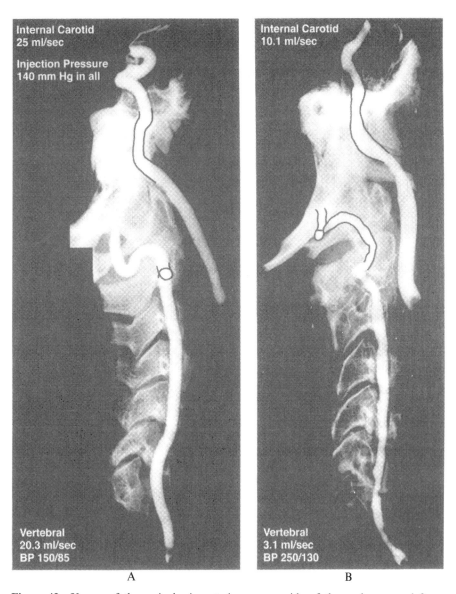

Internal Carotid
25 ml/sec

Injection Pressure
140 mm Hg in all

Internal Carotid
10.1 ml/sec

Vertebral
20.3 ml/sec
BP 150/85

Vertebral
3.1 ml/sec
BP 250/130

A   B

Figure 43 X-rays of the main brain arteries on one side of the neck removed from two human cadavers, showing the routes of the two arteries in relation to the bones of the neck (vertebrae) and the base of the skull. The vertebral arteries take a twisting looping course from their origin at the top of the chest to their termination inside the skull (at the top of the x-rays). **A** shows a normal vertebral and internal carotid artery in a 43 year-old woman with a near normal blood pressure. **B** is from a woman of 59 with severe hypertension and gross stenosis of both arteries by atheroma. The perfusion rates for each artery were measured as described in the text. Then a hot solution of gelatin containing X-ray-opaque barium sulphate powder was pumped in and allowed to set while a pressure of 140 mmHg was maintained until the x-rays had been taken.

345

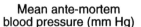

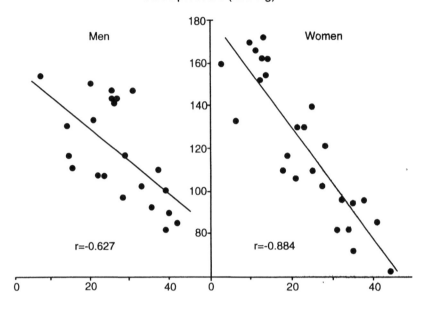

Figure 44 Correlation, in 22 male and 26 female cadavers, between the maximum rate of fluid flow in both vertebral arteries added together, at a standard pressure of 140 mmHg in all cases (as described in the text) and the mean blood pressure recorded in the hospital notes during life. The correlations for both men and women are highly significant. (Data from data of Dickinson CJ & Thomson AD, *Clin Sci* 1960;19:513–538).

The results were very exciting. We found that there was a close inverse relationship between the fluid-carrying capacity of the arteries, especially of the vertebral arteries in the neck, and the blood pressure in life, which a kind friend (Jack Howell) got independently for us from the hospital notes (Fig. 44). An equally close correlation was also apparent between the blood pressure recorded during life and the number and extent of visible lumps (plaques) of atheroma in the vertebral and basilar arteries supplying the brain stem. This measurement was simple to make once the brain had been removed from the skull. Similar comparisons of kidney artery calibre at the time of necropsy showed only a moderately close association with blood pressure during life. Similar measurements on the main leg (femoral) arteries showed almost no correlation between ante-mortem blood pressure and femoral artery fluid carrying capacity.

Scientists recognise that correlations and associations, however close, prove nothing. All one can say is that if someone was looking for a cause of essential hypertension, narrowing of the arteries supplying blood to the hindbrain would answer well. Although it is now generally accepted that narrowing of hindbrain arteries is closely associated with essential hypertension, most people would conclude that high blood pressure has caused the arterial narrowing rather than the other way round. This view cannot be faulted since in several situations hypertension can be shown to increase the deposition of atheroma and thus potentially make arteries narrower.

Apologia pro vita sua

It is a strange and sometimes uncomfortable feeling to find oneself, as I do in respect of the cause of essential hypertension, holding views which almost no one else accepts. But providing that a scientist has not committed the capital scientific crime of falsifying or inventing data, he can be respected if not believed if he can stand by his ideas and defend them in argument. Often there is no universally accepted theory to explain some phenomenon. Several theories seem plausible. This then creates an intellectual battlefield in which each group of scientists supporting a particular theory competes with other groups supporting different theories. Each group tries to find logical flaws and contradictions in alternative theories. Such contests can be very exciting, though it is sad when emotional proponents of a disproved theory cannot accept defeat.

The close involvement of the nervous system in hypertension, especially in its initiation, is now better recognised than it was at the time of our necropsy study. But as I mentioned earlier, many people think that psychological factors are much more important than physical factors. And many of those who reject psychological theories of essential hypertension give pride of place to the kidneys rather than to the brain. Readers of my next chapter will realise that although the brain can certainly raise blood pressure in the short term by increased sympathetic nervous activity, hypertension can only be sustained if the kidneys collaborate. They certainly have the means to do so. The sympathetic nerve supply to the kidneys can cause constriction of the small renal arteries. Furthermore, the secretion of the hormone vasopressin by the posterior pituitary gland at the base of the brain controls water handling by the kidneys. Both brain and kidneys must be involved in sustaining hypertension. But dispute continues to reign over which is the prime mover.

Most current ideas about the cause of hypertension are centred mainly on the circulating chemicals which alter the calibre of blood vessels and on the receptor chemicals with which they interact. Each year seems to bring new discoveries of 'vasoactive' chemicals – which alter the calibre of blood vessels. In the 1930s a protein from the kidneys (renin) was found to raise blood pressure when infused into animals. In the 1950s and 1960s this was observed to work by releasing a small polypeptide called 'angiotensin', which was at the time the most potent blood-pressure-raising material known. In 1988 another more potent polypeptide ('endothelin') was identified. This was produced by the cells lining blood vessels. At the time this was the most powerful blood vessel constrictor substance that had been identified. But in 1999 an even more potent chemical ('urotensin-II') was discovered (more accurately, rediscovered). It is very likely that more as yet unknown blood-pressure-controlling mechanisms will be identified in the future, as the 'curve of discovery' on p. 337 implies.

Many attempts have been made to link essential hypertension with genetic or acquired differences in some of these circulating chemicals and their receptors. During these investigations a number of specific single gene defects causing high blood pressure have been identified. But in the great majority of cases we still do not know what has gone wrong.

Animal models

In various centres, notably in Japan, the USA, New Zealand and Italy, attempts have been made to breed hypertensive rats so that the causes of high blood pressure could be better studied. By measuring the blood pressure of a group of rats and progressively mating the ones with the higher blood pressures with each other, inbred strains of hypertensive rat have been created. The best known was introduced in Japan more than 30 years ago, by Aoki and Okamoto. It is internationally known by and assigned the name 'SHR', which stands for 'spontaneously hypertensive rat'. It was derived from a parent strain, the 'Wistar-Kyoto' (WKY) rat, by selective inbreeding. I was present some years ago at the Fifth Annual International Symposium in Kyoto commemorating the creation of this rat. The traditional Japanese banquet was introduced by the singing of a song, with English words, celebrating the scientific contributions of the rat in question. The words and music may have been banal, but the occasion was bizarre, unique and unforgettable!

This rat strain has proved immensely useful for testing blood-pressure-lowering drugs. But I don't share the current universal enthusiasm for assuming that study of SHR tells us much reliably about the cause of human essential hypertension, even though – for example – there is a link between SHR and insulin resistance (the latter phenomenon known to be associated with essential hypertension). Grafting a kidney from a SHR into a WKY rat can raise the blood pressure of the WKY rat, and replacing the kidneys of a SHR with a WKY kidney lowers blood pressure. This may tell us a lot about rat hypertension. But even though some comparable observations have been made in man, they do not necessarily prove anything about the initiation of essential hypertension. They do not prove that essential hypertension has its origin in the kidneys.

Children with higher than average blood pressures tend to get higher than average blood pressures as adults, a phenomenon referred to as 'tracking'. But the effect is small. Essential hypertension usually starts to show itself in the third and fourth decades. Spontaneous hypertensive rats behave differently. The blood pressure of SHR begins to diverge substantially from that of WKY from the time of birth. There are many other differences between rats and humans in respect of blood pressure measurements. The strong current interest in the inbred hypertensive rat has skewed hypertension research very strongly away from man and towards the rat model. It seems to me more helpful to concentrate on the possible causes of blood pressure elevation in man which appear in the third and fourth decades.

None the less it is fascinating that although brain arteries in the spontaneously hypertensive rat are not affected by atheroma, they are smaller than in the parent WKY strain. Consequently, tying off a main brain artery of an inbred stroke-prone hypertensive rat produces much more extensive damage to the brain than tying off the equivalent artery in a rat with a normal blood pressure. This allows me to speculate that just possibly the hypertension of the inbred hypertensive rat may have something to do with its inadequate brain blood supply, as I have envisaged might be going on in essential hypertension in man.

Why does drug treatment of hypertension protect against strokes?

One particular reason why my views about structural lesions of brain arteries underlying essential hypertension are unacceptable to most people is that lowering blood pressure protects against strokes. This protection is well established. It is indeed the main reason for treating high blood pressure with drugs. The risk of strokes caused by arterial rupture and bleeding into the brain (cerebral haemorrhage) will obviously be less if the blood pressure is reduced by drugs. This is easy to understand. But the majority of strokes are not caused by bleeding but rather by cerebral infarction (Latin: *infartus* = something stuffed in, i.e. something obstructing cerebral blood supply). 'Infarct' is a technical medical term which is used to mean death of a tissue because of a critical reduction of local blood flow. It may be due to a local blood clot, or to an embolus – a clot formed elsewhere and swept in by the flowing blood. Although it seems paradoxical, drugs lowering blood pressure have been observed to protect both essential hypertensive humans and spontaneously hypertensive rats against cerebral infarction. I shall consider the reasons for this in Chapter 34.

Conclusion

To do justice in a brief review to all current ideas about the cause or causes of high blood pressure is impossible. I have summarised my own heretical views in two books and in many published articles. But someone wanting to explore in depth the better-established theories about this fascinating topic should consult a large multi-author review where all the vastly different views of different authors can be sampled.[5]

Hypertension is an extremely common condition. It can be effectively treated by a bewildering array of different drugs. Pharmaceutical companies are intensely interested in the cause of essential hypertension, in case its understanding will lead to better drugs being introduced. So it seems very unlikely that future research into this fascinating field will be curtailed by lack of money!

Summary

High blood pressure in the main arteries of the body is partly genetic, probably involving many genes. It is also partly environmental, being influenced by diet, especially salt intake. The main cause or causes of hypertension are unknown in most cases. Hypertension has a deleterious effect on health and lifespan, both of which are reduced in proportion to any sustained elevation of blood pressure.

Many possible causal mechanisms are currently under investigation. The inbred hypertensive rat (SHR) is the focus of much research. I doubt whether this animal is a good model for man. Human essential hypertension does not usually show itself until the third or fourth decade. It is accompanied by arterial disease, especially of the brain circulation. We do not know at present whether the arterial disease is cause or effect. If it is cause, it probably operates through the 'Cushing' response – the control of which is located in the brain stem. Cerebral arterial atheroma provides a plausible structural basis for elevated basal blood pressure in hypertension.

This is only one theory among many. There is no agreement among investigators about the cause of essential hypertension, though there is growing recognition that the central nervous system plays an important role. However, the kidneys are also necessarily involved in sustaining hypertension of any cause. Many people believe that the kidneys are more likely than the brain to initiate essential hypertension, for reasons which will be examined in the next chapter. The disagreements and uncertainties reflect one of medicine's greatest current mysteries.

32

HYPERTENSION FROM THE KIDNEYS

In the last chapter I summarised what is known about so-called 'essential' hypertension – high blood pressure of unknown cause. Although I emphasised what I believed to be the predominant role of the brain, I also recognised that most of the single causes of hypertension which have been identified involve the kidneys in some way. Indeed, many researchers believe that the kidney is the chief culprit even in essential hypertension, though this is hotly disputed. In this chapter I shall concentrate on those situations where sustained high blood pressure can reasonably be described as having a renal (Latin: *ren* = kidney) cause, even though the precise mechanisms involved may be disputed. I must apologise again for this chapter being somewhat autobiographical because I have been personally as interested in renal as in essential hypertension. But I will try to provide an unbiased account.

The functional anatomy of the kidneys

The two kidneys lie at the back of the upper abdomen on each side of the vertebral column. Each comprises approximately one million similar units known as 'nephrons' (Greek: *nephros* = kidney). Each nephron contains a 'glomerulus' (Latin: *glomus* = ball, of yarn or wool), so named because it is a closely packed ball of capillary blood vessels. These hold back cells and protein molecules in the blood flowing through them but let small molecules in solution – glucose and urea, and metal ions like sodium and potassium – pass out through their walls. The capsule which surrounds each glomerulus collects the fluid filtered off from the blood (the glomerular filtrate: see Fig. 45). This is still under a positive pressure, which drives it along a convoluted tubule. Each tubule joins up with tubules from other nephrons. Eventually the larger tubules (collecting ducts) empty into the pelvis (reservoir) of each kidney, from which urine flows into the bladder, via the ureters.

Vast quantities of blood pass through the kidneys each day (about 150 gallons) and similarly vast quantities of fluid are filtered out into

353

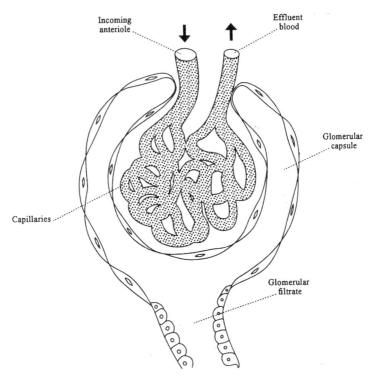

Figure 45 Diagram of a glomerulus – one of the million nephrons within each human kidney – showing the incoming (afferent) arteriole bringing blood to the glomerulus, and the outgoing (efferent) arteriole taking blood away to supply the tubule system.

the tubules (about 40 gallons). Almost all of this is reabsorbed back into the bloodstream, leaving a residue of urine of only 2–3 pints (about 1200 cc) daily for an average fluid intake. One day's glomerular filtrate contains more than 2 pounds weight of salt, but almost all of this is also reabsorbed from the tubules, together with the water. This leaves only about $\frac{1}{2}$ ounce weight of salt (15 g) to be excreted in the urine each day. Over long periods of time the urinary salt excretion is the same as the amount of salt in the diet, less the amount lost in sweat, other secretions and in faeces.

The processes of salt and water reabsorption require energy. At rest about one fifth of the total energy consumption of the body is expended by the kidneys, mostly by the chemical processes actively reabsorbing salt from the glomerular filtrate. The whole process seems incredibly wasteful of energy, but it allows extremely flexible adjustments of kidney function in response to changes in diet and to inter-current disease.

Kidney diseases raising the blood pressure

Richard Bright, a physician at Guy's Hospital in London, reported in 1836 that some people suffering from kidney disease had a pulse which was 'full and hard'. When the sphygmomanometer was invented an association was quickly recognised between kidney disease and high blood pressure. Almost any kind of kidney disease can be associated with hypertension, but it is often difficult to prove in most cases that the disease is responsible for raising the blood pressure. Most medical kidney diseases affect both kidneys. Both organs obviously cannot be removed to see whether they are causing hypertension, because at least one functioning kidney is essential for life. However, a raised blood pressure can often be brought back to normal, for a time at least, by replacing diseased kidneys with one normal one.

Apart from narrowing of the main renal artery, the commonest serious kidney diseases accompanied by high blood pressure are various forms of chronic glomerulonephritis. These will be further discussed in the next chapter. In these diseases the delicate filters of the kidneys become inflamed, damaged, and eventually destroyed. When the kidney of someone in an active phase of glomerulonephritis is examined under the microscope (which can be done in life by taking a minute biopsy specimen with a needle) the filters of the kidney (the glomeruli) are thickened. Inflammatory cells are abundant and the small arteries leading to the glomeruli are narrowed. Life can continue even if only 10% or even fewer kidney units are still working. Thus the greater parts of both kidneys have to be destroyed before there is any life-threatening failure to excrete the body's waste products. One clue to glomerulonephritis is 'proteinuria', the appearance of undue quantities of protein in the urine. This is caused by breaks in the glomerular basement membranes, i.e. in the filters themselves.

The end stage of chronic glomerulonephritis looks very much like the end stage of severe untreated essential hypertension. In both cases the failure of the excretory function of the kidneys can lead to death from renal excretory failure unless a kidney transplant can be done in time. Most patients with long-standing glomerulonephritis have a raised blood pressure, sometimes even before there is substantial damage to the glomeruli.

The definitive animal experiments on renal hypertension were done by Harry Goldblatt. When I lived for a year in Cleveland, Ohio, I

355

heard Goldblatt deliver his famous lecture describing how he came to create hypertension in dogs by interfering with the blood supply to their kidneys. He was a pathologist who had looked through the microscope at slices of kidneys from people who had died from complications of high blood pressure. He had observed that all the small arteries leading to the glomeruli were narrowed. Their muscular walls were thickened. He thought that perhaps constriction of the blood supply to the kidneys might have in some way caused high blood pressure. He wanted to imitate nature experimentally, but realised that he could not possibly put constricting clips on all the many thousands of minute arteries in each of the two kidneys. So he devised a marvellously ingenious but simple experiment. Under a general anaesthetic he exposed both kidneys of dogs, then put constricting clips across both main kidney arteries so that the blood flow would be reduced, but not actually cut off. (Cutting off all blood supply to a kidney would obviously just make the kidney die.) The blood pressure of dogs with constricting renal artery clips rose and stayed up. If he took the constricting clips off, the blood pressure fell back to normal. Goldblatt reckoned that he had got an exact model of sustained high blood pressure in man. Many people still agree with him. His experiments have been duplicated in many mammalian species. Main renal artery stenosis (Greek: *stenos* = narrow) is one of the best recognised causes of high blood pressure in man.

Causes of renal hypertension

At least three renal mechanisms can raise the blood pressure. All appear to be simple, yet the more closely one looks at any of them, the less simple they become. I shall describe them briefly under three headings:

1. Failure to excrete salt and water adequately;
2. Overproduction of the blood-pressure-raising hormone 'renin';
3. Failure to produce enough of a blood-pressure-lowering hormone, e.g. 'medulli(pi)n'.

Failure to excrete enough salt and water

Destruction of many kidney nephrons by disease or by an inadequate blood supply will obviously reduce the amount of blood filtered. But at the same time much less fluid and salt will be reabsorbed from the convoluted tubules because of 'osmotic diuresis' (p. 480). This is due to the high concentrations of dissolved materials in the blood and in the glomerular filtrate. These materials are protein waste products, mainly urea. This is the situation in the early stages of progressive kidney disease. The daily urine volume is substantially normal. It is in balance with fluid intake. Only in the later stages of kidney disease does the urine volume decrease.

If someone with renal excretory failure continues to drink and eat normally the body will start to accumulate excess water and salt once about 90% of all the nephrons have been lost and kidney function is down to 10% of normal. At this stage there may be what used to be called 'dropsy'. The medical term is oedema – swelling of the ankles by fluid under the skin and which can be indented and moved about by gentle pressure. Tissue fluid is not static. It is in a state of dynamic equilibrium with the circulating blood. If salt and water are retained in the body the volume of the blood also increases. By a process which is not fully understood even today this leads to a rise in blood pressure. A simple way of explaining what is happening is to look at Figure 29 (p. 234), which summarises the observations that Jon Thompson and I made when we perfused excised rabbit kidneys with blood at different pressures.[1] The higher the perfusion pressure the faster the excretion of water and also of salt. In life the curve is steeper still. It is easy to see how the body might compensate for failing to excrete salt and water by putting up the arterial blood pressure supplying the kidneys. This would then allow the usual dietary intake of salt and water to be excreted. Stability would be regained.

Severe excretory failure of the kidneys has to raise the blood pressure. If it didn't, the retained fluid would make the body swell up. Harmful waste products would accumulate. But why does an increase in the volume of the blood raise the arterial blood pressure?

I have had the inestimable privilege during the last 40 years of friendship with Arthur Guyton, the former Professor of Physiology and Biophysics at Jackson, Mississippi, who died in 2003. I always regarded him, as many others did, as the greatest and most original circulatory physiologist in the world. We first met in 1961 when I made a pilgrimage to see him in Jackson. We met on many occasions since, in London and at international meetings around the world. He enjoyed arguments as much as I did. He always insisted that the kidneys were the ultimate long-term arbiters of blood pressure because they had 'infinite gain', i.e. in the long-term, blood pressure level had always to be determined by kidney function. Kidney function would in the long run overwhelm all other stabilising mechanisms. The hyper-tension of blood volume expansion was the consequence of what Guyton called 'whole body autoregulation'. This is complicated to

357

explain, but it follows old observations in Holland of the hypertension which can follow eating too much liquorice, which was in use at the time for the treatment of peptic ulcers. Liquorice contains a chemical which makes the kidneys retain salt and water. Guyton's arguments are set forth clearly in his books and articles.[2] Most people have accepted his views, though the curious involvement of the nervous system in this type of hypertension remains a mystery. I was never able to persuade Arthur that the brain might be in charge and able to overrule the kidneys! The truth remains for future generations to determine.

Guyton's classic experiment is worth mentioning. In its simplicity and elegance it is a match for Goldblatt's renal artery clips. Under general anaesthesia Guyton and his colleagues removed one kidney from a dog and also cut out two thirds of the bulk of the remaining kidney. After recovery from the anaesthetic the dog continued to drink water and eat normally. Its blood pressure remained normal. But when salt was added to the drinking water, and nothing else was changed, the blood pressure rapidly rose and remained high until the extra salt was withdrawn, after which blood pressure went back to normal.

Armed with the knowledge which this and comparable experiments provides, doctors treating advanced kidney disease pay great attention to their patients' intake of salt. No one can doubt that overload of the body with salt can cause hypertension, even though some of the details still need to be worked out. Curiously some people are sensitive to salt excess and easily get high blood pressure whereas others seem to be resistant. Similar differences have been noted in different strains of rat. A well-known English professor of medicine, the late George Pickering (whom I have already mentioned in another context) was notably dismissive of the idea that eating salt could raise blood pressure. At lunch I have myself watched him sprinkling lots of salt on his food without a care in the world. He was lucky to have had a genetic constitution which could easily excrete excess salt.

Although changes in blood volume in Guyton's dog experiment were undoubtedly the eventual cause of changes in blood pressure, the blood volume changes were obviously due to the extra salt. If the concentration of salt in the blood rises there is increased thirst. The posterior pituitary gland in the brain sends a chemical message to the kidneys to retain water until the concentration of salt is normal again. Thus, salt and water go hand in hand, though water follows salt rather than the other way round. The medical treatment of excessive fluid accumulation, such as occurs with heart failure, (Chapter 21) usually involves giving drugs (diuretics) which make the kidneys excrete more salt and water.

Renin and angiotensin

Adjacent to each outer glomerulus in each kidney is a tiny collection of cells known as the 'juxta-glomerular apparatus'. This is a ductless gland which secretes, into the blood flowing through it, two hormones. One is concerned with red blood cell formation (erythropoietin). The other is importantly linked with blood pressure control. It is a protein called 'renin', which is an enzyme (a catalyst) which turns an inactive circulating material produced mainly in the liver (angiotensinogen), into a small polypeptide (angiotensin I) which is further changed by another (converting) enzyme into 'angiotensin II', one of the most powerful blood-pressure-raising agents known. There is a true story of the derivation of this hybrid name. Two rival groups of scientists were working on the same material at the same time, one calling it 'angio-tonin' and the other 'hypertensin'. They met at breakfast while both were attending an international meeting, split their differences, and agreed to call the substance 'angiotensin'.

One way of making the kidney produce large amounts of renin is to restrict its blood supply, e.g. by putting a constricting 'Goldblatt' clip on the main renal artery. This sharply raises the blood pressure of any rat, rabbit or dog in which this has been done. I have seen the comparable experiment in nature when a blood clot detached itself from the heart wall of one of my patients and almost completely blocked one main kidney artery. As in the animal experiments, blood pressure rose rapidly and only went back to normal after the offending clot had been removed.

Angiotensin II is a small polypeptide (p. 476) containing eight amino-acids. When infused into the bloodstream of any animal, it constricts arteries and raises the blood pressure. This has been established in human volunteers as well as in animals. Figure 46 is a personal record of the effects on blood pressure of continually infusing pure angiotensin II at a high rate into a rabbit's leg vein over a period of three days. The blood pressure rose to a plateau where it remained until the infusion was stopped.

Everything then seemed simple and straightforward. The hypertension caused by narrowing of the main kidney artery is a well-recognised cause of sustained hypertension in animals and in man. It seemed reasonable to ascribe it to a circulating excess of renin and angiotensin. But there was a snag. Careful measurements of the amounts of renin or angiotensin in the blood, either of animals or man with hypertension and narrowed renal arteries, showed that the amounts present were not enough to raise the blood pressure significantly. So people started looking for some other factor.

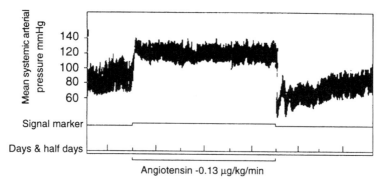

Figure 46 A six-day record of the mean blood pressure of a rabbit made with a servo-manometer. During the 3 days indicated by the signal marker angiotensin II was infused intravenously at a high constant rate. The blood pressure went up rapidly by about 40 mmHg, remained steady for 3 days, then dropped immediately when the infusion was stopped. Damped oscillations with a 4-hour period continued as the blood pressure slowly returned to its control level over the ensuing 2 days.

While pondering this apparent anomaly I had the idea that maybe renin secretion was only switched on when the perfusion of blood through a kidney was reduced and that it was turned off again when blood pressure rose. Perhaps this might explain why there did not seem to be enough renin and angiotensin present to account for the hypertension. I thought that perhaps once an animal had got used to having a raised blood pressure it could bring other mechanisms into play to keep the blood pressure up. To test this hypothesis I constructed a somewhat complicated piece of hydro-electric equipment which continuously sampled a conscious rabbit's blood pressure and which made the intravenous infusion rate of angiotensin II inversely proportional to the animal's blood pressure at any moment.

The effects were spectacular. It was just about the most exciting piece of research I have ever carried out. Over a period of 2–3 days the delivery rate of angiotensin went steadily down at the same time that the blood pressure steadily rose. Later Jim Lawrence and I[3] found that it was simpler just to infuse angiotensin at a very low ('sub-pressor') rate, below that which initially produced any detectable rise of blood pressure. Over the next few days the blood pressure progressively rose. One of our records is shown in Figure 47. Richard Yu and I subsequently found that these sub-pressor infusions of angiotensin had in some way activated the sympathetic nervous system.[4] I thought that this might be because angiotensin had constricted the brain arteries (as it is known to do). I tried to prove this by infusing angiotensin at very

360

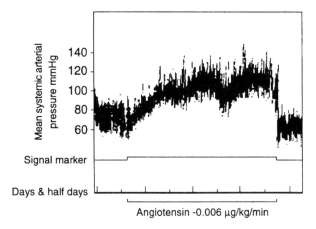

Figure 47 A 4–5 day record made in the same way as in Figure 46, but showing the contrasted and different effect of infusing a *low* concentration of angiotensin at a rate which had no immediate effect on blood pressure. The average blood pressure slowly climbed up by about 35 mmHg over 3 days, but dropped sharply when the infusion was turned off.

low rates directly into the arteries supplying the brain stem in rabbits. This also proved to be a spectacular experiment. It raised blood pressure tremendously, though not in the way I had anticipated. The experiment was serendipitous. The underlying hypothesis was mostly incorrect. The main effect of infusing angiotensin into the arterial supply of the brain stem was a direct stimulation of nerve cells (neurones) in the centres controlling the sympathetic nervous system, rather than an indirect effect mediated through arterial constriction.[5]

> Recent work has established that angiotensin II has important effects on heart function, independently of its power to constrict arteries. In addition to the well known conversion of angiotensin I to angiotensin II by the enzyme known as 'angiotensin-converting enzyme' (ACE), another converting enzyme known as ACE2 has different effects. Some of these antagonise the constricting effects of angiotensin II and improve heart function.[6]

Other mechanisms of renal hypertension: The 'depressor' system

Although salt and water overload and/or renin oversecretion explain most forms of renal hypertension, other observations show that the central part (medulla) of normal kidneys secrete a blood-pressure-lowering factor ('medullipin').[7] Damage or removal of this part of the kidney can raise blood pressure, and (rare) tumours secreting medullipin can reveal themselves by excessively lowering blood pressure. Lack of medullipin probably contributes to hypertension in many cases of renal disease.

Other mysteries of renal hypertension

Perhaps my explanations of those renal hypertensive mechanisms on which I have worked myself have made them seem unduly simple. Alas, this is not so. I have only given the barest outline of an enormous subject. A host of different materials – the steroid hormones and a chemical from the heart increasing the kidneys' excretion of salt ('atrial natriuretic factor') – indirectly influence blood pressure. The well-known heart drug digoxin is now known to have close chemical and pharmacological similarities with a naturally occurring circulating material identical or almost identical with the plant derivative 'oubain'. This material affects kidney as well as heart function. The relationship between angiotensin and the central nervous system is only beginning to be explored, as we realise that angiotensin is itself an important neurotransmitter within the brain.

The way in which an animal gradually adapts to a blood-pressure-raising stimulus (such as the low-dose angiotensin infusion already described) involves many changes. Over long periods, small arteries gradually get narrower. Heart muscle becomes thicker and many other changes occur which allow hypertension to be sustained with little evidence remaining of its initiating factor. These adaptive changes make it extremely difficult to decide which change is primary, and which secondary.

The study of renal hypertension has been of immense clinical value. The many animal experiments which have revealed the underlying mechanisms have resulted in the synthesis of angiotensin converting enzyme inhibitors (e.g. captopril) and of 'angiotensin receptor blocking drugs' (ARBs, e.g. losartan). These are useful in many conditions other than renal hypertension, e.g. in heart failure and diabetes. The story continues to unfold. Plenty of mysteries remain to be solved.

Summary

Kidney disease is often associated with high blood pressure. Three mechanisms (at least) may be responsible: renal excretory failure, especially of salt and water; overproduction of renin and hence of angiotensin; lack of production of medullipin, the renal medullary hormone.

Renal excretory failure expands the volume of circulating blood which leads to hypertension by a process which has been described as 'whole body auto-regulation'. Although there may be very little renin circulating in many varieties of renal hypertension, renin generates angiotensin, a powerful hormone raising blood pressure. Angiotensin exerts a slowly developing, partly neurogenic, action which increases over many days. Consequently, very small amounts of angiotensin acting over many days may eventually sustain high blood pressure. In addition, the central part (medulla) of each kidney produces a blood-pressure-lowering factor, medullipin. Deficiency of this material may also play a part in producing 'renal' hypertension.

33

KIDNEY FAILURE: CHRONIC GLOMERULONEPHRITIS

In the last chapter I described the anatomy and overall function of the kidneys. I mentioned that each human kidney contains about a million units (nephrons) tightly packed together. Each nephron contains a filter (glomerulus) inside a capsule. Each is supplied by arterial blood under pressure. The filtrate passes to a collecting system of convoluted tubes (tubules) which join up and empty their final product (the urine) into the bladder. The energy for the filtering process is supplied by the heart, which pumps up the blood perfusing the kidneys to some 3 feet of water pressure (about 90 mmHg). Some 40 gallons (170 litres) are filtered off from the bloodstream every day. Most fluid is taken back into the bloodstream as the filtrate passes along the kidney tubules. 'Renal' (kidney) failure is defined by a reduction in the rate at which waste products are filtered off from the blood by the glomeruli. This is the 'glomerular filtration rate' (GFR).

Glomerular filtration rate is expressed as the volume of blood cleared of some easily measured waste protein product in a fixed interval of time. GFR can be most accurately measured using a substance – the starch-like plant product inulin is the traditional standard – which is neither secreted nor reabsorbed by the tubules. The technique is tedious and time-consuming. It requires special measurement techniques for inulin, which has to be continuously infused to achieve a level concentration during the procedure. Other substances, including radioactively labelled synthetic compounds (EDTA and DTPA), have also been used. But glomerular filtration rate is most often assessed indirectly from the concentration in the blood of some body constituent filtered by the glomeruli, which is not absorbed by the tubules, and which builds up as GFR falls. Creatinine (a nitrogen-containing waste product derived from proteins) is most often used. Measurement of blood urea concentration is less accurate because it is affected much more by diet than is creatinine. A normal value for plasma creatinine is about 120 µmol/l in both sexes (1.0 mg per 100 ml). This corresponds to a GFR of 120 ml/min: that is, at this rate of glomerular filtration 120 millilitres of plasma would be entirely cleared of creatinine each minute. Students often find the concepts of glomerular clearance and glomerular filtration rate difficult to grasp. The concept seems artificial. Each functioning glomerulus filters off some creatinine. No glomerulus filters off all creatinine coming to it. But we can describe the average function of all glomeruli as if some were doing all the work and the others none.

Lung function is described in a comparable way (Chapter 1) by imagining that some alveoli are ventilated but not perfused with blood (this is the 'dead space'), some are perfused but not ventilated (this is the 'venous admixture'), and some have ventilation perfectly matched to perfusion.

The normal GFR in a fit young adult is about 120 ml per minute. It rises during consumption of a high protein diet and falls when protein intake is restricted. After age 30 it falls gradually throughout life as functioning nephron units are gradually lost. By the age of 80 the average GFR has fallen to about 70 ml/min. But since life can be maintained with only 10% or less of kidney function, the usual rate of attrition of initially healthy kidneys poses no threat to life.

In the first stage of 'chronic' (i.e. longstanding) kidney failure the only measurable abnormalities are a decrease in GFR and a small rise in the concentration of various protein waste products in the blood. At this stage a patient may not have any symptoms or complaints. When the GFR has fallen to about 30 ml/minute (plasma creatinine concentration about 400 μmol/l) – a situation described as 'early' renal failure – there may be a few mild symptoms such as impaired appetite or tiredness. Someone with a GFR between 10 and 15 ml/minute can usually enjoy a reasonable lifestyle, with the help of various compensatory and adaptive mechanisms. Especially if the kidney failure has come on very gradually a patient may assume that tiredness and loss of appetite is just due to the ageing process. But someone with a GFR below 10 ml/min (plasma creatinine concentration above about 800 μmol/l) – a state described as 'late' renal failure – really starts to feel ill. High concentrations of urea and other waste products in the blood cause nausea and vomiting. A common symptom in people with a GFR below about 30 ml/minute is passing a lot of urine (polyuria) and often having to get up at night to pass urine. This seems anomalous, but it results from damaged kidneys being unable to concentrate urine adequately. It leads to increased thirst and may lead to serious dehydration in hot surroundings.

High blood pressure is often associated with and sometimes caused by an impaired blood circulation to the kidneys, as I have discussed in the last chapter. But even minor degrees of kidney filtration failure – not bad enough to cause any symptoms – increase the average rate of discharge of impulses by the sympathetic nervous system. This may raise the blood pressure and may also increase liability to arterial disease. In neither case do we entirely understand the underlying pathological sequence of events.

Breathlessness in chronic kidney disease can be caused by anaemia, which may also be due to kidney disease. The kidneys normally secrete into the bloodstream the hormone 'erythropoietin' (Greek: *erythros* = red; *poiesis* = making), which stimulates the bone marrow to increase the rate at which it is making red blood cells. Recently there has been much publicity about competitive athletes caught giving themselves injections of 'EPO' (i.e. erythropoeitin) to increase their blood concentration of haemoglobin and thus the oxygen-carrying capacity of their blood.

'End-stage' renal failure usually means that the GFR is around 5 ml/min (plasma creatinine concentration greater than 1200 μmol/l). It is associated with a large variety of unpleasant symptoms, particularly from the gut. Morning nausea, loss of appetite (anorexia), and vomiting are characteristic. There may be bone pain and undue itching of the skin. Many years ago, in days before artificial kidney treatment was available, I watched some five of my patients die of terminal renal failure, in hospital. I remember how helpless I felt at that time, able to relieve a few of their symptoms but unable to arrest or reverse their disease. Death came from fluid overload and lung oedema, but also from sudden cardiac arrest due to potassium intoxication (hyperkalaemia) and from inflammation and fluid secretion into the pericardium (the fibrous bag which contains the heart).

The most dramatic patient with end-stage renal failure I have ever seen was a Sudanese man called Omer Beleil. He had qualified as a doctor in Khartoum and came to Britain for further surgical training. When I first met him he was 29 years old. He had already gained the English FRCS diploma, winning the Hallett prize against worldwide competition. He was having further training in neurosurgery at University College Hospital in London. The reason I feel that I may properly mention him by name is that after he had got better he wrote and published in the USA his autobiography, entitled *Two Lives*,[1] describing his life before and after his kidney transplant.

One day, in 1968, he had felt slightly unwell, tested his own urine and found an excess of protein in it. He came to consult me at University College Hospital in London, where we were both working. The waste products in his blood were only slightly raised. The X-rays of his kidneys looked normal. But to make an accurate diagnosis I decided to 'biopsy' one of his kidneys (i.e. take a tiny piece of tissue out under local anaesthesia, with a hollow needle). I was horrified when our pathologist reported that the specimen showed very severe

367

chronic glomerulonephritis (inflammation of the glomeruli). Omer and I both knew that this disease would be present in both kidneys, that it would rapidly progress and that there was no available treatment. The prospects for a foreign national getting long-term dialysis or transplantation in London at this time were negligible. Omer consulted his wife and resolved to return to Sudan, so that he might die in the bosom of his family before he reached end-stage kidney failure. He flew back home with his wife and daughter. I did not expect to see him again.

A few months later I was phoned by the Professor of Medicine in Khartoum to say that he had put Omer on a flight back to London. The Sudanese Embassy collected him from Heathrow and brought him straight to me at University College Hospital. He arrived almost moribund, extremely short of breath, with pink froth bubbling from his mouth. His lungs were grossly congested with blood and fluid. We put a catheter in his abdominal (peritoneal) cavity and flushed through large volumes of a strong sugar solution – a procedure known as 'hypertonic peritoneal dialysis'.[2] His breathlessness improved within an hour or two. A few days later, as we had no facilities at that time in my hospital for the long-term management of people with terminal renal failure, I transferred him to the care of Stan Peart at St Mary's Hospital. He was given further artificial kidney treatment there, followed by a kidney transplant from a cadaver. Unfortunately this failed to work properly, but Omer's brother most generously donated one of his own kidneys, which was sucessfully transplanted.

Omer Beleil lived nearly twenty more years, had a son, and abandoned neurosurgery for renal transplant surgery. He became in due course Professor of Surgery, Dean of the Khartoum Medical School and eventually Vice-Chancellor of the University.

I have performed many renal biopsies myself and have looked after many people with chronic renal failure. The outlook for such patients is much better now than it used to be, but the UK has lagged behind Europe. All doctors want to save lives, but none can be so certain of doing so as those who look after people with end-stage renal failure. I remember being astonished in Heidelberg twenty-five years ago to hear that a German finding himself threatened by imminent death from chronic renal failure could successfully demand and get chronic dialysis treatment from the State as of right. Things are better now in Britain, but there is still an urgent need to find out more about the causes of progressive glomerulonephritis, so that it may be prevented or arrested before it reaches an irreversible stage.

The significance of protein in the urine

As blood flows through the million or so glomeruli in each kidney, water and dissolved material pass through the semi-permeable glomerular membranes into the tubule system. Particles such as red blood cells and large protein molecules are too big to get through the microscopic holes (pores) in the glomerular membranes. Furthermore, some protein molecules such as albumin are negatively charged and are repelled by negative charges on the surface of the glomerular capillary membranes. But if the delicate filtering membranes of the glomeruli are damaged, or lose their electrical charge, proteins and even whole blood cells may leak out of the glomeruli, reach the collecting system and appear in the urine.

The great majority of kidney diseases in some way involve inflammation and lead to an excess of protein appearing in the urine, as in Omer Beleil's case. Chronic renal failure occurring without any protein excess in the urine is unusual. It strongly suggests that the kidneys themselves are probably normal but that there is some problem in their blood supply, e.g. because of large artery narrowing or an impacted blood clot, or because of low blood pressure due to extensive blood loss.

Epidemiology of chronic renal failure

Severe chronic renal failure is rare in children, but its incidence gradually increases during adult life. Current estimates suggest that in the UK about 150 people in every million will reach end-stage kidney failure each year. It is about twice as common in undeveloped countries as in Europe and North America, though there are no overwhelming differences in the incidence and types of chronic renal failure across the world. Because renal transplantation and medical therapy are so successful in keeping people alive, the national financial burden of renal disease is steadily increasing. The prevalence of end-stage renal failure (i.e. the absolute number of people with a kidney transplant, or receiving regular dialysis) has been growing by about 5% per year in all developed countries. It has not yet reached a plateau.

Some form of glomerular disease is present in more than a third of patients with end-stage renal failure. Most of this is 'glomerulonephritis', i.e. inflammation of the glomeruli, but diabetes (see Chapter 14) accounts for about a fifth of all cases. The kidneys seem specially susceptible to damage from many chemicals, from virus and bacterial infections and from damage by the body's own immune mechanisms.

Causes of chronic kidney failure

Two main kinds of chronic renal failure are easy to understand and can hardly be classified as medical mysteries. I have mentioned failure of the kidneys' blood supply, a situation often referred to as 'pre-renal' renal failure. For example, I have seen the level of creatinine rise above 750 μmol/l in a man during the week following his severe heart attack, when the blood pressure was low and he was passing very little urine. But after heart function recovered, kidney function also returned to normal. I have also seen many situations, mostly following protracted vomiting or diarrhoea, in which waste products in the blood rose to damaging levels simply because of severe depletion of salt and water, with a consequent reduction in circulating blood volume. I have also inadvertently brought this situation about myself and have seen it develop several times in hospital by overenthusiastic use of a strong 'diuretic' drug such as frusemide. When this happens a physician has to swallow his pride, admit his error, and put up an intravenous catheter to infuse salt and water as fast as possible, to save his patient's life.

Another obvious cause of longstanding renal failure is obstruction to the outflow of urine. In men this is almost always due to progressive enlargement of the prostate gland. It is extremely common. Few men reach their eighties without at least some symptoms of enlargement of the prostate. Symptoms may begin at a much younger age. Women have no structure comparable to the prostate gland. They seldom get 'post-renal' (i.e. obstructive) kidney failure; but I have seen two cases of chronic renal failure in women caused by blockage of both ureters (the tubes leading from kidneys to bladder) by a spreading cancer of the ovary. In undeveloped countries where cancer of the neck of the womb (cervix) is the commonest cancer in women, death is often caused by kidney failure from local spread of that cancer to obstruct the ureters.

Although specific kidney diseases sometimes predominantly involve the tubule system, diseases of the glomeruli are much more common. Glomerulonephritis (inflammation of the kidney filters) is the main cause of 'renal', as opposed to 'pre-' or 'post-' renal failure. But before discussing specific causes of glomerulonephritis, I want to draw attention to an aspect of kidney physiology which is often overlooked but which may explain why kidney function tends to decline with time, and why it declines so quickly and relentlessly when a certain stage has been reached.

Glomerular hypertension

In the 1980s, Barry Brenner[3] in the USA drew attention to the overwhelming importance of the pressure inside the glomerular capillaries and to the damaging consequences of too high a pressure (glomerular hypertension). Glomerular pressure depends on the resultant of inflow pressure (i.e. arterial blood pressure at the aorta), the resistance of the 'afferent' arterioles (i.e. the very small arteries bringing blood to the glomeruli), the resistance of the 40 or so folded capillaries inside each glomerular capsule, the resistance of the 'efferent' arterioles (the vessels taking blood away from the glomeruli), and the pressure in the kidney veins taking blood back to the heart. The functional anatomy is summarised diagrammatically in Figure 45 (p. 354). Most of the details of kidney function have been worked out in animals, mainly rats. It is possible by means of ultra-thin needles or glass micropipettes to sample fluids or blood at every point in rats' nephrons and to estimate flow rates.

Such studies have shown that afferent and efferent arterioles each contribute about the same resistance to blood flow. The walls of both sets of arterioles contain circular muscle which can narrow the vessels when it contracts under the influence of its nerve supply or circulating chemicals. The nerve supply of the arterioles and the sympathetic neurotransmitter chemical (noradrenaline) can constrict all renal arterioles. Some circulating materials, notably glucose, dilate afferent arterioles selectively, thus increasing glomerular pressure. (This is probably the main factor contributing to kidney damage in diabetes.) Drugs which selectively dilate efferent arterioles and reduce efferent resistance, without having much effect on afferent arterioles (notably the so-called ACE inhibitor drugs) have the opposite effect. They lower glomerular pressure and reduce the leak of small protein molecules like albumin. If the glomerular pressure is not lowered too much – so that filtration ceases – such drugs give the kidneys powerful protection. Medical treatment of high blood pressure is well known to protect against strokes, as I shall discuss in the next chapter. But it also gives some protection against progressive kidney failure[4] by lowering glomerular capillary pressure.

Normal glomerular capillary pressure is about 30 mmHg – less than half the pressure in the aorta and major arteries. This is finely balanced against the flow resistance of the efferent arterioles and the effluent pressure in the veins. In addition, the osmotic pressure of the plasma impedes glomerular filtration. It is a force tending to suck fluid out of the glomerular capsule back into the bloodstream. Since the glomeruli are passive filters, a rise in glomerular capillary pressure can obviously

371

compensate for a decline in the number of functioning kidney units. There is much evidence that simple removal of functioning renal mass, e.g. by cutting out one kidney (nephrectomy), raises the pressure in the glomeruli of the remaining kidney and allows normal GFR to be regained – but at a price.

After one kidney has been removed the remaining kidney grows bigger. Some 'message' must presumably pass to the remaining kidney, instructing it to get bigger and increase the average pressure in its glomeruli. We do not know where the message arises. It is tempting to think that it comes from some organ or structure which detects impaired GFR, probably by the blood concentration of some waste product. Regulation of GFR could be entirely local if the afferent arterioles were the sensors, but somehow this seems improbable. It seems to me much more likely that the brain is in control. Through its sympathetic nervous innervation of the renal arterioles it has all the means necessary to control average glomerular pressure. I would therefore guess that the sensor lies somewhere in the brain, but I have no idea in what part.

Investigation of slow long-term physiological changes is difficult. But it could be rewarding if a way could be found to switch off some of these potentially damaging compensatory reactions. We already know how beneficial ACE inhibitor drugs can be in many situations, notably in diabetes.

The ingredients of a horrible vicious circle appear once renal failure has reached a certain point. Most patients with GFRs less than 25 ml/minute will eventually need long-term dialysis or transplantation, whatever was the original cause of the kidney damage. At this stage progression of renal failure cannot usually be stopped even if its original cause has been removed. Relentless progression towards terminal renal failure can be slowed down by restricting dietary protein, but physicians nowadays are reluctant to advise this because it leads to deterioration in so many other parts of the body and makes the patient less able to take the stress of transplant surgery.

Glomerular capillaries have more than ten times the number of sieve holes per unit area than capillaries elsewhere in the body. This property, and their situation – lying loosely within a capsule – probably makes them uniquely vulnerable to high pressure injury, compared to capillaries in all other organs and tissues. Any undue rise in intraglomerular pressure can lead to increased leak of protein through the glomerular capillary walls. This can in turn damage the tubules downstream.

Many otherwise useful drugs can damage the kidneys. Even the humble aspirin is not all that humble. It is an extremely powerful drug. There is strong suspicion that aspirin and other analgesics like acetaminophen can under some circumstances cause or aggravate chronic renal failure by damaging the kidney tubules.[5]

Chronic glomerulonephritis

The other major mystery in chronic renal failure is the initial causation of glomerular inflammation, which eventually leads to infiltration by inflammatory cells with swelling, obstruction and ultimately complete failure of filtering function. We know that certain cytokines are released from circulating monocytes, especially 'TNFα'.[6] This is a protein that seems to have no function other than to destroy tissues with which it comes into contact.

Viruses or bacteria infecting the kidneys arrive through the bloodstream. The enormous flow of blood through the renal glomeruli gives every opportunity for damaging agents to settle there. It is not always the immediate damage by infecting agents that leads to chronic renal failure but often the body's immunological reactions to them. Some circulating antigen + antibody complexes are large molecule aggregates which stick in the glomerular capillaries. When this happens in capillaries elsewhere it doesn't matter much because the body's repair processes will in due course remove the material. But in the kidneys, solid material which accumulates inside glomerular capsules may not be able to escape.

'Acute nephritis' (acute post-streptococcal glomerulonephritis) is an example of a rapidly developing immune response by the body to an infective agent. It is a disease predominantly of childhood which follows a week or two after a throat infection with group A Type 12 streptococci bacteria. These contain antigens (chemicals able to stimulate immunological defence reactions) which resemble parts of the proteins in the basement membranes of glomerular capillaries. The defence reaction – the generation of antibodies against the bacterial invaders – has the unfortunate side effect that the body finds its defensive armoury turned upon itself. The glomeruli may not themselves be infected by the bacteria. They become inflamed because they are attacked by the body's own defensive antibodies. Full recovery usually follows an attack of acute glomerulonephritis, but in a few cases the inflammation of the glomeruli does not clear up and the stage is set for relentless progression to chronic renal failure.

Nearly a century ago Ernest Goodpasture, an American physician, described kidney disease associated with the 1919 influenza epidemic.

'Goodpasture's syndrome' – shorthand for 'anti-glomerular basement membrane antibody disease' – is now used to describe rare cases of rapidly progressive glomerulonephritis accompanied by bleeding into the lungs. Its immediate cause is the production of antibodies which the body has generated against collagen and other proteins in the basement membrane of glomerular capillaries. We do not know what the (presumptive) infecting organism is. Mice can develop a comparable disease when immunised with a particular collagen, a structural protein.[7] The kidneys may also be damaged in systemic lupus erythematosus (p. 97) a disease also of unknown cause, in which antibodies are generated against the genetic material DNA but which probably also react against components of the glomerular filters.[8]

The commonest of all chronic nephritides is probably that associated with deposits in the glomeruli of a circulating protein (immunoglobulin A) combined with an antibody. The resultant disease is known as 'IgA nephropathy'.[9] It has a high incidence of between 5 and 40 new cases per million population per year, in different populations and in different parts of the world. In nearly 50% of cases this is a progressive disease which leads to end-stage renal failure.

IgA nephropathy has a strong genetic component, associated particularly with chromosome 6.[10] We do not know the trigger event, nor why some people should be genetically susceptible. There has been some interesting Japanese evidence that the common upper respiratory tract bacterium *Haemophilus parainfluenzae* may stimulate production of an IgA antibody which is also directed against kidney glomeruli.[11] It has many features in common with an uncommon and strange disease (Henoch-Schönlein purpura) which I shall discuss in Chapter 39.

There is an interesting relationship between certain virus diseases which specially affect both kidney and liver (notably hepatitis C, and to a much smaller extent hepatitis B). The manifestations of hepatitis C virus infection of the kidneys include membranoproliferative glomerulonephritis, associated with unusual circulating antibodies which precipitate in the cold.[12] Exactly how HC infection causes infective-immune glomerulonephritis is a complete mystery. Perhaps unravelling the causation of IgA nephropathy in mice by Sendai virus infection may shed light on the mystery.[13] If we could understand exactly how human virus infections damage the kidney, the way might be open for prophylactic virus immunisation.

Not only viruses but many bacterial infections can lead to what might be called 'infective-immune' glomerulonephritis. Another factor which needs to be considered is exposure to hydrocarbons (e.g. benzol).[14] These have been shown in animals to cause damage to the kidney glomeruli. Another possible contributory factor is exposure to heavy metals, especially gold – but the evidence for this is weak.

The 'hepato-renal syndrome'

In more than 50% of all people dying from liver failure, whether caused by alcohol, virus or bacterial infections, there is bad kidney function as well. This particular 'double whammy' has been named the *hepato-renal syndrome*.[15] It can even occur without jaundice when there is extensive accumulation of fluid in the abdominal cavity (ascites). Patients may die of the kidney failure even though the liver failure has been successfully treated. Opinions differ about the cause: e.g. low intraglomerular pressure, damage from bile salts, excessive sympathetic nervous constriction of the kidneys' blood supply or release of damaging cytokines. What is particularly fascinating is that despite patients having all the symptoms and signs of kidney failure, the kidneys themselves may be structurally quite normal. If normal blood pressure is restored and appropriate drugs given to improve the blood supply to the kidneys, or if the liver disease has been successfully treated by a liver transplant, full normal kidney function is usually restored. It would seem therefore that bad liver function can in some way affect the kidneys, but we do not know how.

Summary

Each human kidney has about a million individual units. Each unit contains a passive filter (the glomerulus) which lets through water and small molecules in solution. These pass to a system of collecting tubules which lead eventually into the bladder. At rest about one fifth of the heart's output passes through the kidneys. Vast quantities of fluid are filtered out from the bloodstream each day. Most of this is selectively reabsorbed in the tubules.

The main function of the kidneys is to excrete the non-gaseous residues of the diet – chiefly nitrogen and phosphate. These accumulate in the blood when renal function is inadequate. They cause symptoms when function falls below 20% of normal. If it falls below 5% of the normal value, life can only be maintained by artificial kidney treatment or by a kidney transplant.

Most chronic renal (kidney) failure is due to inflammation or destruction of the glomeruli. This has many causes, including bacterial and virus infections. Infections may bring in chemicals which resemble parts of the kidney, especially the glomeruli, and switch on the body's own immunological defences, with circulating antibodies and defensive blood lymphocytes. These may make kidney damage worse. When some critical proportion of kidney function has been lost – probably about 75% – the compensatory mechanisms, especially increased pressure in minute blood vessels (capillaries) in the remaining glomeruli start off a vicious circle which leads slowly but inexorably to complete failure of kidney function. 'Glomerular hypertension' is well recognised in diabetes and is one of the main reasons for renal failure in that disease.

The link between infections and glomerular inflammation is sometimes clear, but in many cases, especially in virus infections (e.g. by hepatitis C virus) we do not yet understand the link between the infecting organisms and the kidney damage. The kidneys are also susceptible to poor liver function, which can make the kidneys fail even though they are structurally entirely normal.

34

STROKES AND HIGH BLOOD PRESSURE

The brain and spinal cord are ensheathed by a thin layer of a colourless watery fluid ('cerebrospinal fluid'). This is contained within a delicate membrane appropriately described as 'arachnoid' (Greek: *arachn* = spider's web; *oid* from *eidos* = resemblance). Over the surface of the arachnoid membrane lies a much tougher fibrous cover, the 'dura' (Greek: hard).

Most strokes are caused either by artery obstruction or bleeding within the brain itself. Such strokes are classified as 'intracerebral'. Bleeding can also take place inside the skull but outside the substance of the brain. Such bleeding is then described as 'extracerebral'. Any collection of blood within the rigid skull, whether it is inside or outside the brain itself can obviously compress and damage soft brain tissue. Such haemorrhage is classified as 'subarachnoid', 'subdural' or 'extradural' according to the space into which the blood has first leaked. With the technical facilities now available in most hospitals, extracerebral strokes are easy to diagnose, mainly by special X-rays which use the technique of 'computed axial tomography' (done by a 'CAT' scanner).

In years past I have several times seen blood leaks outside the brain mistaken for intracerebral haemorrhage. I have also seen a subdural haematoma (a lump of old blood clot) and on another occasion a congenital malformation of blood vessels mistaken for a brain tumour. Diagnostic mistakes of this kind are not made nowadays. Modern techniques have made much of the clinical diagnostic skill of former generations of neurologists redundant. But I still treasure the memory and excitement of watching the late Michael Kremer make several difficult and astonishingly accurate neurological diagnoses at the Middlesex Hospital in London, using only careful history-taking, bedside observation and simple clinical tests.

Collections of blood within the skull may be due to trauma, such as boxing injuries and road traffic accidents. Some arise by blood leaking from a defective brain artery with unduly weak walls (a so-called 'berry aneurysm'). Such conditions are present from birth and hence are described as congenital (Latin: *congenitus* = born with). Berry aneurysms are like miniature time bombs. Their thin walls can rupture without warning, causing the serious condition 'subarachnoid haemorrhage'. When an aneurysm has been recognised accidentally on an X-ray, or after a minor leak of blood, it can often be repaired. Such rare conditions do not appear – to me, at least – to rank as major medical mysteries. But common spontaneous strokes really are mysterious, as I shall explain.

Spontaneous intracerebral strokes

Intracerebral strokes comprise most 'cerebrovascular' diseases, i.e. diseases of brain blood vessels. A stroke can be due to part of the brain dying through lack of blood (technically, this is a 'cerebral infarct'), or less commonly, to compression of the brain by uncontrolled bleeding into its substance (a 'cerebral haemorrhage'). A big stroke, however caused, can be the most devastating misfortune to befall anyone. It may completely paralyse one half of the body. When it affects the dominant side of the brain (the left side in right-handed people) it can also make speech difficult, hesitant or even impossible. Within a few minutes a mentally and physically active individual can become completely helpless, unable to move normally or to communicate thoughts and feelings. Strangely, the sufferer from a stroke often may not realise what has happened to him until he tries to execute some familiar movement, such as getting out of a chair, or enunciating a word. He then finds that he is simply unable to move one side of his body, or to utter the word or phrase he wants. When I ask a patient who is speechless after a stroke: 'Do you know exactly what you want to say, but it just won't come out?' my patient always nods vigorously.

A big stroke is not just a personal disaster. The treatment and later management of strokes is reckoned to cost the National Health Service in the UK about two billion pounds each year.

Blood supply to the brain

Although it only weighs around 3 pounds ($1\frac{1}{2}$ kg) the adult human brain needs a huge blood flow – ($1\frac{1}{2}$ pints ($\frac{3}{4}$ litre) per minute). This provides oxygen, glucose and other nutrients and removes dissolved waste gas (carbon dioxide) and other metabolic products. When blood supply fails, things go wrong quickly. Complete failure of blood supply (e.g. from cardiac arrest) causes loss of consciousness within about 20 seconds and irreversible brain damage after about 4 minutes.

Blood gets to the front of the brain by passing from the heart up the two carotid arteries and to the back of the brain by the two (smaller) vertebral arteries (Fig. 20, p. 139). The word 'carotid' comes from Greek: *karos* = heavy sleep. Compression of both carotid arteries was known for thousands of years to produce coma, which was looked on as a form of heavy sleep. The carotid arteries lie deep inside the neck, on either side of the windpipe (trachea). They are well protected. It is impossible to cut both arteries by a single knife stroke without also severing the trachea, as many unfortunate people attempting suicide have found. The vertebral arteries are even better protected because they lie actually within the bones of the neck.

The effects and severity of a stroke depend on the site and extent of that part of the brain which has been suddenly deprived of blood and has thus become unable to function. Loss of so-called 'motor' function (the ability to move muscles) is the most obvious symptom of a stroke, but loss of function can also impair coordination of movement, or the appreciation of sensations such as touch or passive movement of a limb. Pain is not usually a problem.

Epidemiology

Strokes have an annual incidence between 1 and 2 per 1000 population in North America and Europe. Some 450,000 people in the USA and about 100,000 in the UK have their first stroke each year. In the UK cerebrovascular diseases account for 10 deaths per 100,000 population at age 40, but 1000 per 100,000 at age 75. Across the world, stroke is the fourth leading cause of death. In developed countries it is the third most common, after coronary heart disease and cancer.

The most important association of stroke is with high blood pressure, which I discussed in Chapter 31. As Figure 48 shows, the risk of someone having a stroke is strongly and directly related to their blood pressure level.[1] Since many strokes are due to artery obstruction and since artery obstruction is also the cause of most heart attacks, we might suppose that high blood pressure would also be closely related to the risk of having a heart attack. So it is – but the relationship is not nearly as close as it is with stroke. Lowering blood pressure by drug treatment gives only slight protection against heart attacks, but good protection against strokes.

The same applies when comparing populations. High blood pressure and stroke always go together. For example, Japanese and Chinese people used to have a high incidence of hypertension and also a high incidence of stroke, but a relatively low incidence of coronary artery disease and heart attacks. Some Japanese men may have been misdiag-

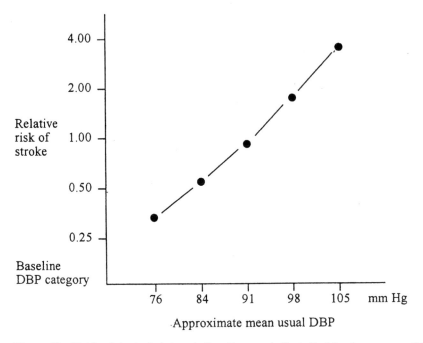

Stroke and usual Diastolic Blood Pressure (DBP)
(in five categories defined by baseline DBP)

Figure 48 Epidemiological data relating the usual diastolic blood pressure of large numbers of individuals to their risk of having a stroke. The data were extracted from published studies which recorded stroke events in 843 people over a standard period of time. Taking a diastolic blood pressure of 91 mmHg as giving a stroke risk of 1.0, the ordinate scale at the left side shows the relative risks of having a stroke with diastolic blood pressures above and below 91 mmHg. Redrawn from data of MacMahon, et al. *Lancet* 1990; 335: 765–774.

nosed in the past as having died from a cerebral haemorrhage when in fact they had died from brain artery obstruction, because dying from bleeding into the brain was once thought to indicate previous intellectual superiority! Over the last 50 years the situation has changed a bit. Stroke incidence has declined in Japan. Is this because the Japanese are eating less salt? Or are they taking more effective drugs to lower blood pressure? Or are many of them also taking 'statins' to lower blood cholesterol concentration? Or are they also taking drugs which inhibit clotting in arteries? Some people are doing all these things. It is difficult to know which is doing most to prevent strokes.

Many investigators have identified environmental factors that tend to raise blood pressure and which are thus inevitably associated with stroke, e.g. a high consumption of salt. Although smoking has no important effects on blood pressure it has a strong positive association with stroke. This may be partly because smoking is a cause of arterial disease. It may also increase someone's liability to blood clotting. When I have failed to persuade someone with high blood pressure to stop smoking – by stressing the dangers of lung cancer – I have sometimes succeeded by describing the misery that a big stroke can inflict. It is much worse even than a lingering death from lung cancer.

Genetics

I have discussed in Chapter 31 the genetic aspects of hypertension. Suffice it to say that genes are responsible for about half of any individual adult's blood pressure, the other half being due to environmental influences. Often both interact. Some people can eat lots of salt without suffering any rise in their blood pressure. We have comparable models in animals. In the USA LK Dahl bred two strains of rat to be either salt-sensitive or salt-insensitive, in respect of their blood pressure. The difference became genetically established and was passed from parents to offspring. The most spectacular animal model of stroke and severe hypertension we now have is the 'spontaneously hypertensive rat, stroke-prone' (SHRSP), developed from the original rat strain (SHR) which I described in Chapter 31. Some 6 months after birth or even earlier, rats of the SHRSP strain develop very high blood pressure and usually die from a stroke, which can be either a massive infarct or a massive haemorrhage. Further selective inbreeding has created an even more hypertensive stroke-prone rat whose hypertension develops into the so-called 'malignant' phase, with inflammation of small arteries and early death.

Causes

So far it all seems simple, at least in respect of bleeding into the brain. One might think that high blood pressure must tend to rupture the small delicate brain arteries. But this overlooks the virtual impossibility of putting the walls of normal small brain arteries under high enough tension to tear them open. The studies of Pierre Simon, Marquis de Laplace (1749–1827) explain why. His formula or 'Law' states that the tension in the wall of a sphere or tubular vessel depends on the distending pressure multiplied by the diameter. The small diameter of brain arteries powerfully protects them against being burst by high pressure. (Think how difficult it is to start to blow up a small balloon, compared with the ease of blowing it up further once the balloon is already distended.) Between the heart and small brain arteries of 50–200 microns (about one tenth of a millimetre) in diameter – the order of size most at risk in hypertension – artery wall tension falls about 10,000 fold. People have tried to rupture human brain arteries at post mortem by tying into a large artery a hollow cannula through which fluid can be pumped at high pressure to stretch all the arteries, down to the very smallest. No leaks occur even with pressures as high as two atmospheres (1520 mmHg)! Even arteries from previously hypertensive individuals are almost equally difficult to rupture. So how is it that human beings can die from a spontaneous massive haemorrhage into the substance of the brain when the blood pressure in life seems to be nowhere near high enough?

Even when the brain is examined within a few hours of death from a massive stroke it can be very difficult to find the precise source of bleeding, or to identify which small artery has been obstructed. One reason is the phenomenon of thrombolysis (p. 215). This is why sometimes a portion of the brain can have died from lack of blood even though at the time of a post mortem examination there seems to be no clot obstructing any artery.

When the tissues in and around a cerebral haemorrhage are examined there are characteristic small artery changes. These comprise the deposition of homogenous fatty material ('lipohyalinosis'), associated with larger artery narrowing by deposits of cholesterol-rich lumps of atheroma. In addition, there is often increased coagulability of the blood. No one knows for sure the cause of lipohyalinosis in small brain arteries, but much evidence points towards recurrent ischaemia (Greek: *ischo* = keep back; *haima* = blood) – i.e. insufficient blood supply to maintain adequate nourishment of the walls of the artery. Although such a process might be sudden, lipohyalinosis is more likely to be the end result of many repeated episodes in which blood supply has been inadequate. This could happen in several situations. For example, most people's blood pressure falls a lot when they go to sleep. If the main brain arteries are obstructed by atheroma some parts of the brain may be critically starved of blood. This is difficult to prove, but the consistent and strong association of lipohyalinosis of small arteries with narrowed or occluded larger arteries of supply is strongly suggestive.

I should mention one theory about the cause of cerebral haemorrhage which at one time excited a lot of interest: that bleeding came from the

382

rupture of microaneurysms – tiny blind sacs on the smallest cerebral arteries. These were first described 150 years ago by the famous French neurologist Charcot and his colleague Bouchard, who examined sections of human brains after death. However, new techniques of microscopy have cast doubt upon Charcot's observations, which appear to have been artefacts of microscope slide preparation.[2] According to the American neuropathologist IR Caplan these apparent 'microaneurysms' have never been clearly identified as responsible for cerebral haemorrhage. (As an aside, I tried many years ago to find whether their appearance could be produced by an episode of severe cerebral ischaemia, which I induced by elevating cerebrospinal fluid pressure to a high level in anaesthetised rabbits. This produced borderline as well as manifest cerebral infarction, but nothing resembling the lesions described by Charcot.)

There is no doubt that prolonged ischaemia can make small arteries liable to rupture. More than 150 years ago scientists examining the brains of people who had died from a brain haemorrhage noted that there was often an adjacent area of softening – the first manifestation of a cerebral infarct. Massive brain haemorrhage can easily be produced in animals by first blocking off the blood supply to the brain for, perhaps, 20 minutes, then releasing the block again. Presumably this sequence can also occur on a small scale. In addition, a sudden rise of blood pressure can send even large arteries into a state of spasm which can take many minutes to wear off. It may last long enough to cause permanent damage and death of brain tissue. The inner walls of blood vessels synthesise powerful constrictor substances (e.g. 'endothelins') and can release them when the blood vessels are damaged or deprived of blood. The spasm produced by even very small amounts of local endothelins can last long enough to produce a brain infarct.

A common situation is that a tear or split on the surface of a lump of atheroma in a diseased brain artery makes the blood clot at that point. This then causes an infarct which may or may not bleed, depending on the extent of the local blood supply. As I have already emphasised, an obstructing clot may soon lyse, certainly within a few hours. Very few people ever die instantaneously of a massive stroke unless there has been an associated heart rhythm disorder. It is usually a matter of 2 or 3 hours, during which blood oozes out of the damaged small blood vessels and gradually compresses the brain, leading to headache, loss of consciousness and eventually paralysis of the breathing control centres in the brain stem.

I have watched this relentless sequence – helplessly – on many occasions. The worst was on Christmas Day many years ago, when I was looking after a young man with acute myeloid leukaemia who had an almost complete deficiency of the sticky elements in his blood (the platelets) which play an important role in local blood clot formation. He started to get a bad headache mid-morning and his neck became stiff. By midday he was unconscious and unrousable. By mid-afternoon he was dead. His breathing had stopped as the continued oozing of blood fatally compressed the respiratory centres in his brain stem.

Large artery disease as a cause of strokes

People talking about cerebrovascular disease are nearly always thinking about arteries inside the skull. Figure 20 (p. 139) shows the layout of the arteries at the base of the brain. These can be seen at a post mortem examination once the brain has been lifted away from the skull. But the larger brain arteries, which have relatively much more extensive atheroma deposits than the small arteries, are not inside the skull at all. They run deeply in the neck and are not easy to examine, even after death.

I became interested in neck arteries when studying human cadavers with the late Drew Thomson, as I mentioned in Chapter 31. We looked at the main brain arteries of 94 people who had many different blood pressures recorded before death. Some had infarcts and some haemorrhages when their brains were examined. Using a very simple measurement technique, we found that the brain arteries of people who had died with strokes of all kinds were much narrower than those of people who had died from other causes.

The vertical scale at the left of Figure 49 is the rough and ready measure we made of the fluid-carrying capacity of all four main brain arteries in the neck, added together: two internal carotid and two vertebral arteries. Drew Thomson and I tied cannulas into each artery at its origin inside the chest, then relaxed each artery fully by flushing it with aqueous ammonia until the flow could not be further increased. We then measured the rate at which water flowed through each artery under a constant standard pressure head of 140 mmHg (equivalent to a blood pressure in life of about 180/120 mmHg). The water flowed out into a jug held inside the open skull. The flow rate for each of the four arteries was calculated using a graduated jug and a stopwatch. It was a simple though rather gruesome experiment, but the results were very exciting. William Osler, a former Professor of Medicine in Baltimore and later the Regius Professor of Medicine in Oxford, is reputed to have said that there was always a place in medicine for anyone who had attended 50 necropsies. I certainly found it most satisfying to be

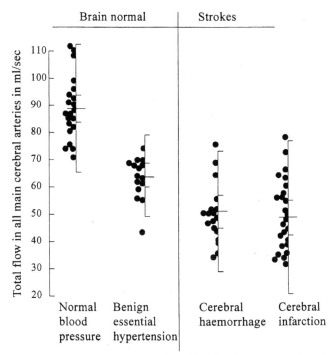

Figure 49 Data from the necropsy study described in the text, showing the measured maximum flow rates in the two internal carotid and the two vertebral arteries (all added together) in four groups of cadavers. From left to right, these are: (1) those with normal blood pressure before death; (2) those with benign essential hypertension (raised blood pressure recorded in life); (3) those dying with stroke due to brain haemorrhage; (4) those dying with a cerebral infarct. Note that there was no significant difference in neck artery calibre between the last two groups, but those who had essential hypertension during life had main cerebral arteries whose fluid-carrying capacity was much reduced, though not as much as in the group with strokes.[5]

able to throw light on diseases of the living by examining the dead, without harming any living creature.

The results of all the cases we could classify, shown in Figure 49, suggest that the large arteries in the neck would often have contributed a very substantial resistance to blood flow during life. Subjects previously hypertensive had much reduced flow rates in our test system. The neck arteries must have contributed an increased resistance to blood flow in life. People who had died with strokes had lower flow rates still. But there was no difference in the overall resistance of the four main arteries in people who had died with cerebral haemorrhage and those who had died with uncomplicated cerebral infarcts.

385

This confirmed many post mortem observations during the last 200 years.[3] Spontaneous bleeding into the brain often occurs in an area or adjacent to an area of 'softening'. Softening of the brain is the first obvious manifestation of an infarct. After the dead brain has been cleared away by scavenger cells over the ensuing weeks, the infarct becomes 'cystic' (Greek: *kystis* = bladder: i.e. it turns into a fluid-filled cavity). A brain with multiple infarcts can look like gruyère cheese. The parts of the brain particularly affected by infarcts (notably a part of the mid-brain known as the internal capsule) are also those parts in which haemorrhage most often occurs.

When the heart stops pumping, after death, the pressure in all blood vessels falls to a low level which bears no relation to the pressures present in life. But at the time of post mortem examination it is possible to estimate roughly whether an individual had previously been hypertensive and if so, how high the blood pressure had been. This is because high blood pressure enlarges the heart and increases the thickness of the walls of its main pumping chamber (the left ventricle). The total heart weight is usually increased. The higher the blood pressure in life, the heavier the heart is after death. Drew Thomson and I extracted from the post mortem records of the Middlesex Hospital the heart weights of 335 people who had died with strokes. Men have bigger hearts than women, but when we compared in each sex the heart weights of those who had died with brain haemorrhages or with brain infarcts there was no significant difference, although most stroke victims had hearts that were bigger and heavier than the normal accepted range.[4]

The large plaques of atheroma visible in the main neck arteries could have been sites of local clot formation. In Chapter 31 I reproduced X-rays from two cadavers in the series that Drew Thomson and I studied at the Middlesex Hospital in London. Each X-ray showed the carotid and vertebral arteries from one side of the neck. The arteries were first dilated with ammonia and washed through. They were then filled with an (X-ray opaque) barium sulphate suspension in a hot gelatin solution, under a pressure of 140 mmHg. The barium sulphate/gelatine was allowed to cool and set while the pressure was maintained. We then took X-rays of the necks to show the course of each artery (Fig. 43, p. 345). The arteries from the severely hypertensive woman showed almost complete obstruction of one vertebral artery and gross narrowing of the internal carotid artery on the same side. The other woman had lower blood pressure and near normal neck arteries.

When Drew Thomson and I measured the fluid-carrying capacity of these two arteries in our whole series of cadavers, we found no difference between the average calibre of arteries of people dying with brain

386

haemorrhage and those dying with brain infarction (Fig. 49).[5] The neck arteries in people who had died with strokes of either kind were much narrower than those in people who were known to have had low or normal blood pressure.

Transient ischaemic attacks

A common precursor of a cerebral infarct is the so-called 'transient ischaemic attack' (TIA). This is usually caused by a clump of platelets (the sticky elements of blood) or a small blood clot impacting briefly in a small artery, thus preventing blood from getting to the tissues that the artery supplies. The person affected might find himself suddenly unable to move a limb or to speak. The distinction from a completed stroke is that the attack passes off in a short time, e.g. within half an hour.

Sometimes the arterial obstruction can be directly seen at the bedside. It is possible to look at someone's retinal arteries at the back of the eye with an ophthalmoscope, an instrument which makes use of the 15× magnification that everyone's own cornea and lens provide for an examiner. During a TIA it has several times been possible to see a blockage in an artery supplying the retina or part of it. It has also sometimes been possible to see the blockage (a small blood clot or white collection of aggregated platelets) swept away in the flowing blood at the same time that normal sight is restored. TIAs are not uncommon. They have an annual incidence of about 5 per 1000 of the population over 60.

A small regular dose of aspirin is an almost sensationally effective treatment to prevent TIAs in most patients. It works mainly by reducing the stickiness of platelets. The anti-clotting agent warfarin is also effective preventive therapy (prophylaxis) against clotting in the brain blood vessels. So far large trials have not shown it to be any more effective than aspirin.[6] Unfortunately large doses of warfarin have caused many deaths through bleeding into the brain. Warfarin is more risky than aspirin and is not yet established as the better prophylactic agent.[7] When there is associated disease of the internal carotid artery, with clots forming on its wall, TIAs may also be stopped by replacing the diseased or narrowed segment of artery with a 'stent' or bypass.

The protective effect of lowering blood pressure

I mentioned in Chapter 31 that lowering blood pressure protects against strokes – not only against bleeding into the brain, which is easy to understand, but also against cerebral infarction. Roughly speaking, the lower the blood pressure the lower the risk of stroke. This comes as no surprise to laymen. Nor does it to the majority of doctors who believe that it is the high pressure which bursts arteries. But it did surprise Drew Thomson and me after we had made our post mortem observations of the grossly narrowed brain arteries in hypertensive people. I will explain why.

High blood pressure and stroke risk

I must acknowledge that the observations and opinions I have expressed in this chapter, and have more fully summarised in a recent large review,[8] may be regarded by some people as unduly bizarre and speculative. But there are many anomalies when one is looking for simple and straightforward explanations for strokes. Although some drugs which lower blood pressure improve brain blood flow, even though they lower the pressure available to send blood through the brain, there is no doubt that lowering of blood pressure, by any means, protects against infarction of the brain. The choice of drug or drugs seems relatively unimportant.[9] Deliberate lowering of blood pressure appears to protect against cerebral infarction even when the initial blood pressure is not higher than normal. One might assume that lowering blood pressure would reduce blood flow through the brain and thus make death of brain tissue (an infarct) more rather than less likely. Why do stroke-prone spontaneously hypertensive rats (SHRSP) succumb to massive cerebral infarcts about as often as they succumb to massive cerebral haemorrhage? How can we make sense of these apparent anomalies?

We know that blood pressure can be reduced a lot before cerebral blood flow starts to fall at all. This reflects the property of the cerebral circulation known as 'autoregulation'. Therefore moderate blood pressure reduction poses no immediate threat to the vitality of the brain. But I shall go further. Lowering blood pressure in most circumstances *increases* the blood flow to the brain. When I first wrote my monograph *Neurogenic Hypertension* I collected from the published literature seven sets of observations in man in which total cerebral blood flow was measured at the same time that blood pressure was reduced by hypotensive drugs or spinal anaesthesia. In all the reports, contrary to what commonsense might predict, reducing blood pressure *increased* total cerebral blood flow. This was even the case when blood pressure was lowered by deliberate bleeding.[10]

Blood pressure in hypertensive rats is very variable during 24 hours, as it is also in men and women with severe hypertension. Pressure can go up suddenly. Arteries exposed to sudden peaks of high internal pressure are stimulated to constrict, by a so-called 'myogenic' response. Constriction of brain arteries has been directly observed in experimental animals (rats) with hypertension. If such arterial spasm continues after blood pressure has fallen, the stage would be set for a potentially critical reduction of blood flow to the affected area, causing cerebral infarction. Thus it seems reasonable to suggest that prevention of spasm by lowering blood pressure should also prevent brain infarction.

The protective effect of statins

Leaving aside the possible anti-thrombotic effects of some of the drugs used to treat hypertension, another protection against stroke can be given by the class of blood cholesterol-lowering drugs known as 'statins'. These provide powerful protection against both stroke and heart attacks – an effect which has been described as 'magical'. There is some evidence that statins may increase the local production of nitric oxide by endothelial cells, lining artery walls. Statins may also stabilise plaques of atheroma and prevent rupture. They may also improve macrophage function.[11] All these possible effects of statins are currently under intensive investigation.

Summary

Intracerebral haemorrhage is not due to the bursting of previously normal small brain arteries under high pressure. There has always been preceding small artery damage, which when repeated on many occasions results in 'lipohyalinosis' – deposits of homogenous fatty material in the artery walls. Intracerebral haemorrhage and cerebral infarction share a common cause, i.e. inadequate blood supply to the walls of small brain arteries. Both are strongly associated with large artery lesions due to atheroma.

Naturally-occurring artery spasm may outlast for many minutes the rise of pressure which originally provoked it. This may threaten ischaemic infarction. Lowering blood pressure, even in people with normal blood pressure, confers a strong protection against stroke, probably mainly by preventing arterial spasm. Under most circumstances it actually increases total cerebral blood flow.

A relatively new class of drugs, the 'statins', can exert a strong preventive effect against stroke, which may be additional to their main action – the reduction of blood cholesterol.

35

PRE-ECLAMPSIA: PREGNANCY-INDUCED HIGH BLOOD PRESSURE

Pre-eclampsia is a common and uniquely human disorder, although a somewhat similar condition has been reported in some patas monkeys. It occurs throughout the world, with an incidence, in different regions, of between 2% and 10% of first pregnancies. It is best regarded as a 'syndrome', i.e. a cluster of abnormalities. In a woman more than 20 weeks pregnant these are (1) a rising blood pressure, (2) excessive amounts of protein in the urine, and (sometimes) (3) swelling of the ankles due to fluid accumulation. The protein in the urine suggests that the filters of the kidneys are damaged and leaky. Very occasionally the other abnormalities occur without an excess of protein in the urine. Although the term 'pre-eclampsia' (P-E) is still in common use, it is a bit misleading, because actual 'eclampsia' is now extremely rare. That word comes from Greek: 'a shining or violently bursting forth'. It is not a bad description of the fits (convulsions) which characterise eclampsia. Good antenatal supervision can almost always prevent fits occurring. However, the term 'pre-eclampsia', meaning a step on the way to eclampsia, will doubtless continue to be used until its cause is discovered.

A woman whose mother or sister has had pre-eclampsia is somewhat more likely to get it herself in her first pregnancy, so there is a significant genetic component. But a recent study of 471 female twin pairs failed to find even one in which the disease had occurred in both members. Lots of women get P-E without any family history of the condition. The pre-existence of a so-called 'collagen vascular disease' (such as systemic lupus erythematosus: p. 374) makes the occurrence of P-E more likely, probably because the placental blood supply[1] may be impaired by the disease.

Epidemiology

Towards the end of a first pregnancy, about one woman in 100, on average, will need to be admitted to hospital because of a diagnosis of

P-E. She will be closely observed. Depending on the severity of the condition she will probably either have labour started artificially (with drugs) or she will undergo a Caesarian section. These manoeuvres will be needed either because of rising blood pressure or because signs of fetal distress start to appear.[2] One in 200 women will require immediate termination of pregnancy for the sake of both mother and child. Pre-eclampsia can cause the death of a baby in the womb, or at the time of delivery. Death of a mother in pregnancy is very rare, but eclampsia is an important cause of it. Eclampsia is not only charac- terised by fits but is also associated with damage to a mother's kidneys, liver, and her blood-clotting system.

It is strange that a condition as serious as pre-eclampsia doesn't usually make a pregnant woman feel ill. High blood pressure can cause headaches, but most commonly doesn't. Kidney damage produces no symptoms at all unless kidney function is very bad indeed. In days gone by, the occurrence of a fit was often the first sign that something was going wrong with the pregnancy. Nowadays prevention of pre-eclampsia, and hence avoidance of eclampsia, is the most important single aspect of care during pregnancy. Simple urine

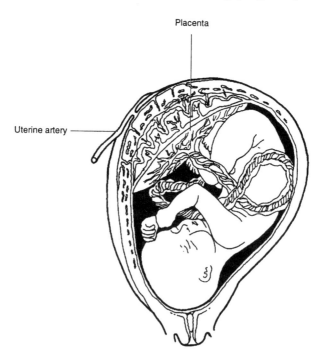

Figure 50 Diagram of fetus, placenta and uterus towards the end of pregnancy.

testing, taking the blood pressure, and checking for undue weight gain are the main requirements. The modest costs of regularly checking these things is best regarded as insurance. Since P-E can appear with startling speed, current attempts to reduce costs by spacing out antenatal checks are misguided.

Since pre-eclampsia is a uniquely human disorder it can only be studied in pregnant women. The ethical and practical difficulties of experiments are formidable. But we know how to cure pre-eclampsia. The essence is to remove the placenta. Unfortunately a fetus is completely dependent on its placenta (Fig. 50). It will die in 15 minutes or so if the placenta is disconnected, e.g. if the umbilical cord joining fetus to placenta is cut or compressed. So cure of pre-eclampsia has to involve removing the fetus as well as the placenta. If the baby is premature, experienced judgement is needed to say how long the pregnancy can be allowed to continue. Usually two weeks is about the longest holding time once P-E is established because it almost never gets better on its own. Sometimes the concern in pre-eclampsia is for the mother rather than the fetus, perhaps because of a disorder of maternal blood clotting or of liver function. But the usual worry is for the fetus.

Cause

The available evidence makes it almost certain that pre-eclampsia is a primary malfunction of the placenta which somehow has bad effects on the mother. All the abnormalities of pre-eclampsia disappear within a few hours or days after the placenta has been removed. The problems almost certainly involve the blood supply of the uterus and placenta. In P-E it seems as if cells derived from the fetus have failed to burrow well enough into the muscular wall of the mother's womb to make sufficiently adequate contact with the spiral arteries which supply blood to the placenta. There may be some deficiency of factors stimulating blood vessel growth even before pre-eclampsia develops.[3] The mother's spiral arteries normally get larger as pregnancy progresses and lose their elastic and muscular coat, but in some cases of P-E this function is defective. The immediate consequence is a restriction of the blood supply to the placenta and hence impaired transfer of nutrition to the fetus.

Lots of clues suggest that a placenta can set off P-E when it is not getting a good enough blood supply. This could be because the circulation of the womb is not fully developed in a first pregnancy, or because there is a extra load on the placenta, e.g. from having to supply blood to twins. Another possibility is that the placental circulation gets obstructed by blood clots. In P-E there is increased production of 'thromboxane', a chemical which constricts arteries and activates platelets – the tiny blood cells concerned in clotting. This suggests that aspirin, which reduces the stickiness of platelets and which gives some protection against coronary thrombosis, might help to prevent P-E. So an enormous number of trials of aspirin have been made. Although collectively these have shown a small but statistically significant protective benefit, aspirin is by no means the answer to preventing P-E.

The placenta in P-E is commonly smaller than in a normal pregnancy. It shows various types of damage, some of an inflammatory nature, some probably due to lack of blood supply and some due to local clot formation. Occasionally the placenta may appear normal on ordinary inspection, with secondary effects including a rise in the mother's blood pressure and a leak in her kidney filters, leading to excretion of much more than the normal trace of protein.

A possible chemical factor?

It seems almost an inescapable conclusion that some chemical material produced by an 'ischaemic' placenta – one with an inadequate blood supply – passes into the mother's body and sets off the various changes. For many years scientists have looked for some such material. Powerful hormones which are known to raise blood pressure (e.g. renin, angiotensin, noradrenaline and endothelin) have not so far been convincingly incriminated. There is some evidence of a deficiency of nitric oxide (which lowers blood pressure) and a deficiency in the enzyme responsible for its synthesis. There may also be a slight deficiency of a hormone called 'adrenomedullin' (a polypeptide which also lowers blood pressure). None of the observed differences in circulating hormones or other factors so far examined can fully explain pre-eclampsia.

There is recent evidence that blood serum taken from pre-eclamptic women increases the permeability to protein of endothelial cells lining blood vessels, whereas that from normal pregnant women and even from women with pre-existent high blood pressure does not.[4] The particular interest of this last report is that the serum factor which causes excessive permeability of endothelium disappears within a few days of delivery, just as P-E does. The authors of the report also produced some evidence that the factor might be an enzyme (protein kinase C) which is an intermediate facilitator of many cellular processes. However, protein kinase C is involved in so many activation processes in so many different cells that the general good health and well-being of most women with P-E is difficult to reconcile with the overproduction of some material involved with so many different actions. I would rather suspect that an excess of protein kinase C is the result of a more fundamental pathological process.

Apart from the placenta secreting some directly damaging material into the maternal circulation, perhaps it can produce something which has an indirect effect, e.g. by acting on the brain or spinal cord. There is already evidence, from direct recording of sympathetic nerve impulses going to leg muscles, that the rise of blood pressure in P-E may be in part 'neurogenic', i.e. brought about by the nervous system. Perhaps the material presumed to be coming out of the placenta in P-E could be something which acts on the brain.[5] In that case, one may ask whether the general increase of sympathetic nervous activity (SNA) observed in P-E can damage endothelium and cause previously normal kidneys to leak protein into the urine. I think this is unlikely because when SNA is increased to the same or to a greater extent in essential hypertension we don't see endothelial damage or large amounts of protein in the urine. But perhaps increased SNA from the brain is due to some chemical from the placenta causing damage to endothelium and leakage in the brain's blood vessels. Perhaps it is this leaked material which increases sympathetic nervous activity and puts the blood pressure up. This seems to me the most likely scenario.

Another suggestion is that there is overproduction of an endothelial 'suppressor factor', derived from a placenta poorly supplied with blood. A factor of this type, suppressing cell growth in tissue cultures, has been identified when endothelial cell cultures are treated with blood plasma derived from women with pre-eclampsia.[6] There is some evidence that an inadequate blood supply to the placenta makes it produce an excess of certain cytokines – such as 'tumour necrosis factor alpha' (TNFα) and 'interleukin-I' (IL-1). When these enter the mother's circulation it is envisaged that they damage the endothelial linings of blood vessels.

In Chapter 16, in the context of obesity, I described the interesting hormone 'leptin', deficiency of which causes gross obesity in man and animals. Leptin concentrations have been noted to be increased in P-E,[7] but whether this makes a significant contribution to P-E is uncertain.

The endothelium of blood vessels seems to suffer the greatest damage in P-E. Instead of being smooth it becomes unduly sticky and unduly leaky.[8] Another potential source of damage is small fragments of placental tissue (so-called 'placental debris'). These can be identified in the circulating blood of most pregnant women, but are present in greater amounts in P-E.

One might envisage that a placenta that is not working properly could make the fetus produce some damaging material which comes back through the placenta and enters the mother's circulation. For various reasons this is rather unlikely. There have been cases in which pre-eclampsia has persisted after the baby has been delivered and has only been cured when a placenta still within the womb has been removed. Confirmation that the placenta is the villain of the piece also comes from examination of the placentas of pre-eclamptic pregnancies. They commonly show 'infarcts' – scars produced by lack of adequate blood supply. Fortunately the fetus itself usually remains healthy providing that P-E is not allowed to get out of control. It is surprising that retarded fetal growth is uncommon.

The striking protection against eclampsia given by magnesium (usually in the form of magnesium sulphate) is greater than that from any other blood-pressure-lowering or dilating drug. This suggests that in some way magnesium – an abundant metal (ion) in the world – is present in inadequate quantities or inactivated in some as yet unidentified way. This is a real medical mystery.

Immunological aspects

So what on earth is going on? One suggestion is that the fetal part of the placenta, which necessarily has fetal rather than maternal genes in its cells, is acting as an antigen – i.e. a material which excites an immune reaction of some sort in the mother. Some cells circulating in a mother's blood can often be identified as having come from her fetus and have even been suspected of causing chronic disease in the mother (e.g. scleroderma). The mother's immune system certainly seems to be involved in P-E.[9] Exposure to chemicals derived from another individual and capable of producing an immune reaction (so-called 'foreign antigens') can eventually give a woman some protection against P-E even though at first they produce an adverse reaction. Previous blood transfusion from an unrelated donor has been observed to reduce the risk of P-E. A previous pregnancy will have exposed a mother to fetal antigens. This may explain why P-E is typically seen in first but not in later pregnancies.

Another way to protect against P-E appears to be the practice of oral sex without a condom. A long period of previous cohabitation with the same partner has also been reported to give protection.[10] However, a second pregnancy with a new partner seems to bring a woman's risk of P-E back to what it was in her first pregnancy. Other observations by the same authors suggest that conception within 4 months of cohabitation has a 50% chance of bringing about pre-eclampsia in an ensuing (first) pregnancy, whereas after one year's cohabitation the chance of P-E drops to about 4%. However, an impressively large epidemiological survey has shown that it is probably not the man's involvement but rather the intervals between pregnancies which is important. When the interval is large, P-E becomes more likely.[11]

Is it possible that there can be an immunological reaction to a specific man's sperm in the vagina? Could this play some part in causing P-E? If so, protection against P-E might be provided by the woman's immune system becoming tolerant of a particular man's sperm. It reminds me of the best example of immunological tolerance of foreign cells. This is the improved survival of kidney transplants in people who have previously had blood transfusions. If all the remarkable immunological observations on pre-eclampsia are correct – and some have been disputed – they could provide a plausible evolutionary advantage for a woman to stick to one partner while she is having children. Perhaps marriage can receive approval from scientists and well as moralists. One may even speculate historically that the institution of marriage itself might have evolved because it gave mothers-to-be the best chance of avoiding pre-eclampsia.

A large recent study has reported that if a woman becomes pregnant by a man who has already fathered a pre-eclamptic pregnancy in a different woman, her risk of P-E is significantly increased. If so, perhaps paternal genes could play some part in causing the condition. The same survey also gave some limited support to the influence of cohabitation already mentioned. Potential antigens in semen need to be itemised, to find whether there is for each a corresponding maternal antibody which increases during prolonged cohabitation with one man. Some really classy chemistry and immunology will be needed!

I am not an obstetrician and have never worked on pre-eclampsia, but the condition has always fascinated me. It is very common and of enormous social and economic importance. If I were now engaged in active research in P-E I should be examining placental extracts for their possible effects on the autonomic nervous system, i.e. those parts of the nervous system which are outside conscious control. If blood serum from women with P-E can be shown consistently and specifically to increase endothelial permeability in tissue culture outside the body, the way would be open gradually to focus down and identify the damaging chemical or chemicals. One would like to know whether the cells lining the blood vessels of the brain might be specially sensitive to placental extracts.

Another growing point of research is obviously going to be the investigation of placental factors controlling blood vessel growth in the later months of pregnancy. Failure to grow new blood vessels properly evidently accompanies inadequate placental function. But whether this is a primary event impairing blood supply, or whether reduced blood supply impairs blood vessel growth (angiogenesis) is debatable. Many different factors converge to stimulate production of vascular endothelial growth factor (VEGF: p. 75). So pre-eclampsia might be due to failure to produce enough VEGF or enough of one of its chemical receptors. Alternatively, P-E might be due to a circulating factor inhibiting the growth of new blood vessels into the placenta. Some of the factors that might be involved were described in Chapter 7. There has been much recent interest in the possible beneficial effect of supplementing the diet of pregnant women with extra vitamins and/ or anti-oxidants – notably with vitamins C and E.[12]

Summary

Pre-eclampsia (pregnancy-induced hypertension with protein in the urine) is common, especially in the last 3 months of first or twin pregnancies. The mother may also develop swelling of the legs because of fluid retention. If the condition is left untreated it may result in death of the fetus and in extreme cases fits and even death of the mother. Prevention of pre-eclampsia is the main purpose of antenatal supervision.

There seems no doubt that the immediate cause of the condition lies in the placenta. Pre-eclampsia usually resolves in a matter of hours after the placenta has been removed. The placenta usually shows scars of probable infarcts, suggesting impaired blood supply. One theory is that the fetal part of the placenta fails to make good enough contact with the maternal part, and that some material coming from the damaged placenta circulates in the mother, raising her blood pressure and damaging her kidneys. We do not know what this material is. Much evidence suggests that there is some immunological intolerance by the mother's body of the fetus and of its part of the placenta, and that this can set the syndrome off. This might help to explain why pre-eclampsia is less common in second and later pregnancies.

36

PULMONARY HYPERTENSION

The normal pulmonary circulation

As I have already mentioned in my introduction to Chapter 31, the lungs normally present little resistance to blood flowing through them. The pressures of blood in the pulmonary arteries and on the right side of the heart are low (Fig. 40, p. 332). An adult lying flat, at rest, has a pressure in the main veins filling the right side of the heart of only about 3 inches pressure of blood. This is the height to which a column of blood would rise if it was connected to one of the great veins. It is equivalent to about 5 mmHg. The right ventricle of the heart pumps this pressure up to about 12 mmHg, which drives blood through the lungs and into the left side of the heart. The powerful left ventricle pumps up the pressure higher still, to about 90 mmHg.

The pattern of blood flow through the lungs in someone standing upright is remarkable. At rest some 9 pints of blood (5 litres) flow through the lungs each minute. Because the pressures are so low, gravity determines that virtually all the blood flows through the lower half of each lung. Almost none goes through the upper parts. Only during exercise, when the blood flow can increase to about five times its resting value, does blood go through the upper parts of the lungs. This distribution of blood flow probably accounts for the typical location of secondary tuberculous infection at the top of the lungs (the apices) where blood flow is least. It also explains the benefit of supine bed rest. This was cardinal therapy in the old tuberculosis sanatoria. Supine rest increases blood flow in the upper parts of the lungs. It probably gives the body's own defences the best chance to resist the spread of infection.

One way of describing the normal pulmonary circulation is to say that it is like a waterfall. Once blood gets as far as the lungs of an upright subject it just tumbles through, with almost no resistance to its passage to the left side of the heart (Fig. 51). So although the lung blood vessels in a supine adult contain nearly 2 pints (900 cc) of blood, on standing there may be only about half this amount. This explains why people whose heart is failing to pump blood adequately and who

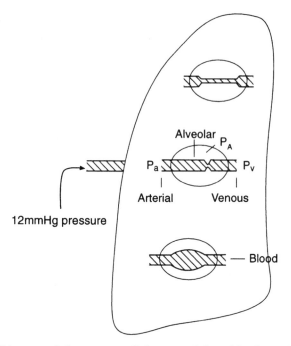

Figure 51 Diagram of three zones of the normal lung blood vessels in an upright subject. In the upper zone the surrounding pressure in the alveoli (P_A) is greater than that in the lung capillaries (P_a to P_v) These are therefore pressed shut, so that little blood flows through the upper parts of the lungs. In the lowest zone the pressure in the pulmonary circulation is everywhere greater than the pressure in the airways and alveoli, so that blood flows freely through the lungs. Blood flow in the mid-zone fluctuates according to the phase of respiration. (Modified from an original diagram by Moran Campbell.)

are breathless from lung congestion when they are lying down get relief from standing or sitting. It also explains why deliberate blood letting ever became a recognised part of medical treatment. When shortness of breath is due to lung congestion removal of blood can actually improve breathlessness. James Boswell, Samuel Johnson's biographer, records that Johnson obtained relief of breathlessness by being bled. However, in most situations blood letting is harmful. In times past it must often have supplied the *coup de grâce* to sick people.

Pulmonary hypertension

When the pressure of blood in the right ventricle and pulmonary arteries rises substantially above its normal 5 inches (10 mmHg) in a resting supine subject, the individual is said to have 'pulmonary hypertension'. This is of a different order from high blood pressure in the rest of the body ('systemic hypertension'). An acceptable definition of pulmonary hypertension is *a pulmonary artery pressure consistently at or above 25 mmHg at rest and above 30 mmHg on exercise*. From the description I have already given of the lung circulation it is obvious that pulmonary hypertension can only arise when more than half the pulmonary arteries are blocked, when the average blood-carrying capacity of all the main pulmonary arteries is less than half its normal value, or when the output of the right ventricle is at least twice as great as normal. People with pulmonary hypertension get unduly short of breath on exercise and are sometimes breathless even at rest. Chest pain on exercise is often the first symptom. This probably arises because the heart muscle is not getting enough blood. If the passage of blood through the lungs is seriously obstructed, systemic blood pressure falls.

Long-term changes in the pulmonary arterioles in pulmonary hypertension

Any longstanding elevation of pressure in the pulmonary circulation can eventually cause thickening of the walls of small arteries (arterioles) because of increase in muscle and fibrous tissue. Both changes narrow the arterioles. There is also reduced production of the dilating materials nitric oxide and prostacyclin, and increased secretion of the constricting material endothelin-1.[1] Currently, prostacyclin or one of its analogues seem to be the best treatment to dilate the small pulmonary arteries, though drugs which inhibit the formation of fibrous tissue (e.g. perfenidone) also show promise.

What can raise pulmonary artery pressure?

Sudden blockage of the pulmonary arteries will equally suddenly raise the pressure in the right atrium and right ventricle. Pulmonary embolism describes the situation in which large blood clots, usually formed in the leg veins, pass up into the chest and along a main pulmonary artery until they block it. If several large clots pass into both pulmonary arteries, the lungs will let very little blood through. The victim may die of 'shock' – a medical term which means and defines a potentially lethal reduction in the output of the heart. Pulmonary embolism is the most feared complication of large surgical operations because of its suddenness and potential fatal consequences. Blood clotting in the legs is favoured by lying still for long periods. Not only surgical operations but also long plane journeys are potentially dangerous. People have to sit still, often cramped up. I have seen a previously fit young man who had travelled overnight from Hong Kong brought into hospital in London under my care almost at death's door, because of extensive pulmonary emboli. Fortunately it was possible to give him immediate 'thrombolytic' injections of clot-dissolving material and save his life.

The consequences of pulmonary embolism seem easy to understand, but there is none the less a medical mystery here. Ventilation (the movement of air in and out of the tiny air sacs of the lung) is normally accurately matched to perfusion (the passage of blood through the walls of the air sacs). If ventilation is inadequate, as in asthma (Chapter 2), the blood may not be properly oxygenated as it flows through the lungs. The patient may look blue. If the circulation becomes inadequate because of clots in the blood vessels one would expect such blood as did get through the lungs to be red and full of oxygen, especially because pulmonary embolism causes overbreathing (hyperventilation). Curiously, in pulmonary embolism the effects on oxygen supply are usually just the opposite. Too little oxygen in the blood ('hypoxaemia') is very characteristic of pulmonary embolism. Patients often look blue. The most likely reason is that some chemical factor or material produced by blood clots causes constriction of adjacent lung blood vessels. This could then disturb the normally good matching of ventilation and perfusion. It would be useful to find the cause of the mis-match, if only because the putative factor causing constriction of lung blood vessels might be related to the causes of 'primary' pulmonary hypertension (see below).

A more long-lasting obstruction to the lung circulation is provided by narrowing of the mitral valve of the heart. This lies between the left atrium and the left ventricle. It prevents blood regurgitating from ventricle back to atrium when the ventricle contracts at each heart beat. Acute rheumatic fever, nowadays a rather rare condition, can damage the mitral valve and lead to its narrowing ('mitral stenosis'). Pressure then rises in the left atrium. This increases the pressure in the lung blood vessels and pulmonary artery. The right ventricle has to pump harder. The diagnosis is made by measuring the pressures at different parts of the system, using fine catheters passed up the arteries from an artery in an arm or leg. The defective valve can either be repaired or replaced. There is not usually any long-lasting lung damage if the condition is recognised in time. The pressures all go back to normal.

Widespread lung disease of any cause may make it difficult for blood to pass freely through the lungs. Some degree of pulmonary hypertension is common in severe chronic bronchitis with lung destruction and fibrosis. But this is usually the least of a patient's problems.

They arise from the lung disease itself rather than from any consequential circulatory embarrassment.

There is another mechanical cause of pulmonary hypertension which has much more serious consequences. Certain defects in the heart and blood vessels may let some of the higher-pressure blood from the left atrium, left ventricle or its outflow tract (the aorta) flow directly into the lower-pressure right side of the heart. Such defects appear during fetal life. They are therefore by definition 'congenital', i.e. something you are born with. There may be an atrial septal defect (ASD), a ventricular septal defect (VSD), a patent ductus arteriosus or sometimes even more complex mis-arrangements of the blood vessels or heart chambers. Small leaks of blood from left to right through one of these holes in the heart are of little consequence, but large leaks can cause serious trouble. The heart has to do much more work because the blood transferred back from left to right side has to be pumped on again. At rest the total output of the left ventricle may be twice normal or even more. It is as if someone apparently at rest has a lung circulation more appropriate to brisk walking. The pressure in the right ventricle and pulmonary arteries obviously has to rise once all the spare capacity of the pulmonary circulation is exhausted. Some people with substantial left-to-right shunts of this sort live reasonably normal lives, though with some restriction of strenuous sustained muscular exertion. Unfortunately in other cases – we don't know in which ones this happens – changes gradually take place in the pulmonary circulation and start an inexorable and fatal vicious circle.

When this situation is recognised early, at birth, there is an urgent need to correct the defect, despite all the difficulties and dangers of large operations on tiny babies. Unfortunately after the structural changes in the lung circulation have taken place, correction of the shunt will not bring back normal conditions. Indeed, once the pressures in the right side of the heart rise to levels similar to those in the left side, no shunting of blood will occur. An operation to close the hole in the heart becomes pointless, and may do more harm than good.

Extensive lung disease associated with 'fibrosis' (too much fibrous tissue in the lungs) is often called 'cryptogenic fibrosing alveolitis'. ('Cryptogenic' means 'of concealed or of unknown cause'; 'alveolitis' means inflammation of the very small terminal air sacs of the lungs, the alveoli.) The condition is about twice as common in women as in men. It usually appears in early adult life. The average age for diagnosis is 35. It appears to be an auto-immune disease, but the trigger factor is not known. It affects between one and two people per million of the general population. If it is not treated, or cannot be treated, average survival is only 2–3 years.

Primary pulmonary hypertension

Some unfortunate adults develop 'primary' or 'idiopathic' pulmonary hypertension, meaning pulmonary hypertension of unknown cause, when none of the mechanisms already discussed seems to be in operation. In some cases widespread small clots seem to be the underlying cause. It is sometimes associated with a recognisable disorder of blood clotting. There is also an association with conditions which involve an increased rate of destruction of red blood cells: 'Sickle cell disease' is the best-known example.

But in most cases of primary pulmonary hypertension the small lung arteries get narrower and develop excessive muscle in their walls, even though the small blood vessels in every other body system seems to be normal. Several therapeutic drugs, especially anti-cancer drugs, have been occasionally incriminated in constricting small lung arteries. Cigarette smoke has a small but measurable ill-effect, increasing blood flow resistance in the lungs. Over-use of the appetite suppressors fenfluramine or aminorex has a definite association with pulmonary hypertension and may increase its incidence as much as ten times. These drugs are believed to act by increasing the local concentrations of serotonin (a blood-vessel constrictor material). Another natural substance ('endothelin') is a strong constrictor of arteries. Some improvement in pulmonary hypertension has been obtained with the use of endothelin-receptor blocking drugs such as bosentan, and also with sildenafil ('Viagra').[2]

Most cases are sporadic and no cause can be discovered, though 6% run in families. Linkage of inherited cases to a gene on chromosome 2 at 2q31-32 location has been confirmed.[3] The immediate cause of the condition is an increase in bulk of the inner lining of capillaries and increase in the bulk of muscle surrounding the small lung arteries. In most cases the common cause seems to be an excessive expression of the growth factor angiopoeitin-1, which combines with a receptor known as Tie2. Angiopoietin-1 is present in excess in biopsy specimens of lungs from people with primary pulmonary hypertension. It is obvious that anti-angiogenic drugs such as those I have mentioned in Chapter 7 will be tried in pulmonary hypertension, in the hope that excess blood vessel growth can be curtailed. We do not yet know why angiopoetin should be present in excess and cause this rare but serious disease.

There are also other inherited conditions which can increase the growth of muscle cells surrounding blood vessels.[4]

An interesting report has suggested that a virus infection may be the trigger which sets off 'primary' pulmonary hypertension. A ubiquitous virus, Human Herpesvirus 8 (HHV8) is known to be the immediate cause of a common complication of human immunodeficiency virus (HIV) infection ('Kaposi's sarcoma') as well as of several other growth disorders of lymph glands. In a small series of people with apparent primary pulmonary hypertension, a majority were recently reported to have HHV8 infection in their lungs,[5] whereas patients with other kinds of pulmonary hypertension were not similarly infected. These observations will clearly be intensively followed up. Primary pulmonary hypertension may be rare, but it is a very serious condition which is usually fatal within a few years.

The vicious circle

A vicious circle may come into operation in any of the situations I have described, when the pressure in the right heart and pulmonary arteries is continuously well above normal. Established pulmonary hypertension is a very serious and intractable condition for which no fully effective treatment has yet been devised. Most people with a sustained pulmonary artery pressure at or above $3\frac{1}{2}$ feet of blood (50 mmHg) die within 5 years. It appears that a substantial rise of pulmonary arterial pressure stretches the walls of the smaller pulmonary arteries (arterioles). This supplies a stimulus for their muscular walls to constrict and eventually stiffen. The narrowed blood vessels increase the resistance to blood flow. Reduced availability of oxygen also tends to constrict pulmonary arteries, a reaction which is observed in people living at high altitude.

In the course of time, perhaps over several years, pulmonary hypertension becomes established and ultimately irreversible. Blood clots then often form in the small lung arterioles. This can increase flow resistance still more. Longterm treatment with anticoagulant drugs such as warfarin improves the outlook in most types of pulmonary hypertension even though it does not cure the condition.

There is an interesting contrast between systemic hypertension (Chapter 31) and pulmonary hypertension. Lots of drugs are known to lower blood pressure in most parts of the body. They do this by relaxing the muscular walls of the small arteries. They are in widespread use for treating established systemic hypertension. There is no doubt that such drugs relieve symptoms and prolong life. Unfortunately none of them seems to have much effect on the small arteries of the lungs, at least when the dose is kept below that which would cause total collapse of the circulation. Lots of things have been tried. One of the most interesting is the gas nitric oxide, which is known to cause systemic arteries to dilate. It can be administered by inhalation. Some limited success has been reported, especially in children and the newborn. Unfortunately its effects seem to be rather short-lived. Many other dilating drugs such as hydralazine and nifedipine have been tried, but without well-established benefit. At the present time, epoprostenol (prostacyclin, a chemical produced by the body and which has a powerful short term dilating effect on lung arteries) seems to be the most effective treatment, but it has to be administered continuously by infusing it slowly into a vein. Agents interfering with blood clotting are usually also prescribed, to reduce further damage by local small clots. In some of the worst cases lung transplantation offers the only hope of survival.

Some improvement in long-term survival can be obtained by mechanical means, surgically creating or opening up a hole between the right and left atria. This lowers pressure in the right side of the heart and in the pulmonary artery. Even though this lets venous blood containing little oxygen mix with oxygenated arterial blood, the result may be beneficial overall.

Cause

The site of increased resistance in sustained pulmonary hypertension is the small arteries (arterioles), but they do not seem to have any gross structural defect. It is just that the endothelium and muscle are thicker than normal. It has been suggested that the matrix material surrounding small lung arteries may be abnormal and in some way affect muscular contraction of vessel walls.

If we knew everything about the control of the circulation through the lungs, we might be able to design a drug which would make more blood vessels in the lungs grow or open up more widely. There are local chemicals secreted by cancer cells which help to secure for themselves an adequate blood supply by opening up local blood vessels. I discussed this general topic in Chapter 7. Unfortunately no suitable material with an action on lung arteries has yet been discovered, though extracts from rapidly growing tumours are being tested by infusing them into the pulmonary circulation, to see whether they reduce pulmonary artery pressure.

If I were in the business of designing such a factor I would take a good look at chemicals derived from the gut. My reason for suggesting this will become apparent to those who have read Chapter 22. I summarised there the evidence that the normal liver probably inactivates or destroys some material, in the blood coming to it, which opens up lung blood vessels. Scarring of the liver (cirrhosis) is often associated with short circuits of blood passing through the lungs. It is sometimes also associated with clubbing of the fingers (p. 239), probably because unmodified blood from the venous side of the circulation gets through to the main systemic side. In days before modern diagnostic techniques were available, patients with severe liver disease were sometimes thought to have some form of congenital heart disease because they had signs (undue blueness) suggesting a substantial shunt of blood from the right to the left side of the heart.

My guess is that the normal liver removes some substance or substances which are capable of opening up small lung arteries. Such material is most likely to be derived from the gut, or possibly from the pancreas. I have not the slightest idea what such a substance might be. Apart from the spleen and pancreas, the gut is the only large abdominal organ whose effluent blood drains through the liver. (Blood from the kidneys, for example, drains directly into the large veins taking it to the right side of the heart.) So it might be worth examining a number of extracts from gut or pancreas to see whether they had any dilating effect on lung blood vessels. Although pulmonary hypertension is fortunately rare, it is one of the most distressing conditions because of its relentless progress once a vicious circle has begun.

Summary

The normal pressure in the pulmonary circulation is low. The circulation there behaves as if it was a waterfall, with almost no resistance to blood flowing through the lungs.

Many conditions can raise the pressures in the pulmonary circuit, e.g. congenital heart defects with an abnormal communication between left and right sides of the heart, clots forming in or getting stuck in the pulmonary arteries, or extensive lung disease with scarring. The most serious situation arises when the condition has been both severe and persistent enough to start off a vicious circle, which can reach an irreversible stage. At this point, treatment is difficult. Cadaveric lung transplantation is then the only available cure. Continuous intravenous infusion of prostacyclin is the only moderately effective drug treatment. Some help may be given by surgically creating an atrial septal defect.

Evidence (summarised in Chapter 22) that some material coming from the gut or pancreas may dilate the lung circulation when it passes unchanged through the liver suggests the possibility that such a material might alleviate chronic pulmonary hypertension, a condition which has so far defied effective, convenient and acceptable treatment.

37

POLYCYSTIC OVARY SYNDROME

At birth a female infant's ovaries contain about 7 million germ cells (i.e. potential ova). These are gradually lost, until by age 10 there are only about 300,000 mature egg cells (oocytes) left. Oocytes in the ovaries of fertile menstruating women are contained in miniature sacs (ovarian follicles), one of which grows much larger than all the rest (to about three-quarters of an inch in diameter) each month. In between menstrual periods this large follicle ruptures and releases its contained egg (ovum) into the abdominal cavity – a process known as 'ovulation'. This occasionally causes slight abdominal pain, known as the mittelschmerz ('middle pain'). The ovum is released from the surface of the ovary, which lies physically close to the open entry of the fallopian tube (Fig. 23, p. 152). When all goes well the ovum gets into a fallopian tube where it is available for fertilisation by a sperm. Ovarian follicles disappear rapidly after the menopause and are usually gone by age 50, after which a woman is necessarily infertile. Measurements of the density of the ovaries (by ultrasound) can be used to estimate the number of residual ovarian follicles and hence assess potential fertility.

One considerable unsolved mystery is why only one ovarian follicle grows larger than the rest each month. Presumably there must be some chemical factor, perhaps blood-borne, which inhibits all the other ovarian follicles – those in the same ovary and also those in the opposite ovary – from growing in size once the selected ovum and follicle has started to enlarge.

Although the main function of the ovaries is the storage and programmed release of ova, in adult life the ovaries also secrete and release into the bloodstream 'sex hormones' – mainly oestrogens. Secretion of oestradiol (the main female sex hormone) in a cyclical fashion starts in late childhood.[1] The cycles are controlled from the pituitary gland in the centre of the skull by intermittent cyclical release of luteinising hormone (LH).[2] After 1 or 2 years, regular ovulation starts taking place in the mid-cycle, i.e. between a woman's menstrual periods.

The normal menstrual cycle

Once the normal menstrual cycle has become established, the ovaries take over most control of a woman's reproductive life, by their cyclical secretion of sex hormones. The growth of the endometrium (the lining of the womb) is stimulated by secretion of oestrogens, mainly oestradiol, by the maturing ovarian follicles. At the time of ovulation, the pituitary gland secretes brief pulses of both LH and of another pituitary hormone known as 'follicular stimulating hormone' (FSH). The secretion of LH precedes and may cause ovulation. One or other of these changes reduces the production of oestrogens by the ovaries and switches on the production of progesterone from the corpus luteum in the bed of the ruptured ovarian follicle. This latter change turns off any further oestrogen-stimulated growth of the endometrium. This leaves the womb lining ready either to be shed at menstruation, at the end of the cycle, or to grow thicker to sustain a sucessfully-fertilised egg.

To a cyberneticist such as myself (i.e. someone interested in negative feedback systems), the mid-cycle surges of LH and FSH can be looked at as weak signals analogous to those amplified in a radio set to entrain its intrinsic oscillator with the extrinsic radio signal received from the aerial. Although the signal may be weak, if it is close enough in frequency to the receiver oscillator frequency it may have just enough energy to entrain the oscillator. This then allows its contained amplitude-modulated (AM) or frequency-modulated (FM) signal to be decoded. A woman's initial menstrual periodicity is roughly determined by the ovaries and by the apparently somewhat random choice of which follicle next grows fully. Later, her menstrual periodicity is set by the brain. This is the only organ in the body which has enough information about the outside world to know the best settings for the menstrual cycle. At least, this is my understanding of the system. We know that a group of menstruating females often find their cycles coinciding if they are living physically close together, e.g. in school dormitories. (One suggestion to explain this well-known phenomenon is that 'pheromones' are involved. These are chemicals having a specific smell and which may convey information from one woman to others about the stage of her menstrual cycle.)

The normal menstrual cycle is the most striking of all oscillations in human body systems. A complex series of hormone changes repeats regularly with an average period of 29 days. This cycle length may have became established during human evolution to follow the phases of the moon. But though it is tempting to assume that this explains how the monthly human cycle evolved, one must be cautious. The

410

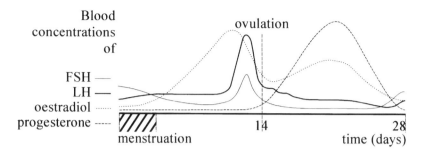

Figure 52 Diagram showing on a timescale of one month the usual hormonal changes in a woman during normal cyclical menstruation. FSH = follicle-stimulating hormone; LH = Luteinising hormone. (Modified from an original by AY Adashi in Clinical Endocrinology: ed GM Besser & A Grossman (2nd ed. 1992). Oxford: Blackwell.)

baboon's cycle extends to about 33 days whether in the wild or in captivity. Maybe the human race has done better than baboons through being more in tune with nature!

The cyclical changes in concentrations of the major hormones throughout a menstrual period is illustrated graphically in Figure 52. We do not know all the factors which bring about the oscillation. Evidence from other systems suggests that the anterior pituitary gland is dominant and controlled by some sort of intrinsic chemical clock. The clock itself resides in the hypothalamus, lying above the pituitary gland in the centre of the skull (Fig. 7, p. 45). By means of its chemical secretions (known as 'releasing hormones') the hypothalamus is in overriding control of many of the body's interacting negative feedback systems.

I have enjoyed making digital computer models of several body systems. One does not usually make new discoveries by these means, but modelling is a good way to clarify one's thought processes and to comprehend how complex systems might interact. I have not personally created a computer model of the ovarian/menstrual cycle, though this has been done by others. But I can give an example from another field of the puzzling way in which oscillating systems can behave. Some years ago I designed a digital computer model of the main components of the human respiratory system. I named this 'MacPuf' for quick reference. The program was written in the high-level language 'Fortran IV' and published complete in book form.[3] As a compiled package it has been supplied to many medical schools around the world. It allows the simulation of many different combinations of functions.

In one 'experiment', I eliminated Macpuf's brain's central drive to

411

respiration but increased its sensitivity to carbon dioxide and to low oxygen tension, and reduced its cardiac output. If these changes were brought about gradually the model would attain a steady state without oscillation. But if a large change was then applied (the illustration in my book was a brief episode of artificial ventilation) the model would then simulate indefinitely, with reasonable accuracy of timing, the phenomenon of Cheyne-Stokes respiration – episodes of zero ventilation alternating at intervals of about a minute with episodes of overbreathing.

To turn from this computer model (which embodies stiff differential equations) to a real clinical situation involving ovarian function: I have seen a young woman, whose periods had stopped because she was not eating enough, still not restarting regular periods even though her weight had gone up from 38 kg to 45 kg. But a single episode of menstruation, induced by giving an oestrogenic hormone and then withdrawing it, restarted normal cyclical periods.

Evolution of the polycystic ovary syndrome

The 'polycystic ovary syndrome' (PCOS) – also known as the 'Stein-Leventhal' syndrome – is the commonest *hormonal* disorder in women, i.e. one which affects the ductless glands. In most countries it affects between 5% and 10% of all women to some degree. Currently about 5 million women in the USA have the condition. The typical history of a woman developing PCOS is that after a few years with regular normal menstrual periods the periods become irregular and less frequent – a situation which has been described as 'menstrual chaos'. Fertility is reduced and ovulation ceases. After the periods have become less frequent they may stop altogether. The woman is then commonly infertile. At the same time she often puts on weight and develops excessive body hair growth in a masculine pattern (virilisation). This latter change is brought about by excessive secretion of testosterone, the male sex hormone. This may also be associated with excessive, non-fluctuating, secretion of the hormone LH by the anterior pituitary gland in the brain. There may also be subnormal secretion of FSH. Many differences from normal in the secretion of hormones during the day have been recorded in PCOS.[4]

Abnormal-looking follicles visible under the translucent capsules covering the ovaries can be seen by ultra-sound imaging. This is the most sensitive diagnostic test for PCOS.

In recent years it has been recognised that women with PCOS usually have increased secretion of and resistance to the hormone insulin, similar to that seen in Type 2 diabetes (Chapter 15).[5] There may also be abnormally high concentrations of fat in blood plasma (hyperlipidaemia). Epidemiological studies have shown that women with PCOS are at increased risk of having heart attacks, high blood pressure and frank Type 2 diabetes.[6]

Cause

The virilisation which is the commonest manifestation of PCOS is certainly caused by excessive circulating male sex hormones (androgens), notably testosterone. Although in women most testosterone is normally secreted by the adrenal glands, in PCOS there seems often to be additional abnormal synthesis of testosterone by the ovaries. There is also reduced ovarian synthesis of oestrogens such as oestradiol.[7]

Although it is now becoming accepted that increased insulin secretion coupled with increased resistance to the actions of insulin are usually present in PCOS, it is not clear whether these changes are causes or results.[8] Resistance to insulin action is associated with a defect in the response of many body cells to insulin, once insulin has combined with its (chemical) receptor. There is a strong suspicion that this defect may be genetically determined. This fits with epidemiological evidence of genetic predisposition to PCOS, a disease which has often been reported to run in families.

But the changes I have described are not found in all cases of PCOS. This makes it likely that PCOS is not a single disorder. It may be one in which several different causes can bring about the same ultimate effect. There is a strong suspicion that high levels of insulin may stimulate the secretion of high levels of testosterone, but also that a reciprocal relationship may occur. If so, this would obviously comprise a potential vicious circle which, untreated, might well get worse and become established:

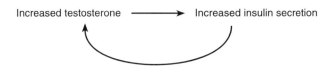

It is notable that the anti-diabetic drug metformin, which increases sensitivity to insulin, can slightly but significantly reduce testosterone concentrations and hence virilisation. Metformin has also been observed to improve fertility by increasing the number of menstrual cycles in which ovulation occurs.[9]

One rare cause of obesity is lack of the hormone leptin, produced by fat cells (p. 169), but it is doubtful whether leptin deficiency plays any part in causing PCOS.[10]

We do not know at present whether PCOS is a single entity, nor whether it is predominantly genetic or acquired. If it is acquired, what is the basic abnormality? There is a need for a hypothesis or theory to explain all the features of the syndrome, but none has yet been proposed or generally accepted. Is the primary disorder in the ovaries themselves? This seems a bit unlikely. In the natural history of PCOS, menstrual and ovarian function usually start normally but go wrong later. Such a sequence raises the possibility that PCOS might be an 'auto-immune disease' (p. 69), though there is at present no direct evidence at all for this. Antibodies directed against ovarian tissue have been reported to be present in many women with PCOS, the levels being as high as those recorded in women with primary ovarian failure.[11]

Most experts doubt whether PCOS can be regarded as an auto-immune disease, particularly since normal cyclical periods can usually be restored for a year or two by treatment. In the past such treatment has involved so-called 'wedge resection' – cutting small wedges of tissue out of the ovaries. Treatment nowadays is equally bizarre. It usually involves making multiple small holes in the surface of the ovary by diathermy (local electrically generated heat). This extraordinary treatment seems able to restart ovulation, correct abnormal rhythms of hormone secretion and partly restore fertility. So there must be a strong suspicion that the underlying disorder in PCOS probably lies not in the ovaries themselves but higher up in the control hierarchy, i.e. in the hypothalamus or pituitary glands.

In the evolutionary history of the human race it is obvious that PCOS must have conferred some survival advantage on women, to have become as common as it is today – despite the inevitable reduction in womens' fertility which comes with it. But the cause of PCOS remains elusive. Maybe we have yet to discover a new hormone whose disordered function can account for the polycystic ovary syndrome.

Effects of treatment

'Wedge resection' of the ovaries or ovarian damage by multiple diathermy lesions can restore fertility and normal menstrual cycles for a year or two. These strange results suggest to me an analogy with the oscillatory behaviour of the computer model of human respiration which I described earlier in this chapter. In that situation regular oscillation was initiated by imposing a single drastic and sudden change on the system. Can disordered menstruation perhaps be regarded as comparable, in that a sudden change can restart regular periods and (presumably) restart regular ovulation? One standard treatment for PCOS has been to give drugs, notably an oestrogen-stimulating drug such as clomiphene, combined if necessary with additional insulin-lowering drugs. In addition, attempts have also been made to restart cyclical menstruation by intermittent timed administration of controlling hormones.

Although several such treatments have been reported to restore fertility, I have not found any clear evidence that any of these treatments, except perhaps metformin, reduce excessive body hair growth. Increased testosterone secretion remains as mysterious as many other aspects of the disorder.

Summary

The polycystic ovary syndrome (PCOS) is commonly associated with infertility, mainly through failure of ovulation. There is also, in most cases, excessive growth of body hair in a male pattern, obesity, and increased secretion of and increased resistance to insulin.

The immediate notable hormonal abnormality is increased secretion of luteinising hormone (LH) from the anterior pituitary gland. Under normal conditions, during late childhood, slow hormonal fluctuations give way to regular menstruation, with mid-cycle ovulation (release of a mature ovum from the ovary). But in PCOS the periods become irregular and ovulation eventually ceases.

The cause or causes of PCOS are still unknown, though some examples of genetic predisposition have been recognised. Deliberate damage to the ovaries has been reported sometimes to improve menstrual irregularity and improve fertility, but these techniques have been largely superseded by hormonal drug treatments.

38

CHRONIC FATIGUE SYNDROME:
SO-CALLED 'ME'

Every general physician (internist) or general practitioner has been consulted by people with the chronic fatigue syndrome (CFS). Unfortunately most patients with this condition prefer to describe themselves as having 'myalgic encephalomyelitis', or just 'ME'. This description is inaccurate. It sounds impressive, but it annoys doctors a lot. The widespread use of the term is one of the reasons why patients often get a raw deal from the medical profession. Doctors resent having to accept a spurious and inaccurate self-diagnosis. Although the condition can often be correctly described as 'myalgic' (Greek: *my* = muscle; *algi* = pain), there is no evidence whatsoever that sufferers have active inflammation in the brain and spinal cord (Greek: *en* = in; *kephal* = head; *myel* = marrow: i.e. spinal cord; suffix '-itis' = inflammation of).

As it is currently defined, CFS implies that for at least 6 months there has been persistent or relapsing fatigue which does not resolve with bed rest and which is severe enough to reduce average daily activity by at least 50%. Other chronic conditions including previous psychiatric disease must have been excluded. There may also have been a gradual onset of symptoms, mild fever or chills, sore throat, tender lymph glands, muscle weakness with pain or discomfort, excessively lengthy post-exercise fatigue, headaches, flitting joint pains, sleep disturbances and minor psychological symptoms. In the last century such a condition was described as 'neurasthenia' (Greek: *asthenes* = weak). 'Weak nerves' is not a bad description of CFS. I shall argue that the fault probably lies in the brain rather than in muscles or glands.

Applying strict criteria for the diagnosis of CFS excludes all but a few percent of people complaining of longstanding fatigue. In most cases of CFS there has been no well-defined or consistent abnormality either on clinical examination or laboratory investigation.

Since short-lasting fatigue follows many different virus infections, is CFS simply a non-specific response to several possible triggers? Many viruses have been suggested as causes of CFS, e.g. Coxsackie B, human herpes virus-6, hepatitis C and Epstein-Barr virus, the latter already well known as the cause of glandular fever. All are common. Evidence of previous infection by one of these viruses can often be found in normal people. There is fairly strong evidence that CFS more often follows glandular fever than follows other febrile illnesses.[1]

An Australian report has provided good evidence of a causal relation between a single exposure to an infecting organism (*Coxiella burneti*) and the later development of CFS.[2] This organism is a very small bacterium (technically one of the 'rickettsiae'). It is endemic in some cows and ewes and infects people who inhale the organisms in an aerosol.

So are CFS patients genetically predisposed to react adversely and excessively to a virus or other infective trigger? Have CFS patients a psychological make-up which renders them specially liable to develop CFS after a minor illness that leaves most people unscathed? If so, is this vulnerable psychological predisposition itself genetically determined? The case remains open. There is some evidence of altered immune mechanisms in CFS, but it is maddeningly inconsistent. CFS has been regarded as 'a non-specific complex of symptoms related to various causal agents able to induce an immune response'. Such a hypothesis is imprecise. It cannot be tested.

Could CFS be due to the accidental ingestion of a poison? For example, an illness known as ciguatera is caused by eating extremely poisonous chemicals called ciguatoxins, which are found in certain Oriental and Caribbean fish. Some of these fish are highly prized culinary delicacies but need careful preparation to remove the poisonous parts. The toxin damages 'ion channels', structures in cell membranes which are exquisitely sensitive to various external agents. Ciguatoxins can damage these structures semi-permanently leading to a chronic condition which is virtually identical with CFS.[3] There is extreme fatiguability and often muscle and joint pains. Unfortunately so far there is no epidemiological evidence that CFS is due to an external poison. No plausibly damaging food item has been identified in the European diet. But it is impossible to disprove the possibility that some common article of food might have toxic effects in unlucky people with some particular genetic make-up.

Is the problem a low blood pressure and inadequately-filled blood circulation, due to lack of steroid hormones, possibly because of impaired function of the pituitary or adrenal glands? There has been intermittent interest in this possibility over several years, but it is disappointing that low-dose cortisol (hydrocortisone) treatment produces only slight improvement in symptoms. This is hardly worthwhile because of the side-effects of suppressing patients' own adrenal gland function. Steroids have a definite non-specific tonic effect in some people but CFS has not been proved to accompany significant pituitary or adrenal gland dysfunction.

Although CFS patients have normal electrocardiograms and normal heart function while they are resting, on exercise they have a reduced oxygen consumption and work capacity compared with matched healthy control subjects. Their maximum heart rate is greatly reduced. Muscle metabolism during exercise shows evidence of impaired energy supply. But an obvious problem in attributing reduced capacity for physical work to a muscle disorder is that it may simply be the effect of prolonged inactivity as well as from reduced central nervous system drive. There is usually no good evidence of any specific muscle defect in CFS. In any case, it is difficult to see why a primary muscle disease should produce mental as well as physical fatigue.

Looking after patients with CFS is frustrating. A doctor can't explain to a patient the cause of the illness. It is unknown. There is little practical help available. The condition often appears to be used as an excuse to give up work, either in the home or outside it, leaving spouse, partner, parent, friend or even child to cope as best they can. Some patients have already had an episode of major depression before the onset of CFS. Although the definition of chronic fatigue syndrome put forward by the Atlanta Center for Disease Control in the USA specifically excludes patients with major prior psychological illnesses, there are often minor psychological symptoms before CFS is diagnosed. Some doctors have regarded the illness as 'often a cultu-rally sanctioned form of illness behavior'.[4] Faced with the evidence of a strong association between CFS and depression some physicians suggest that since depression is a psychological disorder, CFS is likely also to be one.

> This argument overlooks strong evidence that severe depression, espe-cially 'bipolar' depression – that kind which alternates with intervals of maniacal excitement – often responds more successfully to manifestly 'organic' therapy such as lithium than to psychotherapy. This is not sur-prising, in view of the recent spectacular recognition that 10% of people with bipolar depression have a specific gene defect (GRK3) which alters the reactions of their brain cells to the neurotransmitter serotonin.

Central nervous system abnormalities

It is well known that the rate of blood flow in different brain regions changes approximately in parallel with changes in the electrical and chemical metabolic activity of nerve cells in those regions. In CFS most outer (cortical) regions of the brain have reduced blood flow.[5] There is a general reduction in nerve activity, which is confirmed by other evidence of reduced local consumption of glucose and reduced uptake of oxygen. The rate of blood flow at the back of the brain (in the brain 'stem') has also been reported to be reduced in CFS.[6] Apparent abnormalities have been reported in many series of patients having magnetic resonance imaging (MRI) of the brain. Although similar areas can be seen in normal people, they are much commoner in people with CFS,[7] though not all investigators agree.[8]

A recent Scottish study compared 12 CFS patients with 11 age- and sex-matched sedentary controls, under conditions of progressively increasing physical exercise. All the patients showed marked intolerance of exercise when compared with the control subjects. A number of significant differences emerged, especially in relation to the amino-acid tyrosine. This is a rate-limiting precursor of the neurotransmitter dopamine, which was significantly reduced both at rest and at all levels of physical exercise. In addition the rate of turnover of serotonin was increased in the CFS patients compared with controls. The authors suggested that both observations supported the hypothesis that central nervous mechanisms contribute to the increased perception of effort by patients and to their exercise intolerance.[9]

Is there a plausible unifying hypothesis?

No such hypothesis has yet achieved substantial acceptance. All have been lacking in detail. The first thing to say is that the condition does not appear to shorten life. Most of my patients have been in their thirties or forties. So far I know of no necropsy observations. There is often evidence that people with CFS have had previous depression and neurotic personality traits but too much can be made of this. It is only to be expected that a previous psychological disorder would aggravate any symptoms arising from a basic non-psychological cause. The presence of psychological disorder does not absolve us from looking further afield. We have to try to disentangle a possible underlying physical cause from its psychological overlay.

When I was first a medical student I was very keen on psychological explanations for physical symptoms. And I have sometimes had the gratifying experience of patients losing their physical symptoms after psychological counselling. For example, I persuaded a male patient of mine that hopeless marital incompatibility was his underlying problem, not a physical disease. His physical symptoms were immediately cured by divorce. A woman realised that her rejection of sex in her marriage, with consequent physical symptoms, derived from previous childhood sexual abuse by her father. I also recall a young recently married woman running a low-grade fever, confirmed by two weeks' observation in hospital. Nothing was found after extensive tests. But the fever resolved after a simple operation to incise an imperforate hymen which had made penetrative sexual intercourse impossible. So actual physical symptoms, genuine fever in this last case, can undoubtedly be caused by mental anxiety.

On the other hand, I have just as often found physical explanations for apparently neurotic symptoms. I recall vividly a 35-year-old woman who complained of sweating and indescribable sinking feelings after intercourse. The cause seemed to be the sexual habits of her husband who had first to be tied up, beaten and humiliated. This disgusted her. She had consulted psychiatrists without obtaining any satisfaction. A surgeon had removed some of her thyroid gland by an operation on her neck because her 'basal metabolic rate' was elevated, suggesting overactivity of the gland. Her blood pressure was normal and there was no apparent physical abnormality. I was in despair when, after leaving the ward, she returned to my outpatient clinic complaining of the same old symptoms. Unable to think of anything else useful to do, I sent a random urine specimen off to have adrenal gland hormones measured. She proved to have a vast excess of circulating adrenaline. After my surgical colleague Leslie LeQuesne had removed an adrenaline-secreting tumour the size of a tangerine from one of her adrenal glands she lost all her psychological as well as her physical symptoms.

Possible involvement of the reticular activating system

After reviewing as dispassionately as possible all the available evidence, I have come to think that a powerful case can be made that small localised defects in part of the upper brain stem, brought about in most cases by a previous virus infection, might interfere with the ascending 'reticular activating system' (RAS) (Fig. 6, p. 43). In animal experiments this has been shown to raise the level of electrical activity of the brain cortex when it is stimulated. Lesions of the RAS diminish arousal.[10] Brain imaging by 'positron emission tomography' (PET) and by 'single photon emission computerised tomography' (SPECT) shows that patients with depression as well as with CFS have reduced metabolic rate and local blood flow in many areas of the brain cortex, compared with normal subjects. Available data suggest that it is only in CFS that brain stem metabolism is reduced, compared either with

421

normal people or those with depression.[11] These observations fit well with previous work, already mentioned, of reduced brain stem blood flow in CFS. They also fit with the hypothesis that an underlying functional defect in CFS may lie in the reticular formation of the brain stem. If all these observations are confirmed they might lead to the Holy Grail: an objective diagnostic test for chronic fatigue syndrome.

The syndrome of 'post-polio fatigue' is highly relevant. Fatigue disproportionate to neuromuscular paralysis was observed long ago after people had recovered from acute poliomyelitis.[12] It was present every day in these patients and increased as the day went on. Necropsy observations showed damage in the region of the RAS and in its cortical connections. The similarity of symptoms between post-polio fatigue and chronic fatigue syndrome is remarkable. Persistent damage to nerve cells, rather than simply the persistence of viruses at some site, seems a plausible explanation of fatigue and neurological dysfunction, as I envisaged in a comprehensive review.[13]

A striking clinical feature of multiple sclerosis (MS) – a much studied disease (Chapter 3) – is fatigue, which is present in almost all cases. It often precedes any identifiable paralysis. My wife had noticed otherwise inexplicable fatigue, especially in hot weather, several years before she had any neurological symptoms or signs. Later she developed a stiff (spastic) paralysis of the legs. The diagnosis of multiple sclerosis was confirmed by magnetic resonance imaging of her brain. I have seen several patients whose initial symptoms were ascribed to hysteria because nothing could initially be found on examination or after tests. No one seriously suggests that fatigue in multiple sclerosis is psychological simply because it cannot yet be clearly attributed to lesions consistently found in any well-defined site in the brain. But multiple small lesions around the brain ventricles can almost invariably be demonstrated by magnetic resonance imaging. It seems reasonable to suggest that they are in some way the cause of the fatigue that is so characteristic of multiple sclerosis.

The curious disorder known as narcolepsy (p. 49) is characterised by usually brief episodes of sleep, sometimes triggered by laughter or emotion and sometimes accompanied by muscle weakness (cataplexy). This disorder is now known to be due to discrete brain stem lesions, sometimes caused by a previous virus infection, associated with changes in the hypothalamus at the front of the brain. People with narcolepsy often complain of undue fatigue. The condition is another example of an organic brain disease which can produce the same symptoms as those seen in the chronic fatigue syndrome.

At present it appears to be a tenable hypothesis to suggest: (1) that in chronic fatigue syndrome there are multiple small patchily distributed brain lesions affecting the ascending reticular activating system; (2) that the lesions may have been caused by an infective agent, which might be an enterovirus, Epstein-Barr virus or herpes virus-6, perhaps a rickettsial organism; (3) that the syndrome does not require living viruses necessarily to be present in the putative structural lesions, nor for any active inflammation to be present; (4) that lack of activation of the cortex produces the sensation of fatigue, without gross neurological abnormality other than some defects in postural blood vessel control and giddiness.

Even if it proves that an initiating acute illness can only trigger chronic fatigue syndrome in people previously predisposed by their psychological make-up, there are enough clues to justify further studies. The identification of tangible lesions underlying CFS would be immensely valuable to patients, even if it led to no immediate therapeutic advance. And in the confusing scenario which the chronic fatigue syndrome presents, the identification of an organic basis for the illness would provide a more rational basis for therapy than exists at present. I am hopeful that improved regional brain imaging and regional studies of brain metabolism may eventually answer the big question whether tangible brain stem lesions consistently underlie CFS. If so, its psychological manifestations could be the result of those lesions.

Alternatively, perhaps CFS is 'all in the mind', as many physicians believe. It makes a lot of difference who is right. My personal approach has been to say to patients: 'I don't know the cause of your chronic fatigue and I have found no evidence of serious disease in my examination or tests. In my experience most people with your condition gradually improve with time...Come and see me again in 3 months' time, so that I can see how things are going. In the meantime, take as much exercise as you can as long as it is not making you too exhausted.' Rather more specific advice has been given by some psychiatrists who advocate 'cognitive behaviour therapy' which has had some success in a controlled clinical trial. But such successes do nothing to solve the problem of causation. We all know that extreme fatigue can be overcome by extreme effort of will. How can an observer ever know how much fatigue someone with CFS is experiencing and how hard they are trying to overcome it?

Summary

The chronic fatigue syndrome (CFS), sometimes incorrectly called 'myalgic encephalomyelitis' (ME), has been intensively studied during the last 40 years, but no conclusions have yet been agreed about its cause. Most cases nowadays are sporadic. In the established chronic condition there are no consistently abnormal physical signs or abnormalities on laboratory investigation. Many physicians remain convinced that the symptoms are psychological rather than physical in origin. This view is reinforced by the emotional way in which many patients present themselves. Furthermore, there is an overlap of symptoms between CFS and depression. This remains a source of confusion.

There is some evidence both for a previous virus infection and for an immunological disorder in the chronic fatigue syndrome. Many observations suggest that the syndrome might derive from residual damage to the reticular activating system (RAS) of the upper brain stem and to its cortical projections. Such damage could be produced by a previous infection, which is most likely to have been with a virus.

Studies by modern imaging techniques have not been entirely consistent, but many magnetic resonance imaging (MRI) studies already suggest that small discrete patchy lesions can be found in the brain stem and in layers of cells just beneath the brain cortex. There is reduced blood flow in many regions of the brain, especially in the brain stem. Similar lesions have been reported after previous poliomyelitis infections, in multiple sclerosis and in narcolepsy. Chronic fatigue is characteristic of all these conditions. In the well-known post-polio fatigue syndrome, lesions have been identified mainly in the reticular activating system of the brain stem and in its subcortical connections. If eventually similar underlying lesions in the reticular activating system can be identified in CFS, the therapeutic target for CFS would be better defined than it is at present. A number of logical approaches to treatment can already be envisaged.

39

VASCULITIS: TEMPORAL ARTERITIS AND ALLIED CONDITIONS

'Vasculitis' derives from Latin *vasculum* = small vessel (diminutive of *vas* = conveying fluid). The suffix -itis' has its usual meaning: inflammation. The group of vasculitic disorders, collectively referred to as 'vasculitides', are uncommon conditions in which there is inflammation of the walls of blood vessels, especially arteries, leading to consequent ill-effects on the organs or tissues involved. There is local inflammation and death of cells, which may take on an appearance known technically as 'fibrinoid necrosis'. There may also be 'granulomas' (the more correct Greek plural is 'granulomata'). These are microscopic circumscribed areas, firmer than the surrounding tissue. They contain characteristic large single-nucleus cells, sometimes with a few large cells with several nuclei ('giant cells'). Vasculitis may occur (rarely) in rheumatoid arthritis (Chapter 9) and in other allied conditions, but in this chapter I shall confine my discussion to a few of the best known vasculitides. In these, inflammation of blood vessels is the predominant disorder. There have been two helpful recent American reviews of these conditions.[1]

Polyarteritis nodosa (PN)

When the larger muscular arteries are involved the condition is known as 'polyarteritis nodosa', that is, many ('poly-') arteries with inflammation ('-itis') and with lumps or nodes ('nodosa'). Smaller arteries and veins can also be involved in an inflammatory process, which often involves the kidneys severely, sometimes leading to kidney failure. A large number of differently named sub-groups with some common features have been recognised, with exotic names such as Takayasu's arteritis, Henoch-Schönlein purpura, Behçet's disease, Churg-Strauss syndrome and Kawasaki disease. One of the commonest is temporal arteritis (see below). Any of the larger arteries, including the aorta itself, may be affected. Other rather similar conditions predominantly

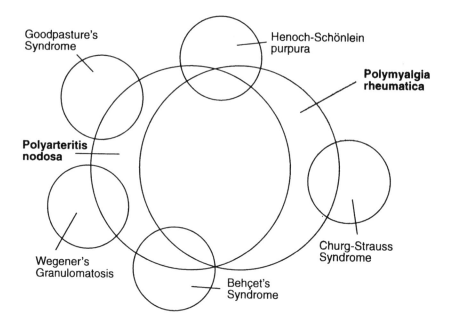

Goodpasture's Syndrome

Henoch-Schönlein purpura

Polymyalgia rheumatica

Polyarteritis nodosa

Wegener's Granulomatosis

Behçet's Syndrome

Churg-Strauss Syndrome

Figure 53 Diagram emphasising the overlap between various vasculitic disorders, affecting blood vessels of different sizes.

affecting small arteries include Wegener's granulomatosis, Good-pasture's syndrome, microscopic polyangiitis (hypersensitivity angiitis) and cerebral vasculitis. Figure 53 emphasises the overlapping features of some of these conditions.

Most of them produce fever, aching in muscles and in joints, with general feelings of tiredness and weakness. In most cases there is widespread involvement of many different organs and tissues. Blood markers of inflammation such as the erythrocyte sedimentation rate (ESR) and the C-reactive protein concentration (CRP) are usually increased. Despite the similarity of these various conditions, when the inflamed vessel walls are looked at under the microscope, their natural histories are distinctly different. Takayasu's arteritis is a rare condition predominantly affecting young women in the second and third decade of life, in Eastern countries. Polyarteritis nodosa is relatively common and mainly affects old people. Many international conferences have attempted classification of these overlapping syndromes. I shall not attempt one of my own, but simply describe the main features of two common conditions and one rare one. These make an intriguing contrast with polyarteritis nodosa (PN).

Temporal arteritis (TA)

Temporal ('giant-cell') arteritis can be regarded as a sub-group of polyarteritis nodosa. It is less severe, frequently burns itself out and seldom involves the kidneys seriously. I have looked after several patients with the condition. The first symptom may be a general feeling of tiredness, with a low-grade fever, headache and weight loss. In classic cases there may also be tender points or actual lumps over the temporal arteries. These run across the outside of the skull across the temple, above the ear. For people over 50 the incidence of the disease is about 20 per 100,000 per year, though there are wide variations in time and place. The disease is about twice as common in women as in men. Though the temporal arteries themselves are not invariably affected and tender enlarged temporal arteries can be felt in less than 50% of patients, the diagnosis is usually and conveniently made by removing a tiny piece of a temporal artery and examining it under the microscope. (The temporal arteries lie only just beneath the skin, so that surgical access is easy; furthermore the blood supply of the scalp is so good that temporal artery biopsy is a harmless procedure when competently performed.)

Many physicians who suspect temporal arteritis will start patients on glucocorticoid ('steroid') drugs such as prednisone as soon as they suspect the disease – sometimes without even doing a temporal artery biopsy, because of the danger of sudden obstruction of the main eye (retinal) artery. This can lead to permanent blindness in the affected eye. I have never felt certain whether steroid drugs simply suppress the manifestations of the disease and allow it to disappear of its own accord, or whether steroids play a part in its eventual cure. The complications of temporal arteritis are due to obstruction of small arteries, especially those in the kidneys, but symptoms may arise from impaired blood supply to many tissues, including those of the brain, gut and other organs.

Polymyalgia rheumatica (PR)

Another condition – polymyalgia rheumatica – (from *poly* = many; *my* = muscle; *algi* = pain) affects a similar age group. It is also associated with the same changes in the blood, aching muscles, fever, and weight loss that are found in temporal arteritis. PR is nearly twice as common as TA. Many people regard them as essentially the same condition. There are epidemiological parallels because the incidence of both diseases tends to rise and fall at the same time. Acute infections often seem to be able to trigger temporal arteritis. In the long run, temporal arteritis usually gets better on its own, as does polymyalgia rheumatica. But I have looked after patients who have needed steroid drugs (usually oral prednisone) for several years to keep the signs and symptoms of disease suppressed. One of my patients with polymyalgia rheumatica had to take steroids for 3 years and one with temporal arteritis needed nearly 5 years of treatment. Both patients were eventually able to stop steroids when their pain and fever remitted and their blood tests returned to normal.

Wegener's granulomatosis (WG)

This condition is much rarer than temporal arteritis and usually begins at an earlier age, sometimes in childhood. The sexes are equally affected. The condition usually appears to start in the upper respiratory tract (that is, the nose and internal nasal passages), sometimes with ulceration and bleeding, together with many of the less specific features of temporal arteritis. Later the lungs usually become involved, producing cough, chest pain and shortness of breath. The kidneys also eventually become involved in most (untreated) cases. Death from kidney failure is sometimes only preventable by a kidney transplant or by intensive immunosuppressive chemotherapy. However, with current treatment – which usually combines the immunosuppressive drug cyclophosphamide with a glucocorticoid steroid such as prednisone – most patients achieve a remission, though relapse is common and may necessitate further courses of treatment.

The definitive tissue diagnosis is usually made by examining a small piece of tissue from one of the nose ulcers under the microscope. Certain changes in the blood – the appearance of 'antineutrophil cytoplasmic antibodies' (ANCA) – are particularly characteristic, though they may also occur in some rarer but rather similar conditions. Antineutrophil antibodies are proteins, produced by lymphatic tissue, which attack and kill 'neutrophils'. These blood cells are described as 'white' because they do not take up stains from certain dyes. 'Cytoplasmic' means 'pertaining to the cell body rather than to the nucleus'. In WG these antibodies attack some of the body's own defensive white blood cells by combining with a particular enzyme (proteinase-3) which is expressed on white cell surfaces.[2] So-called 'immune complexes' are formed by the combination of the circulating antibodies with complement and with particular component parts of the white cells.

Cause

Three causes of vasculitides such as PN, TA and WG are currently being seriously investigated. They are:

1. An infection, which might involve:
   a) viruses,
   b) bacteria,
   c) fungi, and
   d) other larger organisms.
2. An immunological disorder, in which the body has become sensitised to some 'antigen' (i.e. a material which triggers a response by the body's immunological system). Such an antigen could be:
   a) extrinsic to the body (e.g. ingested, inhaled, put on the skin),
   b) intrinsic, i.e. a normal body constituent to which the body has become sensitised, or which has been changed by a somatic mutation.
3. A combination of (1) and (2), in which an infection has precipitated an immunological disorder, either by the organism itself acting as an antigen, or by facilitating access to the body by a damaging antigen, or by changing the antigenic properties of some previously normal cells or tissues in such a way that they become antigens.

Almost all the available evidence favours involvement of the body's immune system in some respect in these conditions, if only because immunosuppressive measures and immunosuppressive drugs make these conditions better, even though they do not cure them.

Since ANCA are so characteristic of Wegener's granulomatosis, we need to consider what could have caused production of these potentially damaging antibodies. One possibility is that the disease has been started by an infection, perhaps by an (as yet) unrecognised bacterium, one of whose cell components is chemically similar to some material in normal blood white cells, perhaps the enzyme proteinase-3 (see above). Then when the bacteria are detected by the body's immunological defences, antibodies are produced. These may then destroy normal defending white blood cells as well as neutralising the (presumed) infection. The fact that no infection has so far been identified means nothing. In the past there have been many infections which went unrecognised for years. *Helicobacter pylori*, a main cause of peptic ulcers, is a good example.

In many respects these conditions resemble rheumatoid arthritis (Chapter 9), but there are several notable differences which point to a different underlying cause. Whereas rheumatoid arthritis typically occurs in children and young adults, temporal arteritis is almost confined to the elderly. It is rare under the age of 50, but becomes commoner with each later decade. Arteritis is not usually seen in rheumatoid arthritis, so that the most dreaded complication of temporal arteritis – blindness – does not occur.

It is very difficult to escape the suspicion that PN, TA and PR are triggered by an infection which induces a harmful immunological reaction in one of the ways I have envisaged. In the case of temporal arteritis or polymyalgia rheumatica the disease usually begins suddenly, within a week or two. It eventually burns itself out after months or years. If it had been induced by a somatic mutation (p. 73), for example, eventual spontaneous cure would not be expected. Unfortunately we have no idea what might be the nature of the infection, nor why it should largely confine its attacks to the elderly. There has been some evidence to incriminate a triggering infection by various organisms, notably *Mycoplasma pneumoniae*. There has also been some suggestive evidence that *Parvovirus B19*, *Chlamydia pneumoniae* or a rickettsial infection might be involved. So far observations have been inconsistent. No known trigger factor can account for all cases.

Wegener's granulomatosis is equally mysterious. Like temporal arteritis it usually starts suddenly, but the indications of a triggering infection are considerably stronger. There is the way it usually starts in the nose, suggesting an air-borne infection. Secondly, the bacterium *Staphylococcus aureus* is found to be living in the nose of some 60% of people with WG. (This bacterium causes boils on the skin and infections elsewhere, but it can live in the nose cavity without necessarily causing any symptoms.) Not all patients with WG carry the organism. Only a few patients carrying the staphylococcus in their nose develop WG, though carriers are more prone to relapses than non-carriers. Thirdly, early cases of WG respond well to the combination broad spectrum antibiotic, trimethoprim/sulfamethoxazole. Unfortunately, even though such treatment may eliminate the staphylococci from the nose, relapses of WG still occur. Indeed, complete cure of Wegener's granulomatosis is exceptionally rare. This makes me wonder if some other, as yet unknown, infective agent not only triggers WG but also perhaps makes it easier for the staphylococcus bacterium to live in the nose. Alternatively, a local staphylococcal infection in the nose might make it easier for some other infective organism to gain a hold.

A painful and unpleasant skin condition known as pyoderma gangrenosum may occur together with Wegener's granulomatosis (as well as with many other inflammatory conditions of uncertain origin, such as inflammatory bowel disease). The association gives a further clue to the possibility of a hitherto unidentified infecting organism being involved in Wegener's granulomatosis. It is also interesting that dapsone and clofazimine (anti-bacterial drugs mainly used to treat leprosy) appear to be helpful in pyoderma gangrenosum, in addition to standard treatment with immunosuppressive drugs such as steroids, cyclophosphamide and cyclosporin.

I cannot finish my account of Wegener's granulomatosis without telling a bizarre but true story. When I was a junior doctor (a 'house physician') in 1953, my chief was Max Rosenheim, who was later elected President of the Royal College of Physicians. He had in his charge a middle-aged woman who was running a fever and who had a blood-stained discharge from her nose. Max made a clinical diagnosis of Wegener's granulomatosis, which was confirmed by biopsy of the ulcer in her nose. At that time there was no treatment known to help Wegener's granulomatosis. The diagnosis was equivalent to a death warrant. The kidney failure to which it appeared to be progressing was uniformly fatal. I therefore asked my chief if I might try some unorthodox treatment. On the assumption that a bizarre infection might be the cause of the disease I administered a full course of an organic antimony preparation (a rather toxic drug which was used to treat certain tropical parasitic infections, notably leishmaniasis). In addition I gave my patient a full course of potassium iodide (because at the time it had a reputation as an anti-fungal agent). To my chief's amazement, and mine, the fever went down and the patient made a full recovery, with no relapse. Everyone assumed that the diagnosis had to have been mistaken, that the patient (an ex-nurse) had been falsifying her temperature readings and that the nasal ulceration was caused by self-induced trauma – despite the firm diagnosis made by our pathologists on the basis of the nasal biopsy. But I have often wondered since this case if some very unusual organism might underlie Wegener's granulomatosis and whether my choice of unconventional therapy might perhaps have cured the patient. Some extremely indolent forms of leishmaniasis are known. As far as I can discover no investigations of antibodies to leishmaniasis or other tropical diseases have been reported in Wegener's granulomatosis.

It would be interesting to make a controlled trial of this therapy. Unfortunately, because combined immunosuppressive treatment nowadays usually controls the disease fairly well (even though it does not cure it) such a trial might be difficult to justify ethically. It is obviously a commonly accepted ethical rule that once any treatment has been shown to improve or control an otherwise fatal condition, it becomes unethical either to withhold that treatment or to administer a dangerous untested alternative.

431

Henoch-Schönlein purpura

This is one of the most interesting small vessel vasculitides. It causes a characteristic skin rash and joint pains. It may also involve the gut, causing colicky abdominal pain. Although there is often both protein and blood in the urine, kidney damage is usually mild and does not progress. It is commonest in childhood, but can occur at any age. There is characteristic deposition of particular (IgE antibody + antigen) immune-complexes in many organs. The disease is unusual in that in most cases cure is spontaneous, after running a short course lasting only a few weeks. I have seen two cases, curiously both in elderly men. It is very difficult to imagine that such a disease is not triggered by an infection arriving suddenly from an external source. It often follows an upper respiratory tract infection. It seems to me very likely that there exists an as yet unidentified organism, which might be a virus or a bacterium and which sets off or triggers the auto-immune reaction which we recognise as Henoch-Schönlein purpura. The relative rareness of the condition makes it difficult to study. It can be confused with more serious conditions such as microscopic polyangiitis.

A patient may suffer from rather general symptoms before the diagnosis can be firmly made. This is a pity because the way in which Henoch-Schönlein purpura usually runs a short sharp self-limiting course might give us important information about the cause of commoner and more serious vasculitides.

Summary

There are many varieties of vasculitis (inflammation of blood vessels), which may affect large or small arteries and to a lesser extent, veins. Temporal arteritis and polymyalgia rheumatica are the commonest conditions. Each runs a course of a few years before resolving, usually spontaneously. Henoch-Schönlein purpura may run a serious explosive course, but in most cases gets better on its own within a few weeks. Polyarteritis nodosa and Wegener's granulomatosis are more serious conditions which do not usually resolve spontaneously. They produce extensive systemic symptoms and organ damage, and usually require continuing immunosuppressive therapy.

In none of the 'vasculitides' I have discussed is the cause known, but many appear to be initiated by an infection in a genetically predisposed individual. They all involve the immune system and respond in various degrees to immunosuppressive drugs.

40

SCHIZOPHRENIA

The word, from Greek (*schizo* = to split; *phren* = mind) encompasses a mixed bag of illnesses. There is no generally agreed definition. The most notable symptoms are delusions, hallucinations and sometimes abnormal behaviour. Since these manifestations can all be found in other disorders, certain symptoms are regarded as 'first-rank' and specially characteristic: e.g. the feeling that other people are reading the victim's thoughts or that his or her thoughts are being inserted or controlled from outside. There may be auditory hallucinations of someone speaking to the victim, perhaps referring to him or her as a third person. There is a lack of logical connected thought. Judgement is impaired. Emotional responses are flattened. In longstanding schizophrenia (SCH) there is commonly apathy and social withdrawal. Surprisingly, long-term memory and consciousness are not usually much affected.

SCH is not uncommon. In different populations and groups throughout the world it affects between 1 in 250 and 1 in 70 people during their lifetime. Apparent geographical differences in prevalence may be due to different criteria for the diagnosis in different parts of the world. In the UK there is at present over-representation of young black Afro-Caribbean men in the category of people diagnosed with SCH, but the reasons for this are not clear. SCH has often been noted to be associated with urban living and has a lesser incidence in people living in the country. In a Danish study the risk of SCH was more than twice as great in town than in country dwellers.[1]

The disease usually begins – or at least becomes apparent – in adolescence or early adulthood. I have personal knowledge of some four young victims, school or college friends of my own or of our children. Typically the first symptom was loss of concentration and intellectual drive in someone previously apparently normal in every way. Two achieved entry to Oxbridge colleges, but started to behave strangely, failed to stay the course and subsequently dropped out. A British survey reported that some 12% of social 'dropouts' were university graduates now living rough on the streets. Some dropouts may have ruined their lives by reckless gambling, overuse of alcohol or of other drugs. But many who are neither reckless gamblers nor drug addicts are individuals with schizophrenia. They might have made a promising start in adult life but were overcome as the disease crept up on them.

The final state of many chronic schizophrenic individuals is one of apathy and withdrawal from social contact. Some 60% of patients with SCH need disability benefits within the first year from the onset of the disease. Some get so depressed about their state that they take their own lives. One of my own school classmates, a very able 17-year-old boy, started behaving strangely, then committed suicide by leading coal gas (then in use in the UK) under his bedclothes. In all, at least 10% of people with SCH commit suicide. This may even be an underestimate because coroners sometimes suppress the diagnosis in their reports, to spare the feelings of relatives.

The disease may develop slowly; but it can also appear as a single episode of inexplicable and perhaps violent behaviour, which may recover almost completely but then recur. Less than 20% of patients make a full recovery after the first episode. Such people present appallingly difficult problems in diagnosis and management if they commit criminal acts. Sometimes it may be difficult to decide if a patient is suffering from acute SCH, from a drug-induced paranoid state, or from some acute medical illness associated with mental symptoms. I recall a friend (and patient) who while febrile from a severe streptococcal septicaemia became absurdly talkative and euphoric. He was convinced that he had 'a yo-yo in my hypothalamus' but his delusions disappeared as his fever subsided. He later became a distinguished endocrinologist. A previously normal elderly man with severe pneumococcal pneumonia climbed out of a fourth floor window on one of my hospital wards and launched himself into space, apparently attempting to fly. Surprisingly, he survived by falling onto the roof of a saloon car, which effectively broke his fall and gave his chest rather violent physiotherapy. He only fractured a small bone in his leg. But other sufferers from acute 'organic' mental disorders such as those which my two patients had are not so lucky.

Pathological changes in the brain in schizophrenia

People used to think that there were no gross pathological changes in the brain in SCH. Ordinary brain X-rays were normal. Anatomical studies of the brain were once described as a 'graveyard' for neuropathologists. The cause of SCH seemed obscure and inexplicable. But recent imaging techniques have changed all this. It is now well established that the brains of people with SCH are on average smaller than those of normal people.[2] At the onset of the disease the fluid-filled ventricles within the brain are larger. Although this suggests that there has been actual loss of nerve cells it now appears that on average neurones are smaller than normal, rather than reduced in number. Structures linking nerve cells together (synapses) are smaller and less abundant than in normal brains.

It has not so far been possible to identify one particular part of the brain as being consistently involved in SCH. There is probably damage to widespread nerve systems. The frontal and temporal lobes of the brain are most often affected. Some authors have noted asymmetries between the two sides of the brain.[3] In some cases reduction of the volume of 'grey matter' (i.e. nerve cells) in certain regions of the brain has been seen to precede the first schizophrenic symptom. As the disease progressed, the volume of brain in the affected regions gradually diminished further.

There is a significantly higher incidence of structural (bony) abnormalities of the face in people with SCH, suggesting that some anatomical changes may have taken place during development.

Genetics

Someone with a first-degree relative (parent or sibling) with the disease has statistically about a seven times greater risk of developing schizophrenia than someone without a first-degree relative with SCH. The risk for someone with both parents having clinically severe SCH is some 47 times greater. Twin studies confirm the importance of genes in determining whether or not an individual develops SCH. Identical twins resemble each other in respect of SCH much more closely than non-identical twins, but most studies show only about a 30% concordance between identical twin pairs.[4] So although the genetic basis of SCH is strong, it is not overwhelming.

Especially in the prefrontal cortex there is a reduction in concentration of a large matrix protein ('reelin') which is concerned with the development of normal brain architecture. A gene known as DISC-1 has been linked with SCH in Scotland and Finland, and several other related genetic predispositions have been identified. There is some evidence of a link of SCH to a gene or genes on chromosome 11, on chromosome 1,[5] and on the X chromosome.[6] A genetics group in Iceland has recently reported a link between SCH and the 'neuregulin 1' (NRG1) gene on chromosome 8. A 'genome scan' – i.e. a fishing expedition without a previous hypothesis or lead to guide it, looking for chromosomes con-

435

taining a gene linked to SCH – has reported possible links with chromosomes 22, 13, 10 and 6.[7] Search continues for a single gene which might have an overwhelming influence on developing SCH, but so far the searches have been inconclusive.

There are some clinical similarities between SCH and the so-called 'bipolar' disorders. Episodes of manic behaviour can be as bizarre as in SCH. However, brain size is not significantly reduced in manic depression, as it is in SCH.

Developmental aspects: Half-way between genes and environment

Since there is only partial concordance between identical twins, in respect of schizophrenia, there must be additional strong non-genetic influences on the disease from the environment. There are several clues to the operation of what may be called 'developmental' factors. Some are difficult to classify. For example, a child's risk of developing SCH is much higher than average if he or she has been conceived by an elderly father. Men between 45 and 49 are twice as likely as men younger than 25 to have schizophrenic children. Evidence from several other diseases suggests that older men have more defective genes in their sperms than young men. Steve Jones, a well-known British geneticist, is passionate that elderly men (he includes himself!) should not be conceiving children, for this reason. It would be interesting to find whether the progeny of a typical group of sporadic SCH sufferers are genetically distinct from the progeny of selected SCH individuals with elderly fathers. I have not so far found any published evidence about this.

It has often been reported that SCH is more likely to develop in babies born in the winter than in the summer months.[8] In one study, children born in early March had a risk of developing SCH that was 1.1 times greater than for those born in early June or in December. Such observations suggest that maternal virus infections during pregnancy could be responsible. It would be unwise to make too much of this. For example, an excessive use of aspirin by a mother might conceivably predispose her fetus to develop small brain haemorrhages.[9] The odds of a child developing SCH have been reported to increase linearly with the number of obstetric complications involving oxygen lack (hypoxia).[10] But since many fetuses have suffered severe hypoxia while in the womb without later developing SCH, lack of oxygen to the developing brain can only be regarded simply as increasing the chance or severity of SCH. It is not a common or important cause.

436

Infections

There have been many observations suggesting that viruses, particularly retroviruses (p. 473, note 6) might cause SCH. Some patients' cerebrospinal fluid (the fluid surrounding the brain) has contained pieces of genetic material (i.e. genes or parts of genes) which closely resemble the genes of some known viruses.

A most promising clue so far suggests that there has sometimes been infection with the Mason-Pfizer monkey virus. Antibodies to this virus have been found in the blood of nearly a third of newly diagnosed people with SCH but very rarely in normal individuals.[11] Borna disease (a RNA virus) affects the brain of some animals and there has been suggestive evidence that it can also infect the human nervous system.[12]

There is an interesting *negative* association between rheumatoid arthritis and schizophrenia: in other words, someone with rheumatoid arthritis is statistically less likely to suffer from SCH than is the average person. We do not know why, but since some of the genetic predisposition to rheumatoid arthritis is linked to the human leucocyte antigen (HLA) system this makes up another piece of evidence suggesting that infection may play a part in damaging the brain and causing schizophrenia. Someone's HLA inheritance seems to affect the chance of him or her getting many of the infectious diseases.

Is there a single cause?

One difficulty in trying assigning a single cause for schizophrenia is that the disease can present itself in so many different ways. Maybe it is several different diseases, rather than one, as has often been suggested. There seems to be a fundamental difference between schizophrenia and psychiatric conditions such as depression and obsessional neurosis. SCH is generally classified as a *psychosis* whereas most of the other conditions are classified as *neuroses*. In most neuroses, however severe, the pattern of thinking remains logical and the patient is usually conscious that his or her mind is temporarily disturbed in some way. This seems not to be the case in most people with SCH. Recent work suggests that many psychotic symptoms such as delusions and hallucinations may be due, in the first place, to the victim being unable to think clearly. Such difficulty, technically described as 'cognitive dysfunction', may precede any frankly psychotic symptoms. This may represent an important revolution in thought about the cause or causes of schizophrenia. It is already beginning to focus attention on disorders of attention, short-term memory, problem solving and decision making, some of which may be identifiable long before frank schizophrenic symptoms appear.

I recall the sequential anatomical studies of Parkinson's disease (Chapter 28). These allowed a particular part of the mid-brain (the substantia nigra) to be identified as the part initially and mainly affected by that disease. But I am not yet convinced that anyone has succeeded in assigning any one single part of the human brain to sensible thinking and to producing crazy thinking when it is damaged, deranged or absent. We need careful long-term neuroimaging studies of teenagers whose parents have SCH. Some of these are going to develop SCH themselves. So it might be possible to observe pathological changes developing in the brain during the course of the disease, as is being done in one current study. As the disease progressed, the volume of brain in the affected regions gradually diminished further.[13] In these patients, the left medial temporal region of the brain was the most severely affected, but there was little consistency between individual patients.

All drugs that increase the concentrations of the natural chemical neurotransmitter dopamine in the brain (e.g. cocaine and amphetamines) increase the chance of someone developing schizophrenic symptoms. So also do some drugs used to treat Parkinson's disease (Chapter 28). All anti-psychotic drugs used to treat SCH diminish dopamine actions by blocking its 'D2' receptor, but the nature of the presumed link has not been established. At present there is both interest, and alarm, that cannabis may provoke symptoms and lead on to frank schizophrenia in susceptible people, especially in those who take the drug when young.

A neat way of summarising the problem of schizophrenia is to say that it is a disease of the brain which is expressed clinically as a disease of the mind. The symptoms and signs seem too diverse to suggest that it can be attributed to defects in any particular region or regions of the brain. With improved imaging of the brain by modern techniques, including CAT scanning and MRI, several anatomical changes in the brain have been found associated with SCH. Unfortunately the changes have not usually been consistent enough to make a coherent story. Perhaps there are really too many different causes of what we lump together as schizophrenia.

Antagonism to science

Most people in the United Kingdom, and in many developed countries, seem to have a strong aversion to science and logic and a strong attraction to mysticism and intuition. Some figures collected by Steven Pinker[14] are extraordinary: for example, the extent to which the observations and conclusions of Darwin, and his concept of evolution by natural selection, are rejected in many American schools. I believe that the pervasive scientific mysticism in the UK mainly reflects the poor teaching of science in our schools. It is very sad that, at a time when science is advancing with such huge and exciting strides, people who consider themselves cultured do not realise that some under-standing of science is a growing part of our culture. Anti-scientific attitudes often get reinforced by unlucky situations or events. For example, classical medicine failed for many years to be able to give any coherent account and explanation for what we now recognise as 'prion' diseases such as scrapie and bovine spongiform encephalo-pathy, in terms of what was known at that time about infections *not* conveyed by unruly desoxyribose nucleic acid (DNA). This failure was pounced on with glee by the cadre of British anti-scientists: 'So you see, scientists don't know everything!'

That is true. It always will be, as all scientists would acknowledge. But it is surely the best possible reason for making observations which might help to explain or comprehend the underlying causes of diseases in terms of current scientific knowledge. Unfortunately opinions about science and medicine not backed by statistically reliable evidence can be not only misleading but positively harmful. I recall the popularity of a book by the late RD Laing called *The Divided Self.* This asserted that the mental manifestations of SCH were due to faults in the way that children were brought up: i.e. the parents were to blame. This caused a great deal of anguish to many parents. The link was never statistically established. But it is another example of the way in which otherwise intelligent people construct and expound theories about causation which fail to stand up to any sort of critical examination.

Summary

Schizophrenia (SCH) describes a condition, or a group of conditions, in which logical thought is suspended, either temporarily or perma-nently. Sufferers cannot concentrate and may exhibit bizarre patterns of behaviour. Some of these are dangerous. Suicide is not uncommon.

The disease may appear to start suddenly, usually in the teens or early twenties, but there may be preceding defects in clear thinking. The symptoms of the disease sometimes recur in a series of relapses, or move gradually into a chronic state. Only about 20% of affected individuals recover completely from SCH.

Although for many years the disease was thought to be purely of psychological origin, modern studies by brain scanning and imaging techniques have revealed that there are usually anatomical changes in the brain, including an actual reduction of brain volume, especially in parts of the frontal and temporal lobes. However, no single part of the brain has yet been identified as specifically affected in SCH.

Genetic factors seem of greatest importance, but some relevant developmental factors have also been identified, e.g. season of birth. There has often been suspicion of an underlying and perhaps causal virus infection, though as yet the evidence is indirect and not directly causal. Drugs affecting the neurotransmitter dopamine, including cannabis, may provoke symptoms and lead to frank disease in susceptible people. Longitudinal studies of currently normal potential victims are urgently needed.

41

FAINTING

The Greek word *syncope* (pronounced 'sin-co-pee') strictly means a 'cutting short' or a swoon, i.e. a sudden loss of consciousness. A faint is a particular kind of syncope. Physicians often describe a faint as 'vaso-vagal' or 'neurocardiogenic' syncope, for reasons which will be explained later.

The most dramatic faint that I have ever seen took place at an international conference in Paris at which a distinguished physiologist was about to deliver a lecture on – ironically – the physiology of veins. He had been seated listening to an appropriately flattering introduction. He stood up, said, 'Mr Chairman, Ladies and Gentlemen ... .' then his voice faded, he passed out and fell to the ground. Although he quickly regained consciousness, he had to abandon his lecture. I took him out to lunch and gave him a lot of salty soup, though he had already fully recovered. He was unlucky. It was a high-prestige occasion; he was tired and nervous; the hall was hot; he had been sitting down for some time before.

What is the mystery? Surely someone faints when the blood pressure gets too low and not enough blood is going to the brain? Correct! But it's not quite that simple. The first thing to note is that people who are lying down flat don't faint. Indeed it is exceptionally rare even for anyone sitting in a chair to faint. The victim of a faint is usually standing up. Someone who is slowly bleeding to death on the ground will just as slowly lose consciousness as his blood pressure slowly falls. In a faint, on the other hand, a lot of things happen very suddenly, within a few seconds. The blood pressure falls sharply. Consciousness is lost. A victim who is standing falls to the ground.

Normal control of the circulation during standing

So let me start by itemising the things that normally happen when someone stands up. Gravity drags some of the circulating blood towards the feet. Elastic blood vessels expand a bit and allow some blood to pool in the lower parts of the body. This reduces the effective

441

volume of circulating blood. The heart can't pump so much blood round. The blood pressure therefore starts to fall. But within a few seconds it comes back to normal because:

1. the fall of blood pressure is detected by pressure sensors in the main arteries and in the heart chambers: these connect to the brain stem via nerves;
2. the brain coordinates the information and sends messages down nerves connected to contractile blood vessels, especially those in the lower parts of the body – the leg veins especially: this makes them contract and squeeze blood towards the heart: the heart therefore fills up better;
3. the brain also sends messages in nerves supplying the heart, making the heart speed up and contract more vigorously.

The control centres in the brain stem are getting all this information continuously, every second of our lives, day and night. The so-called 'autonomic' nervous system (p. 481) automatically brings about appropriate corrective action. It is a classic negative feedback system. If the blood pressure starts to fall for any reason, e.g. standing up, or losing blood, the brain corrects the fall.

What happens during a faint?

During a faint something goes wrong. A reviewer in 1996 commented: 'The cardiovascular system is striving to maintain an adequate blood pressure. What suddenly switches off this compensation...remains one of the most intriguing mysteries in cardiovascular physiology.'[1] Instead of the heart gradually beating faster it suddenly slows right down. Instead of the veins and arteries continuing to contract they suddenly dilate. Consequently, blood pressure falls sharply. The flow of blood to the brain becomes inadequate. The victim loses consciousness and falls to the ground. The faint is preceded by the skin becoming pale and sweaty. There is often accompanying nausea.

The sequence of events has been carefully studied by experiments on normal volunteers on tilt tables. Figure 54 shows on a realistic timescale a diagram of the circulatory changes in a normal young man tilted head-up in a warm room. For the first few minutes (from A to B) the blood pressure was falling slightly, heart rate was gradually increasing and muscle blood flow in arms and legs was decreasing. The blood pressure was being maintained by increased activation of the sympathetic nervous system (p. 481). This corrected the effects of

442

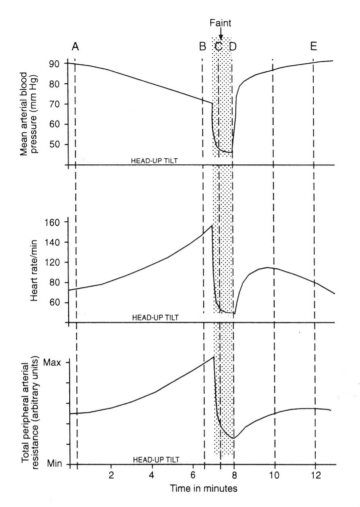

Figure 54 Graphic diagram of the sequence of events (time running from left to right) in the minutes before, during and after a faint, induced in a normal supine adult volunteer by head-up tilting in a warm room. The appropriate compensatory mechanisms were maintaining blood pressure and adequate brain blood supply until the blood pressure fell suddenly and the subject lost consciousness (see text).

gravity by increasing resistance to the flow of blood through the small arteries which comprise the so-called 'peripheral resistance'. Activation of the sympathetic system also constricted veins and increased the heart rate. At point B in Figure 54 the subject complained of nausea. His skin became pale and sweaty. Then suddenly the peripheral resistance fell. Arteries previously constricted suddenly dilated. The heart

443

slowed right down (point C). The blood in the arteries was no longer at a high enough pressure to supply the brain with enough blood. Our subject fainted. Fortunately the whole system started to reverse as soon as he lay flat (point D). The heart speeded up again. Arteries and veins constricted again. Within seconds everything was back to normal (point E).

Such events have often been witnessed by thousands watching military parades in hot weather. It is commonplace for an entirely fit young male soldier, standing stock still, to lose consciousness and fall to the ground as if poleaxed. I have once fainted myself, many years ago, while standing tired and immobile in a hot room. The last thing that I can remember before I lost consciousness was being engulfed by waves of nausea. Before this became actual vomiting I lost consciousness and slumped to the floor. I awoke a few seconds later, feeling entirely well again, though alarmed to find myself on the floor looking up at a ring of anxious faces.

The activities of the autonomic nervous system, especially of its sympathetic division, have been studied during fainting by directly recording nerve impulses from an accessible sympathetic nerve, usually in the leg. This can be done by pushing ultra-thin needles (insulated except at the tip) through the skin and into a nerve trunk. Such records show that until the moment of the faint the rate of discharge of electrical impulses in sympathetic nerves going to arteries supplying the leg muscles progressively increases. This is what makes the arteries constrict. But at the moment of a faint everything reverses. The rate of discharge of impulses in sympathetic nerves gets less and may stop altogether. Blood pressure drops sharply and the heart rate slows. The force of contraction of heart muscle also diminishes. The changes in heart function are mostly brought about by increased nervous discharges in the vagus nerves, which run from the hind brain to the heart. These 'parasympathetic' nerves are also part of the autonomic nervous system, but they have mainly opposite effects to those of the sympathetic nerves. It is possible to remove the cardiac component of fainting by injecting the drug atropine, commonly known as 'belladonna' = beautiful lady, (so-called because it makes the pupils dilate). After giving atropine and tilting someone upright, the heart rate does not slow down. Despite this subjects can still be made to faint.

Fainting has been induced and studied in human volunteers by various combinations of head-up tilt, blood-pressure-lowering drugs, deliberate bleeding, pooling of blood using leg cuffs or lower body negative pressure, and emotional trauma. It may be aggravated by heat, fever, coughing, passing urine or lack of oxygen. The results have been strikingly consistent and conform exactly to the sequence of events shown in Figure 54. The faint itself is accompanied by sweating and by massive secretion of various powerful circulating chemicals (hormones). But however severe it may be, a faint can always be terminated at once by putting the subject flat, or head down, when all the changes reverse within seconds.

Cause

'There is no more dramatic or thoroughly investigated cardiovascular response than the everyday common faint.'[2] The current and now conventional view of its cause was first propounded in 1972. It was suggested that fainting is caused by 'increased activity of the (nerve) receptors located in the left ventricle (of the heart)...with rapid bleeding or pooling of blood, the receptors are excited by an improper squeezing of the myocardium when the ventricles contract vigorously around an almost empty chamber...it seems reasonable to conclude that they (ventricular receptors) are, to a large extent, responsible for triggering this response.'[3] I think that this explanation is wrong, or at best incomplete.

Here is a more recent verdict: 'A link between ventricular receptor activity and the vasovagal reaction (i.e. the faint) is not firmly established. It has not even been demonstrated that there is a net increase in ventricular (baroreceptor nervous) activity after hemorrhage.'[4] Karl Popper has pointed out that although no amount of supportive evidence ever proves a case, a scientific hypothesis may be refuted by a single piece of contradictory evidence. Such evidence is now available. Typical faints have been observed in cardiac transplant patients. Such patients have had both ventricles removed and replaced. All nerves to the ventricles have been cut. In one patient studied, after infusion of a drug which dilated blood vessels 'classic vasovagal symptoms suddenly developed...accompanied by the abrupt cessation of sympathetic discharge. From these observations, we conclude that vasodilator-induced syncope is not always dependent on ventricular baroreceptor activation.'[5] Although heart transplantation removes the cardiac ventricles it leaves behind the posterior walls of the two atria. Many sensory nerve endings in the atria and great veins will inevitably survive. Figure 55 shows the normal human heart viewed from the front. The right and left ventricles (sacrificed before transplantation) are horizontally line-shaded.

The remaining back walls of the two atria and the superior vena cava are left. It is notable that after cardiac transplantation 'afferents from the remnant atria, venoarterial junctions, pulmonary veins...are

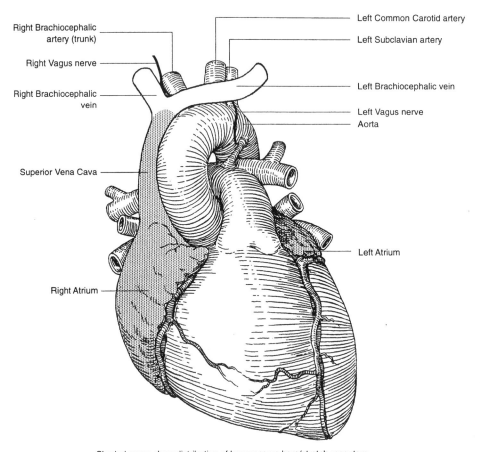

Right Brachiocephalic artery (trunk)

Right Vagus nerve

Right Brachiocephalic vein

Superior Vena Cava

Right Atrium

Left Common Carotid artery

Left Subclavian artery

Left Brachiocephalic vein

Left Vagus nerve
Aorta

Left Atrium

Shaded areas show distribution of low pressure baro/stretch receptors

Figure 55 Diagram of the heart and main blood vessels seen from the front after opening the chest. The horizontal line shading shows the two ventricles, with coronary arteries on their surface. The fine shaded areas – the right atrium, superior vena cava and left atrium – contain in their walls the low pressure stretch receptors (venous baroreceptors). These send nerve impulses up to the brain via the vagus nerves on each side.

left intact.' So why could not vaso-vagal syncope be triggered from these receptors rather than from the ventricles?

Fainting can, as I have suggested elsewhere,[6] be best accounted for by the sudden collapse of inadequately-filled atria (especially the right atrium) and of unfilled great veins. This could send misleading information to the brain, telling it that the heart was over- rather than under-filled. Consequent dilation of arteries and veins would decrease

446

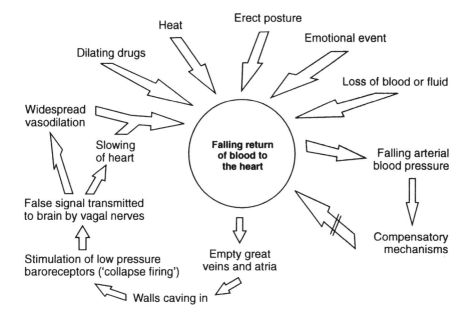

Heat

Erect posture

Dilating drugs

Emotional event

Loss of blood or fluid

Widespread vasodilation

Slowing of heart

Falling return of blood to the heart

Falling arterial blood pressure

False signal transmitted to brain by vagal nerves

Stimulation of low pressure baroreceptors ('collapse firing')

Empty great veins and atria

Compensatory mechanisms

Walls caving in

Figure 56 Hypothetical but plausible vicious circle, showing precipitating factors leading to falling blood pressure and to a sequence of events which – if compensatory mechanisms are not powerful enough – could cause slowing of the heart and widespread dilation of blood vessels, leading to fainting.

right atrial pressure still further and lead to a vicious circle (Fig. 56). This would explain the abrupt nature of the faint.

Many years ago, when working with the late David Whitteridge in the Department of Physiology at Oxford I was recording the electrical activity of nerves in the neck of anaesthetised cats. These were conveying electrical impulses from the heart to the brain. I noticed that there were numerous nerves coming from receptors in the atria and great veins but relatively few from receptors located in the cardiac ventricles. It was easy to increase the rate of discharge of nerve impulses from the right atrium by lightly pressing its front wall with a glass rod, or even with my fingertip. Inward collapse of the atrial wall would therefore be expected to lead to an increase in the rate of discharge of nerve impulses coming from atrial stretch receptors. Even in the more rigid carotid artery it has been observed that when internal pressure falls to zero, or close to it, the discharge rate of the baroreceptors in the carotid sinus wall paradoxically increases. This phenomenon is known as 'collapse firing' of these receptors.

447

My explanation of fainting is supported by a brief report of old observations[7] that when nerve impulses coming from atrial stretch receptors were recorded during experimental haemorrhage the discharge rate notably increased. My emphasis on the low-pressure side of the systemic circulation is also compatible with observations by the late EP Sharpey-Schafer, who made many of the seminal clinical studies of fainting. He noted that congestive heart failure in man, in which the circulation is overfilled and pressure in the right atrium and great veins is greatly increased, gives 'immunity from vaso-vagal syncope' – as my hypothesis would predict.

There is considerable, though not unanimous, evidence which I have reviewed elsewhere that increased nerve impulse traffic from atrial stretch receptors causes reflex dilation of blood vessels and slowing of the heart. So far, so good. But the effects of atrial volume changes on heart rate are less clear cut. Increased pressure in the right side of the heart in dogs and in cats has been recorded as causing slowing of the heart, through a vagus nerve-mediated reflex. In other circumstances opposite effects on heart rate have been observed. However, all the available evidence suggests that the normal physiological response to increased discharge from atrial and atrio-venous baroreceptors is dilation of systemic arteries and veins. This is exactly what happens at the start of a faint. There is no reliable evidence to contradict my premise that the normal physiological response to increased venous baroreceptor discharge, at least at high initial heart rates, is slowing of the heart. This is the other component of the vaso-vagal response.

Though the evidence in favour of my hypothesis is strong, it is not of course conclusive. Indeed, as a follower of Karl Popper, I must accept that there is no such thing as a scientific 'proof' of anything. We have to work at all times on the balance of probabilities given the evidence available at the time. I have tried, so far without success, to persuade someone with the necessary facilities to join me to look by ultrasound imaging of human subjects at the cavity of the right atrium as the faint begins, to see whether it collapses inwards precisely at that moment, as I predict. I also predict that it should be possible for a subject to initiate a faint prematurely by trying to breathe out against resistance, e.g. by blowing up a balloon. This should make the low-pressure atria and large veins in the chest collapse.

Fortunately these are such simple experiments that I am hopeful a definitive answer will soon be forthcoming. In the meantime, the current opinion of most physiologists is still that the cardiac ventricles are primarily involved, and/or that the faint reaction is coordinated in the brain. I am suggesting, in this heretical chapter, that the cardiac ventricles play no important part in initiating fainting and that the brain is getting its misleading information from low-pressure receptors in atria and large veins. But whether I am right or wrong, I hope the reader will agree that fainting is one of the most fascinating medical mysteries around.

Summary

Fainting is a strange reaction which can occur in people standing upright who remain very still, lose blood or in some other way suffer a gradual fall of blood pressure. Suddenly the heart rate (which had been hitherto increasing) slows right down. Systemic arteries (which had been progressively constricting) open up. The blood pressure falls dramatically, within a few seconds. There is then not enough blood going to the brain and the individual faints. Before the faint 'the cardiovascular system is striving to maintain an adequate blood pressure. What suddenly switches off this compensation...remains one of the most intriguing mysteries in cardiovascular physiology.'

I have suggested that 'collapse firing' of low-pressure baro(stretch)-receptors in the right atrium and great veins, and possibly on the left side of the heart as well, is a plausible and sufficient explanation for the sequence of events in fainting. The central effects of such inappropriate information coming to the brain are dilation of systemic blood vessels and slowing of the heart. Activation of ventricular muscle receptors is neither a probable nor a necessary cause of fainting, though it might play an additional part in the response. This hypothesis explains logically why fainting does not occur in the presence of congestive heart failure and why it can still be observed in patients who have had heart transplants.

If at the moment the faint occurs the right atrium and/or great veins do not suddenly collapse inwards, my hypothesis is disproved. The atria and great veins can easily be watched moment to moment by ultrasound imaging, which can show the outline of these low-pressure vessels without even puncturing the skin. So far I have been unsuccessful in persuading anyone with the necessary facilities (tilt table and 3-dimensional ultrasound) to join me to examine the problem, but I live in hope!

42

MOTOR NEURONE DISEASE

I shall review a lot of published work in this last chapter in considerable technical detail. I want to use motor neurone disease (MND) as
an example of the enormous number of interconnecting lines of
evidence which sometimes have to be examined in attempts to understand a common but mysterious condition. I have looked after several
people with the disease, but have never done any personal research on
it. The only advantage I claim for this review is that it starts from no
particular point of view, though inevitably I have developed an
opinion of my own about it. Non-technical and lay readers of this
chapter might be well advised to skip it, but I have included it as an
example of the different ways and paths that medical scientists have
been following, during the last 100 years, while trying to understand a
common human disease. In this chapter I have briefly summarised
their hypotheses.

Motor neuron(e) disease is a progressive and fatal disease of the
spinal cord and/or the brain.[1] It affects both 'upper' and 'lower' motor
neurones (defined in Chapter 3). Figure 3 (p. 32) shows the main nerve
tracts which connect cell bodies in the brain and spinal cord to the
muscles they control. The commonest form of motor neurone disease
is 'amyotrophic lateral sclerosis' (ALS)[2] in which both upper and
lower motor neurones are involved. Less common varieties of MND
are 'progressive (myelopathic) muscular atrophy', in which the lower
motor neurones in the spinal cord are principally involved, and
'(progressive) bulbar palsy', in which the lower parts of the brain
supplying the tongue and swallowing muscles are chiefly affected.
When some famous person is said to have suffered from 'motor
neurone disease' (for instance, the late David Niven, James Mason or
Jill Tweedie) this usually means ALS.

Between 5% and 10% of people with motor neurone disease report
that someone in the immediate family has or had the condition. In
most of these uncommon familial cases the disease is passed on as an
autosomal dominant[3] characteristic. But in the majority of cases the
disease is sporadic. It arises in families which have no similarly
affected relatives. It appears to strike at random. Such sporadic non-

genetic cases make up the great majority. But since familial cases behave clinically in a similar way to sporadic cases, in terms of speed of deterioration and in selectivity of affected neurones, study of familial cases might shed some light on the possible cause or causes of the much commoner sporadic cases.

> It is interesting that certain variants in the gene for vascular endothelial growth factor (VEGF: see p. 452) affect the risk of developing ALS. This new avenue is being actively explored to find whether increasing VEGF concentrations might favourably modify the course of ALS. In the mouse, a gene has been identified which can have specific effects on *motor* nerve function but which does not involve other categories of nerve fibres or neurones in the brain or spinal cord.

Men are about $1\frac{1}{2}$ times more commonly affected by motor neurone disease than women. Somewhere between 3 and 14 people in every 100,000 of the population of the world are affected at any one time. MND is relatively common compared with other neurological disorders. It has an incidence comparable with that of multiple sclerosis(Chapter 3). But the number of sufferers alive at any one time is much less than those with multiple sclerosis, because the life span of MND is so short. All varieties of motor neurone disease account for around one in 100,000 deaths per year in most populations. No notable racial differences have been identified but the disease is commoner in white than in black people. Skilled non-manual workers have the highest incidence, but differences between social classes are small. There are some geographical differences in incidence, though it is not certain whether the disease in Japan and in some Far East islands (Guam in particular) is the same as in other parts of the world.

The clinical course of MND

The disease causes weakness and eventually paralysis of the muscles supplied by the affected neurones. Weakness usually appears first in the leg muscles. Later other muscles concerned with breathing and swallowing may be affected. The eye muscles are usually spared. Death usually results from paralysis of breathing, or from pneumonia. The disease runs an inexorable course. It lasts about $2\frac{1}{2}$ years from first symptoms to death, though longer survivals are possible. Only about 15% of sufferers live as long as 5 years from first diagnosis. The disease seems to progress more rapidly in older than in younger people. Artificial support of breathing, eating and other bodily functions can extend life, though most sufferers choose not to accept such options even when they are available. Intellectual function may become impaired but in many cases it remains normal throughout the illness. Careful studies sometimes reveal minor faults in intellectual functions and language in some patients.[4] Everyone knows of the intellectual scientific achievements of Stephen Hawking, the Cambridge theoretical physicist. Much of his recent work has been done despite his inability to speak, swallow, or move almost any muscle in his body. There is an allied disease in which the typical motor paralysis is associated with dementia from the onset of the illness, but this is less common than classic motor neurone disease.

The disease can strike from the age of about 40 onwards: 62 is the commonest age at death. There may have been a slight increase in death rates from motor neurone disease in the last few decades, but this may be due to better diagnosis and to the increasing age of the population. Although some data suggest that the longer you live the greater your chance of getting the disease, other data suggest that 55–75 are the years of maximal risk and that the risk declines after age 75.[5]

Some studies have suggested that preceding severe mechanical trauma to the head or neck may be commoner in MND patients than in a control population of similar age. Previous vigorous physical activity has also been said to be associated with MND. In animals, head trauma can initiate neuronal damage which can be alleviated with nerve growth factors. In man, the evidence that trauma plays a significant part in motor neurone disease is controversial.[6]

Pathological changes in MND

The cell bodies of motor neurones bear the brunt of the disease. Conduction of impulses in the thin nerve fibres themselves usually remains normal until late in the disease, though a sub-group of ALS patients show conduction abnormalities in their motor nerve fibres early on.

Under the microscope the cell bodies of motor neurones show several abnormalities.[7] Swellings looking like filaments or microtubules are common. These are about one thousandth of the diameter of a single human red blood cell (10–15 nm in diameter).[8] The filamentous swellings are in loosely-arranged bundles (skeins). They are sometimes seen both in motor nerve cell bodies and in motor nerve fibres. They contain a specific protein (ubiquitin) which, when attached to unwanted proteins or protein fragments, marks them down for removal by the so-called ubiquitin-proteolytic pathway.[9] (See also note 3 for Chapter 19.)

Other abnormal collections of material inside cells – so-called cellular 'inclusions' – are almost invariably seen in motor neurone disease, but only rarely in other neurological disorders except for the two common ones described in this book: the neurofibrillary skeins and tangles of Alzheimer's disease (Chapter 19), and the Lewy bodies in Parkinson's disease (Chapter 28).

In motor neurone disease the cellular inclusions known as 'Bunina bodies' are usually visible in lower motor neurone nuclei in the spinal cord and brain stem. The inclusions can be appropriately dyed and identified under the microscope. They are reliable markers of MND when present.[10] They don't look like either viruses or bacteria. Instead they appear to be abnormal collections of proteinaceous material, some of which is ubiquitin. This is known to bind strongly to the metal element aluminium, though concentrations of aluminium are not increased in nerve cells in ALS. The presence of discrete Bunina bodies containing ubiquitin suggests that they comprise material which has been marked down for degradation and removal, but which cells cannot process normally. This therefore accumulates and damages nerve cells.

A better understood type of abnormal cell inclusion is found in nerve cell nuclei in 'Huntington's disease' in man and in the genetically-engineered mouse which is bred to expresses abnormal (mutant) Huntington's genes. Huntington's disease resembles motor neurone disease only in that it is a relentlessly progressive human brain disease of middle age. It is associated with dementia and bizarre muscle movements. It is an hereditary disease in which the genetic fault gives rise to an excess of so-called 'triplet repeats' of the CAG code in the DNA of a specific chromosome (the short arm of chromosome 4). This instructs the cell to make a protein which is abnormally lengthened by a string of glutamine residues. The protein cannot be metabolised normally. It therefore accumulates as intracellular particles which eventually damage or destroy nerve cells.[11] This may be due to aggregation of the particles themselves or to aggregation with other proteins. Despite its combination with ubiquitin, it seems that cells cannot process the unwanted material. Several other conditions causing nerve or muscle disorders are also caused by the 'triplet-repeat' type of genetic fault, but there is no evidence of a similar fault in sporadic motor neurone disease.

Chemically and under the electron microscope[12] Bunina bodies resemble the structure inside cells known as the 'rough endoplasmic reticulum'. (Although the Latin word *reticulum* means a net, the endoplasmic reticulum is really more like a collapsed balloon, with a cavity surrounded by a membrane. It is concerned with the folding and processing of newly synthesised proteins.) Other 'hyaline' (Greek: *hyalos* = glass; i.e. glassy) ubiquitin-containing inclusions may also be present. These have been reported in both familial as well as sporadic motor neurone disease. All these cellular inclusions might suggest that neurones in MND have been suffering from excessive protein degradation, but the concentrations in spinal cord tissue of all known enzymes concerned with protein degradation appear to be normal.[13] The presence of intracellular inclusions in MND suggests that nerve cells are producing insoluble lumps of protein which cannot be broken down by cellular enzymes. It is reasonable to assume that such inclusions interfere with nerve cell function and are the immediate cause of symptoms.

Affected neurones seem to become apoptotic.[14] The body is somehow signalled to accept this form of cell death. Apoptosis does not provoke an inflammatory response. There has been some evidence that apoptosis-promoting gene(s) may be overactive in MND, but nothing to suggest why they should be switched on. The cytokine TNFα is increased in the cerebrospinal fluid of MND patients. It may mediate or accelerate neuronal cell death.

Cause

A recent reviewer wrote: 'A unifying hypothesis will have to explain the diverse geographical occurrence, clinical features, and selective vulnerability and relative resistance of different neuronal populations in the disease...Viruses, metals, endogenous toxins, immune dysfunction, endocrine abnormalities, impaired DNA repair, altered axonal transport, and trauma have all been etiologically linked with ALS, but convincing research evidence of a causative role for any of these factors is yet to be demonstrated.'

Many investigators have pointed to resemblances between three common neurological disorders which all occur at a similar time of life: motor neurone disease, Alzheimer's disease (Chapter 19) and Parkinson's disease (Chapter 28). Two of these diseases have several times been observed in the same patient. The epidemiological resemblances have suggested that all three conditions might result from defective resistance of cell constituents to oxidative damage from 'free radicals'[15] – highly reactive chemicals produced during metabolism (see below). In Alzheimer's disease the protein ubiquitin accumulates inside cells as it does in MND, but it is contained in so-called 'neurofibrillary tangles' rather than in hyaline or skein-like inclusions.

The way in which previously normal individuals can be struck down by these diseases in their fifties or sixties has suggested the possibility that age-related attrition of neurones may be superimposed on some subtle damage arising early in life. Such a theory may eventually prove to be true, but it is rather unhelpful since there is no obvious way in which it can at present be tested.

A specific enzyme defect

There is now much evidence that familial cases are linked to point mutations in the gene which codes in nerve cells for a specific enzyme, a
protein catalyst called 'copper-zinc superoxide dismutase' (Cu/Zn SOD).
The enzyme concerned is one of a family which helps to inactivate and
disable highly reactive and potentially damaging 'free radicals', chemicals
produced during reactions involved in extracting energy from foodstuffs.
Technically, free radicals are chemical species containing one or more
unpaired electrons. This makes them highly reactive. The most damaging
is the hydroxyl radical, but a number of other chemical species are also
important. There is evidence of hydroxyl radical damage to brain neurones in many cases of dementia, though not in all the neurodegenerative
diseases. One important school of thought, impressed by the clinical and
pathological similarities between Parkinson's, Alzheimer's and motor
neurone disease, has suggested that in all three conditions nerve cells are
damaged by the accumulation of superoxide radicals.

The human gene for Cu/Zn SOD resides on chromosome 21 in the
21q22.1 band.[16] Each molecule of the enzyme concerned contains one
zinc and one copper atom. These are intimately concerned with the
enzyme's chemical function. Many different mutations have been recognised. Most result in a dominant type of inheritance of motor neurone
disease, but an autosomal recessive variety has also been recognised.[17]
On the face of it, it is odd that many diverse differences in the protein
structure of an enzyme can give rise to the same clinical manifestations.
Many minor alterations in protein shape can interfere with the metal
binding sites in the molecule.[18] It is strange that such a biochemical
disease should often show itself in heterozygotes, i.e. in people whose
cells contain only a single copy of the defective enzyme. In most situations of this sort half the normal amount of an enzyme will usually only
produce mild if any symptoms. A recent extraordinary observation is
that mice in which Cu/Zn SOD has been removed ('knocked out') by
genetic manipulation appear to be entirely normal. It may therefore be
that it is not the impaired removal of superoxide by defective Cu/Zn
SOD which causes neuronal damage in MND, but rather the acquisition
of a toxic gain of function by the mutant protein. Alternatively, perhaps
the defective Cu/Zn SOD protein is abnormally prone to form damaging
aggregates (see below).

The selective vulnerability of motor neurones in the presence of SOD
mutations is only a relative phenomenon. It is not a 'black-or-white'
affair. Careful examination has shown abnormalities in other parts of
the nervous system, e.g. in pathways concerned with sensation rather
than movement.

Human genes can be grafted into mice, creating so-called 'transgenic' animals. Human neurofilament genes inserted into mice make

the animals develop neurological defects and abnormal filamentous swellings in nerve cells resembling those of human ALS.[19] Other transgenic mice have been created having the mutation in the gene coding for superoxide dismutase-1 which causes human familial MND. These mice also develop neurological defects resembling ALS.[20]

As mentioned above, an interesting recent suggestion has emerged from these studies – that mutations in the Cu/Zn SOD gene may have created an inverted, anomalous and toxic *gain* of function rather than a loss of function. Instead of mopping up damaging free radicals perhaps the altered enzyme might actually produce free radicals. Various hypotheses can explain how a gain of enzyme function might arise and how abnormal handling of free radicals by mutant SOD1 might increase the formation of highly damaging peroxynitrite or hydroxyl free radicals. Cellular toxicity might result from release of copper or zinc. Perhaps abnormal protein deposits could result from aggregation of a defective SOD1 protein. Concentrations of the SOD1 enzyme have been measured in brain and in various other tissues in sporadic MND. They are not abnormal, though a related free radical scavenger enzyme (glutathione peroxidase) may be reduced in ALS.

Horses carry a gene closely similar to the human Cu/Zn SOD gene. They can also suffer from an inherited condition similar to ALS.[21] Motor neurones in their spinal cord show abnormal structures in nerve cells which resemble Bunina bodies, though these are not the same as in man. Unfortunately the superoxide dismutase gene in these diseased horses appears to be identical with that in normal animals, so horse ALS is clearly not the same condition as human inherited motor neurone disease.

Motor neurone disease runs in families in 5-10% of cases. Mutations in the superoxide dismutase gene account for 20% of familial cases and for about 2% of all cases of MND.[22] But neither in the human sporadic cases of MND nor in inherited motor neurone disease in horses is there commonly a recognisable defect in the enzyme, although a few specific mutations have been reported in apparently sporadic human cases. A technique known as 'linkage analysis' has revealed that human chromosomes 2q and 9q may contain gene mutations, some of which may underlie some rare forms of juvenile MND. But no genetic predisposition has so far been identified in the great majority of human MND sufferers.

Other possible causes

Many investigators have speculated that MND might be caused by some mineral deficiency, e.g. of calcium, magnesium, copper or iodine; but mineral supplementation has no effect on the disease. The largely negative findings 'suggest that generation of free radicals from exogenous chemicals is not important in ALS, and further that the neurone (as compared with other cell types) is poorly protected against the toxicity of hydrogen peroxide'. It is striking that the motor neurone disease seen in Guam and related Pacific islands is associated, like sporadic MND, with Bunina bodies and skein-like 'inclusions' inside cells.[23] No one yet knows why these structures appear. If they are simply produced when motor nerve cells degenerate and can appear in various different varieties of motor neurone disease they may not necessarily tell us anything at all about its underlying cause. On the other hand, Bunina bodies are virtually diagnostic of MND and are almost never seen in other neurodegenerative conditions.

Auto-immune dysfunction

Many diseases in man are 'auto-immune' – that is, caused by the body reacting against its own cells and tissues in a damaging way. In some people dying from ALS an excess of lymphocytes has been seen in the spinal cord, suggesting immunological damage.[24] Degeneration of motor nerve cells can be produced by inoculating animals with spinal cord 'grey matter'. This contains the cell bodies of lower motor neurones and provokes an immune reaction ('auto-immune grey matter disease') which damages both upper and lower motor neurones, producing muscle weakness similar to that of MND in man.[25] The foci of damage in the recipient animals' spinal cords look similar to lesions of MND in man. However, the evidence for a comparable immune reaction in human MND is not strong. It is possible to show the presence of antibodies and increased chemical neurotransmitter release in mouse motor neurones after injecting mice with serum from ALS patients, but not after injecting serum from normal people.[26] This also suggests that an immunological reaction could be damaging. But this is a long way from creating an animal model of motor neurone disease. Most human auto-immune diseases respond in some degree to so-called 'immunosuppressive' drugs such as steroids and azathioprine, but such drugs have been given for a year to ALS patients with no discernible benefit.

Multifocal motor neuropathy with conduction block is a rare condition with some features resembling MND, though MND can be distinguished by the absence, until late stages, of nerve conduction block. MMNCB is presumably immune-mediated. The neurological features of motor weakness and paralysis often improve spectacularly with high doses of immunoglobulins.[27] Unfortunately motor neurone disease is not improved by this treatment.

Virus infections

Since acute poliomyelitis (formerly called 'infantile paralysis') is known to be due to an infection with the polio virus, which particularly attacks lower motor neurone cells in the spinal cord, it is natural to speculate that some similar virus might selectively attack upper as well as lower motor neurones and cause MND. However, searches for poliovirus infection in ALS have so far drawn a blank.[28] In any case, poliomyelitis has now been gone from the developed world for almost a decade because of the great success of vaccination. MND incidence has not altered during this time.

Inoculating monkeys with another virus (technically a 'togavirus') has produced neurological defects resembling ALS.[29] Some genetically susceptible wild mice develop a progressive motor neurone disease, after a long latent period, when infected by a specific virus[30] – but no comparable virus has been identified in human MND. One objection to invoking a virus cause of MND is its natural history. MND is a relentlessly progressive condition. Although an acute attack of polio-myelitis can be devastating, once the patient has recovered the pattern of muscular paralysis usually remains constant for the rest of life. None the less, other viruses are capable of producing a grumbling rather than an acute infection (e.g. hepatitis C). As I discussed in Chapter 3, multiple sclerosis may well be triggered by a low-grade persisting virus infection acquired decades before the disease becomes clinically manifest.

Deficiency of nerve-growth or nerve-protective factors

Another chase which seems to have petered out is the investigation of various nerve growth factors – chemical stimulants which cause neurones to grow and to sprout fibre connections. So far there is no evidence that the known nerve growth factors are deficient in MND.

Instead of incriminating some damaging neurotoxic factor, is MND due perhaps to the absence of some neuroprotective factor? During development of the brain and spinal cord some neurones are cleared away by apoptosis while others are stimulated to grow, by chemical 'neurotropic' factors, of which at least four separate ones have already been identified.[31] This avenue is still being actively explored. There is current interest in gene products called 'Brn-3a' which appear to give nerve cells in culture some protection against apoptosis. Indirect protection of nerve cells is also given by angiostatic factors such as those discussed in Chapter 7, because the survival and growth of nerve cells is only possible if cells retain an adequate blood supply. One of the growth factors mentioned above is a protein called 'ciliary neurotropic factor' (CNTF) which has been observed to improve the survival of several types of nerve cell cultured outside the body. It has been tried experimentally as a possible treatment for motor neurone disease.[32] Unfortunately it has too many adverse side effects. But its distribution in the body of MND patients has thrown up the surprising finding that it is present in unusually high concentration in the skin, perhaps as a response to the disease process. There is a curious observation that patients with MND almost never get bedsores, even though they are grossly enfeebled towards the end of their lives and lie still for long periods. It has therefore been suggested that CNTF may in some way protect against bedsores.

Extrinsic toxic agents

Various metals have been suspected of being causal agents of MND, e.g. lead, aluminium, selenium and many others. Some seem to be taken up selectively by motor neurones, making them plausible causes of MND, e.g. inorganic mercury.[33] Unfortunately there is no evidence of excess of mercury or of any other element in the brain, apart from aluminium. Acid rain can liberate large amounts of aluminium in a bioavailable form.[34] So far all searches for environmental aluminium have been negative, though it is interesting that chronic inflammation of the spinal cord resembling MND can be produced in rabbits by long-term low-dose administration of aluminium. Aluminium toxicity in man has been seen in some patients with kidney failure inadvertently given aluminium. It involves bone and blood disorders as well as disorders of the nervous system. Since motor neurone disease is not directly associated with either bone or blood disorders, aluminium toxicity seems unlikely to be its cause.

Could the neuronal damage be due to a common external organic damaging agent? Two examples of neurotoxic materials causing human disease are lathyrism and cassavism. These two conditions are both examples of irreversible spastic paralysis caused by eating staple diets of grass pea and cassava root, respectively. Mildewed sugar cane can produce brain damage and muscle disorder. The cycad seed kernel, containing the neurotoxin cycasin, is thought to have a role in causing the variety of Parkinsonism/dementia-associated ALS which is found in the Western Pacific.[35] A clue to the possible involvement of such an agent is that spouses of affected patients appear to have an increased risk of ALS. Deficiency of calcium and magnesium has been suggested as perhaps magnifying the neurotoxic effects of harmful dietary constituents.

One report has suggested an increased incidence of motor neurone disease in farmers. Considerable impetus has been given to the search for an ingested toxic factor in MND by the discovery that an agricultural chemical called MPTP can produce in man a picture virtually identical with the common neurodegenerative condition known as Parkinson's disease. In 1942 in Italy there was an epidemic of combined lower and upper motor neurone damage, without sensory loss, which closely resembled ALS. The condition was eventually traced to organophosphate poisoning from a rubbish dump close to a farmyard. But once the affected patients were isolated no further neurological damage ensued, though the disability persisted.[36]

Poisoning by some specific article of diet does not adequately account for the progression of the disease. I have watched several sufferers from MND towards the end of their lives. They remain in hospitals or hospices, on standard diets. Despite this they continue to deteriorate relentlessly. I think therefore that MND is most unlikely to be due to a limited exposure to a toxin over a short time period. Organic compounds of mercury may be an exception. Bacteria can transform inorganic mercury into a fat-soluble organic form (methyl mercury),[37] which can induce neuronal apoptosis.[38] A single exposure to dimethyl mercury has been recorded as having caused long delayed brain damage in man. Perhaps we have yet to identify a poison which has the same progressively damaging effects as does dimethyl mercury. Cases of intolerance to specific foods (e.g. peanuts) are well known. It therefore remains remotely possible that motor neurone disease might be caused in a few specially susceptible individuals by some common article of diet, such as potatoes. Continuing exposure to or ingestion of a common environmental or dietary factor could perhaps explain the relentless way in which motor neurone disease behaves even in a protective hospital environment. Although this seems to me most unlikely, it is exceedingly difficult to disprove.

The 'excitotoxic' theory

This currently popular theory implies that motor neurones are being damaged by being driven to discharge excessively. Activation of neurones involves a series of complex chemical reactions leading to the entry of calcium ions into cells and to the release of calcium bound to an intracellular structure, the endoplasmic reticulum. The many observations of increased calcium concentrations in neurones and in motor nerve terminals in ALS are compatible with excessive activation. Aberrant electrical excitation of heart muscle fibres in a circus manner is well known. It leads to failure of coordinated cardiac contraction and can even cause death by 'ventricular fibrillation'. One might therefore envisage the possibility that there is a comparable abnormal circus excitation going on in the brain in MND. If so, an increase in local metabolic rate and regional blood flow would be expected. But overall glucose consumption and cerebral blood flow are both less than normal. Regional blood flows in the frontal and anterior temporal regions and in the sensori-motor cortex are all reduced in MND. On these grounds I do not believe that aberrant excessive circular excitation could possibly account for MND. Indeed, unless excessive neuronal activation could be identified in the early stages of motor neurone disease, before neurones were supposedly 'exhausted', excitotoxic theories seem (to me) to be non-starters.

On the other hand, there is some evidence that MND patients do have excessive release of the ubiquitous excitant chemical neurotransmitter 'glutamate'.[39] Excessive glutamate release might somehow have exhausted motor neurones. There is some evidence that glutamate transporters (chemicals which remove glutamate from the junctions between nerve cells, thus terminating its excitatory effect) are deficient in ALS. Reduced activity of these transporters seems the likeliest cause for a (compensatory) increased concentration of glutamate in the fluid surrounding the brain (the cerebrospinal fluid). One of the active principles of the cycad seed is an amino-acid which is a low potency activator of glutamate-requiring receptors. Observations of this kind have led to a trial of a drug (riluzole) which partly blocks glutamate release at nerve terminals, thereby decreasing the rate at which motor nerve cells discharge electrical impulses. Riluzole has been thought to protect nerve cells from glutamate-induced damage. In an early trial in ALS, treated patients with ALS survived longer than untreated ones.[40] Several later trials have confirmed some beneficial effect. This same drug is also being tested for its possible benefit in Parkinson's disease, another neurodegenerative condition. There is also current interest in lithium, the chemical element which is extensively used to treat depression, especially manic-depression. Lithium is also thought to work by interfering with glutamate action.

Does the cycad seed give us further clues about motor neurone disease? Cycasin, its toxic constituent, has been observed to interfere with glucose transport across cell walls, or into vesicles (minute fluid-filled bladders) inside cells.[41] Neurones are not supplied with nutrients directly from the bloodstream and do not make direct contact with blood vessels. The cells lining brain capillaries (endothelial cells) are

462

joined together at so-called 'tight junctions', which limit the diffusion of water and small molecules between cells. Such junctions in brain blood vessels are up to 100 times tighter than those between endothelial cells elsewhere in the body. This property seems to derive from them having nerve cells close by. Nerve cells appear to have the ability to make the junctions between blood-vessel-lining (endothelial) cells tighter and less permeable, possibly by secreting one or more cytokines such as bradykinin, serotonin, substance-P or interleukins.

Nutrients and oxygen get into nerve cells via the glial cells. These cells comprise the connective tissue of the brain. They may be 10 or even 100 times more numerous than neurones. The largest are the star-shaped astrocytes which have processes making contact with many other glial cells and with neurones. Smaller glial cells (the oligodendrocytes) have fewer and smaller connecting processes. The cells are named from their appearance under the microscope: (Greek: *oligo* = few; *dendron* = tree). The smallest but most numerous cells are the microglia.

When I was a student no one seemed to know what lymphocytes did, even though they comprised more than a third of all the white cells of the blood. Their vital role in immune protection was only revealed several years later. In the brain there are far more glial cells than there are neurones, so glial cells must be immensely important.[42] We have very little idea exactly what they do. As Thelma Lovick put it recently in a review, 'Behind every successful powerful neurone is a fleet of astrocytes whose contribution (to cleaning, feeding nurturing and repairing neurones) has, until recently, gone largely unrecognised'. Glial cells can modify neuronal function, e.g. by altering the local concentration of calcium and of neurotransmitters such as glutamate. As I mentioned in Chapter 19, the neurofibrillary tangles which characterise damaged neurones in Alzheimer's disease are also seen inside glial cells. Perhaps in MND damaged glial cells become functionally inadequate in handing on glucose or oxygen.

The human brain in adult life is unique, amongst other organs, in relying exclusively on glucose for its energy supply. In fetal life, and in the newborn, the brain can use other sources of energy, particularly ketones – breakdown products of fat as well as of carbohydrates. In an indirect way I discovered that the brain also uses these alternative fuels in individuals with established and severe high blood pressure, as well as in degenerative cerebrovascular disease.[43] Since the adult brain can evidently adapt to use fuels other than glucose, might MND be helped by deliberately increasing the concentration of ketones in the blood? I have tried to find out whether diabetes, especially Type I, in which ketone excess is often present, gives any protection against

MND, but the evidence is against this.[44] One old observation is interesting: reduced glucose metabolism was demonstrated in structurally normal brain cortex in motor neurone disease, with normal neuronal numbers. This suggested that in MND some neurones 'exist in a state of neuronal nonfunction, rather than cell death'.[45] The suggestion has also been made that ALS might be due to an inadequate blood supply, for which there has been some evidence,[46] but this has yet to be confirmed. I find it difficult to believe that it can be a major factor. There are quite gross differences in the symptoms, signs and prognosis of motor neurone disease and of disease of cerebral arteries.

Recent work has shown that the rate of turnover of energy supplies in the human body is very rapid. Virtually all energy-requiring activities, such as muscle movement, glandular secretion or neuronal excitation, are fuelled by adenosine triphosphate (ATP). Its contained energy is released when it loses one of its three phosphate groups and becomes adenosine diphosphate (ADP). ATP can be regarded as a powerful rechargeable battery whose contained energy can be released at body temperature. Curiously the analogy is less far-fetched than it sounds. Energy is released by oxidative reactions in mitochondria, hundreds of which minute bodies are found in every cell of our bodies. Mitochondria extract energy by, in effect, burning up foodstuffs. Each mitochondrion uses the energy so produced to build up a negative electrical charge inside it of one tenth to one fifth of a volt. This charge can be regarded as a storehouse of energy. In the human adult at rest it can be calculated that ATP equivalent to half the body weight (35 kg) is synthesised and broken down each day. Since the brain consumes about one fifth of the total energy breakdown of the body at rest, one may conclude that about 7 kg (15 pounds weight) of ATP is synthesised by mitochondria in brain cells and broken down each day. Looked at this way it would seem that the brain's energy supplies must be extraordinarily robust. It is surprising that the energy supply fails so rarely.

Resemblance to the prion diseases

Several points of resemblance between MND and the spongiform encephalopathies are noteworthy: the dual pattern of inherited and sporadic cases; the uniform prevalence of MND in different populations; the late onset of the disease, suggesting a long incubation period; neuronal loss without much inflammation; the link with copper through Cu/Zn SOD; the specific copper-binding sites in normal prion protein (which contains copper). But all attempts to produce neuronal damage in animals by inoculating fresh MND necropsy material have failed. No lesions were seen in mice during 600 days of observation after inoculating them with human diseased neuronal material.[47]

It is not unlikely that a shape change in the protein structure of Cu/Zn SOD may have interfered with its function, specifically in the way in which body constituents bind to the zinc which forms part of the protein.[48] Such a possibility might seem ridiculous, except that the example of the prion diseases comes again to mind. In prion diseases such as scrapie in sheep, bovine spongiform encephalopathy (BSE) in cows, kuru, Creutzfeldt-Jakob disease (CJD) and fatal familial insomnia in man, it appears that a normal body 'prion' protein product (PrP^c) is somehow changed in molecular spatial structure (though not in its chemical constituents) and folds into an abnormal protein shape (e.g. designated as PrP^{sc} or PrP^{cjd}). The protein's abnormal molecular shape prevents it being cleared away by protein-degrading enzymes (proteinases). The abnormal protein then accumulates in nerve cells, perhaps by a process akin to crystallisation, and damages them.[49]

If insoluble protein aggregates are toxic and damaging, there may be a common factor in all diseases involving misfolding of newly synthesised proteins.[50] Several neurodegenerative diseases other than MND – notably Alzheimer's (Chapter 19) and Parkinson's disease (Chapter 28) – share some epidemiological similarities. All are characterised by accumulation within nerve cells of abnormal lumps of protein combined with ubiquitin. Another neurodegenerative condition (Huntington's disease) is also associated with abnormal structures inside nerve cells. In this case the protein 'huntingtin' is combined with ubiquitin.

Could Bunina bodies and intracellular skeins, containing ubiquitin and other molecules, also contain structurally altered protein – without necessarily accumulating in large quantities as, for example, the starchy protein amyloid does in Alzheimer's disease? It seems possible that there might be a conformational change in the non-metallic part of one of the superoxide dismutase enzymes. A mutation of Cu/Zn SOD1 in mice has been reported to lead to rapid neurological deterioration.[51] Tests with appropriate antibodies suggested that the glial cells of these mice contain both SOD1 and ubiquitin, and that motor neurone cells contain SOD1.

Negative observations during attempts to transmit human MND to other species (usually mice) do not rule out MND being a protein-conformational disorder. Although some prion diseases can certainly 'infect' individuals of a different species from the one in which the prion disease first occurred, it may well be that there are good immunological reasons why human NMD tissue will not grow in mice. Perhaps a much longer time span than those currently envisaged is needed. Perhaps normal mice possess some factor which inhibits mouse proteins (but not BSE material) from flipping over into the damaging and self-replicating conformation that underlies human MND.

Deliberate experimental inter-human transmission is obviously unethical. But researchers need to look out for any situations in which – for example – a neurosurgical operation was performed on someone not known until later to have MND, and in which the same surgical instruments were used on another individual. Prions can be extraordinarily stable. Prion infectivity can resist boiling. Most surgeons are aware how difficult it can be to prevent prion transmission from one individual to another. They now insist on having brand new surgical instruments for all neurosurgical operations.

Misfolding of proteins

Although proteins can have exceedingly complex three-dimensional structures, all proteins are synthesised in ribosomes within cells as one or more long chains of polypeptides. Reversible folding and unfolding of a single protein molecule was first observed in a small protein (acyl phosphatase). Since then the 3-dimensional study of protein structure has advanced at great speed. We are beginning to understand the ways in which proteins either assemble themselves, or are assembled with the aid of so-called chaperone proteins (see below). Sometimes assembly starts first into modules, which later join up. We know that the process is subject to quality control, so that aberrant foldings are reversed or removed. Some complex misfoldings can not only give rise to abnormal plaques or lumps inside cells, but also to 'fibrils' – extremely fine tubular crystalline structures. Both are seen in Alzheimer's disease (Chapter 19). These presumably damage nerve cells. It is a reasonable presumption that Bunina bodies or their precursors impair nerve function in motor neurone disease.

It is now recognised that some so-called 'heat shock proteins' (hsps) – proteins whose synthesis is enhanced by stresses such as a rise in temperature – act as 'chaperones'. This delightful word describes their function of controlling the appropriate folding of protein chains, during or immediately after their synthesis, thus preventing their sticky surfaces becoming glued together and aggregating.[52] Chaperones are usually found in the endoplasmic reticulum inside cells.[53] Chaperones have hydrophobic surfaces which recognise and bind to the exposed hydrophobic surfaces of improperly-folded proteins, thus preventing them aggregating with other similarly misfolded proteins and causing damage. Presumably cells have a greater than normal need for chaperones when rapid replacement of proteins is needed after stresses such as temperature elevation. This would explain why their synthesis is enhanced by such stresses.

One possible functional defect in motor neurone disease might be that in sporadic MND (the common form) a normal chaperone protein is deficient, or perhaps changed so that its normal assembling function is deranged. This might then account for the abnormal collection within neurones of proteinaceous material, forming Bunina bodies (specific for MND). Defects in genes coding for neurofilaments have also been found to be associated with MND.[54] Consequential aggregates of neurofilament proteins could be a main causal factor in MND. One notable observation has been made of affected neuronal populations in Alzheimer's disease and MND. The affected neuronal populations are anatomically interconnected, suggesting that a damaging agent such as a virus or an abnormal protein might pass from affected cells to unaffected ones.

To my mind, one of the most compelling reasons for thinking that MND is a protein-conformational disorder is that although in familial MND cases (with positively identified mutations in the Cu/Zn superoxide dismutase-1 gene) the supposedly 'defective' enzyme has normal biochemical activity in cell culture. In transgenic mouse studies it can still apparently cause neuronal damage similar to that seen in human motor neurone disease. When we also take into account that even a single copy of the defective Cu/Zn SOD 1 gene can result in a dominant form of inheritance, normal expectations of genetic biochemical disorders are confounded. Doctors have long been familiar with the situation where a homozygous disorder causes disease, whereas an individual heterozygous for the condition is a 'carrier' who may suffer a little from minor aspects of the full-blown disease or may be entirely normal. Sickle-cell disease and fibrocystic disease are examples. By contrast, an unfortunate individual carrying only a single copy of the abnormal but still functional Cu/Zn SOD-1 gene may suffer and die from clinically typical motor neurone disease.

Some unanswered questions

Do motor neurones use more energy than other neuronal types? If so, a general defect in neuronal function might pick them out.

Is there mitochondrial exhaustion in MND? Mitochondrial DNA is particularly susceptible to oxidative stress. Mitochondrial metabolism is a major source of potentially damaging free radicals. In addition, there is a normal age-dependent damage to and deterioration of respiratory enzymes.

467

If it is true that the Japanese get less MND than most other races because they carry a higher frequency of the mitochondrial Mt5178A gene, which seems to predispose to longevity, is there an inverse relationship between Mt5178A and MND?

Can the high prevalence of MND in the Western Pacific, especially in the island of Guam, be explained by some local factor, such as the supply of trace elements, deficiency of calcium or magnesium, or an excess of some toxic metal, e.g. lead or mercury?

Are the abnormalities reported in glutamate and glycine transport in MND relevant to its causation?

Is there any evidence that before glucose consumption and electrical activity start to fall (as they are known to do in MND) there is a period of time in which both are increased – as might be expected by the 'excitotoxic theory'?

Deletions of the neuronal apoptosis inhibitory gene NAIP or another related gene are associated with proximal spinal muscular atrophy in childhood but so far no similar mutations have been found in MND. What other genes might control neural apoptosis?

Ubiquitin-positive skein-like inclusions, which may be precursors of Bunina bodies and Lewy-body inclusions, are seen in ALS neurones. This suggests that nerve cells may be in an early stage of neuronal degeneration. But if so, why does MND seem to be 'all-or-none'? We don't see 'mild' cases at all (I think): this makes exhaustion of enzyme chains less likely.

There is a striking contrast between MND and organophosphate poisoning. A conformational change in a protein might explain the inexorable progression of MND, as already suggested. In organophosphate poisoning the neurological signs and symptoms stopped once the toxin had been removed. Is it fair to take the persistence and progressively damaging course of MND as evidence pointing more towards a virus cause or a prion? Or is it that the more abnormal prion protein is present in nerve cells, the faster more can be formed – as happens during ordinary crystallisation?

Why do almost all the genetic mitochondrial disorders involve neural problems? Is this because of the immense energy requirements of the brain?

Do Bunina bodies contain Cu/Zn SOD? Is this why they are virtually specific for ALS? Could a prion-like process lead to loss of function of this dismutase inside cells? If the dismutase is in Bunina bodies, then perhaps, despite nerve cells having otherwise normal cell constituents, might the enzyme be non-functional?

Is the recently identified NF-H mouse gene (also identified in MND) damaging, by making neurones produce too many filaments?

468

The Brn-3A transcription factor is a powerful stimulant of nerve filament growth. Is this overexpressed in MND? If not, why not?

What do glial cells do? Why are there so many of them? Why cannot neurones get their energy supplies directly from nearby blood vessels without the intervention of glial cells?

NOTES

Chapter 1 Emphysema and chronic bronchitis

1. The 'peak flow' corresponds to the tangent to the steepest part of the downslopes in Figs. 2A and 2B. Martin Wright, then working for the British Medical Research Council in Harrow, devised an instrument which could measure peak flow directly, at the bedside or in the clinic. 'Wright' peak flow meters are now in use all over the world.
2. Dornhorst AC. Respiratory insufficiency. *Lancet* 1955; 1: 1185–1187.
3. Barnes PJ. Chronic Obstructive Pulmonary Disease. *New Engl J Med* 2000; 343: 269–280.
4. Carrell RW, Lomas DA. Alpha-1-antitrypsin deficiency – a Model for Conformational Diseases. *New Engl J Med* 2002; 346: 46–53.
5. Tynan K (1987). *The life of Kenneth Tynan*. London: Weidenfeld & Nicholson.
6. Lee HS, Yap J, Wang YT, et al. Occupational asthma due to unheated polyvinylchloride resin dust. *Br J Indust Med* 1989; 46: 820–822.
7. Moisan TC. Prolonged asthma after smoke inhalation: a report of three cases and a review of previous reports. *J Occup Med* 1991; 33: 458–461.
8. Nielsen J, Fahraeus C, Bensryd I, et al. Small airways function in workers processing polyvinylchloride. *Int Arch Occup Environ Health* 1989; 61: 427–430.
9. Falk H, Portnoy B. Respiratory tract illness in meat wrappers. *J Am Med Ass* 1976; 235: 915–917.
10. Kogevinas M, Antó JM, Sunyer J, et al. European Community Respiratory Health Survey Study Group. Occupational asthma in Europe and other industrialised areas: a population-based study. *Lancet* 1999; 353: 750–754.

Chapter 2 Asthma

1. 'Allergy' refers to the liability of man and other animals to develop irritant or harmful responses to the same foreign substances after repeated exposures.
2. Florence Nightingale – the famous and influential nurse who in 1854 transformed the treatment of wounded British soldiers in the Crimean war – had learned (correctly) that although plants produce oxygen in the light, they consume oxygen in the dark. She therefore recommended that flowers should always be taken out of hospital wards during the night.

She must have lacked a feeling for relative gas volumes. But her reputation ensured that this extraordinary practice survived in the UK until about 1960!

3. Bach J-F. The Effect of Infections on Susceptibility to Autoimmune and Allergic Diseases. *New Engl J Med* 2002; 347: 911–920.
4. Weiss ST. Eat Dirt – The Hygiene Hypothesis and Allergic Diseases. *New Engl J Med* 2002; 347: 930–931.
    Braun-Fahrlander C, Riedler J, Herz U, et al. Environmental exposure to endotoxin and its relation to asthma in school-age children. *New Engl J Med* 2002; 347: 869–877.
5. The human body contains about 10^{14}(100,000,000,000,000) individual cells. Almost all cells have a nucleus containing 46 microscopic thread-like chromosomes (Greek: coloured bodies). Under the microscope each of these looks different and each has been assigned an identifying number. They are present in pairs. One of each pair comes from the individual's father, one from the mother. Chromosomes are made up of double-stranded twisted strings of DNA (deoxyribose nucleic acid). Certain sections of DNA (exons) contain a code which can be transmitted to other structures ('ribosomes') inside the cell but outside the nucleus. There the code is read and specific proteins are made. The coding sections of DNA are known as 'genes'. At present the entire sequences of genes in all the human chromosomes have been painstakingly worked out, through international collaboration. This 'human genome project' has identified and located the chemical structure of all the (approximately) 35,000 human genes. It is now possible to find what protein each gene codes for, thus giving clues about its function.
6. Platts-Mills TA, Tovey ER, Mitchell EB, et al. Reduction of bronchial hyperreactivity during prolonged allergen avoidance. *Lancet* 1982; 2: 675–678.
7. Schreck R, Albermann K, Baeuerle PA. Nuclear factor kappa B: an oxidative stress-responsive transcription factor of eukaryotic cells. *Free Radic Res Commun* 1992; 17: 221–237.
8. Brunekreef B, Holgate ST. Air pollution and health. *Lancet* 2002; 360: 1233–1242.
9. Terada N, Maesako K, Hiruma K, et al. Diesel exhaust particulates enhance eosinophil adhesion to nasal epithelial cells and cause degranulation. *Int Arch Allergy Immunol* 1997; 114: 167–174.
10. Barnes PJ. Pathophysiology of asthma. *Br J Clin Pharmacol* 1996; 42: 3–10.
11. Lipworth BJ. Leukotriene-receptor antagonists. *Lancet* 1999; 353: 57–62.
12. ISAAC. Worldwide variation in prevalence of symptoms of asthma, allergic rhinoconjunctivitis, and atopic eczema. *Lancet* 1998; 351: 1225–1232.
13. von Mutius E. Infection: friend or foe in the development of atopy and asthma? The epidemiological evidence. *Europ Resp J* 2001; 18: 872–881.
14. 'Auto-immune' implies that the body's mechanisms that normally defend

472

it against attacks by micro-organisms turn against itself and generate defensive antibodies or T-cells which can damage normal body constituents.

15. Yemaneberhan H, Bekele Z, Venn A, et al. Prevalence of wheeze and asthma and relation to atopy in urban and rural Ethiopia. *Lancet* 1997; 350: 85–90.

16. Dagoye D, Bekele Z, Woldemichael K, et al. Domestic risk factors for wheeze in urban and rural Ethiopian children. *QJMed* 2004; 97: 489–498.

Chapter 3 Multiple sclerosis

1. The last 'e' is omitted in the USA and many other places, with the expected change in pronunciation.

2. Magnetic resonance imaging (MRI) provides much more detailed information about body structures than can be obtained from ordinary X-rays or even from a computer-aided tomogram (CAT scan) in most situations. It is especially valuable in providing images of the living brain. The head is placed in a strong magnetic field which can suddenly be changed in strength or direction, setting individual molecules of body tissue in resonant motion. This can provide a magnetic image of the part examined. No harmful X-radiation need be used. Unfortunately the equipment required for MRI is complicated, bulky and expensive to install and to maintain. However, it is particularly valuable in diagnosing and assessing MS because the lesions of MS do not show up in X-rays.

3. Gale CR, Martyn CN. Migrant studies in multiple sclerosis. *Prog Neurobiol* 1995; 47: 425–448.

4. Whereas bacteria are minute single-celled living organisms, viruses are smaller. They can be thought of as inanimate packets of nucleic acid and other chemicals, which after entry to a body cell can stimulate it to produce more of the virus's own material.

5. McHatters GR, Scham RG. Bird viruses in multiple sclerosis: combination of viruses or Marek's alone? *Neurosci Lett* 1995; Chapter 18.

6. A name given to a virus which gets into a cell by the back door, so to say. One of its components is a facilitating protein (an enzyme) – 'reverse transcriptase' which can insert its own genes into the genes of the host cell. These then instruct the microscopic structures inside cells (ribosomes), which synthesise proteins, to make more copies of the virus. Thus the infection is perpetuated.

7. Perron H, Garson JA, Bedin F, et al. Molecular identification of a novel retrovirus repeatedly isolated from patients with multiple sclerosis. The Collaborative Research Group on Multiple Sclerosis. *Proc Natl Acad Sci USA* 1997; 94: 7583–7588.

8. The 'T-'lymphocytes make up a substantial proportion of the 'white'

473

cells of the blood, i.e. those not containing the red pigment, haemo-globin. After appropriate priming they directly attack foreign cells or foreign material. The 'B-' lymphocytes exert their protective function indirectly by producing soluble proteins (antibodies) which combine with and inactivate potentially damaging chemicals or cells. Their protective action is thus exerted at a distance, whereas T-lymphocytes are themselves participants in immune reactions by secreting powerful chemical 'cytokines' (Greek: *cyto* = hollow/cell; *kine* = movement). These substances can diffuse from one cell to another and excite reactions there, after combining with a specific 'receptor'. A receptor is a chemical which is embedded in the outer membrane of a cell, but has parts of its molecule projecting inwards as well as outwards. This allows a chemical coming from outside a cell, and which combines with the external part of the receptor, to influence internal cell function without itself entering the cell.

9. An antigen (Greek: *anti* = against; *gen* = to produce) is a chemical compound or part of an organism which can induce an immune reaction when it enters or comes into contact with appropriate receptors on the surface of body cells. A group of natural antigens known as the 'human leucocyte antigen' (HLA) system plays an important part in natural resistance and susceptibility to infections of many different kinds. The production of components of the HLA system is controlled by an indivi-dual's inherited genes. Antigens already in the body before birth are described as 'auto-antigens'. Multiple sclerosis has a strong association with certain HLA groups. This suggests that the condition may be one of the so-called 'infective/immune' group of diseases, in which an external infecting agent so closely resembles some human tissue or organ that the circulating antibodies and defensive lymphocytes which the body produces to combat the infection react in a damaging way against its own tissues or organs. Antigens present before birth are accepted as part of 'self' and do not excite immune reactions. The well-known chemi-cals determining blood groups 'A' and 'B' are examples of antigens which can cause transfusion reactions in people who have antibodies against them. (I used to be puzzled to know why people with blood group A had antibodies to the Group B antigen, and vice versa. I thought that this was because blood group antigens are present in saliva and that the universal practice of kissing new-born babies exposed them to a wide variety of antigens. But I later found that blood group chemi-cals are ubiquitous enough to make this mechanism superfluous!).

10. Romagnani S. T-cell subsets (Th1 versus Th2). *Ann Allerg Asthma* 2000; 85: 9–18.
11. Miller DH, Khan OA, Sheremata WA, et al. A Controlled Trial of Natalizumab for Relapsing Multiple Sclerosis. *New Engl J Med* 2003; 348: 15–23.
12. Trapp BD, Peterson J, Ransohoff RM, et al. Axonal transection in the lesions of multiple sclerosis. *New Engl J Med* 1998; 338: 278–285.

Chapter 4 Sleep and sleep disorders

1. Gaultier C. Cardiorespiratory adaptation during sleep in infants and children. *Pediatr Pulmonol* 1995; 19: 105–117.
2. Madsen PL, Vorstrup S. Cerebral blood flow and metabolism during sleep. *Cerebrovasc Brain Metab Rev* 1991; 3: 281–296.
3. Gottesmann C. Neurophysiological support of consciousness during waking and sleep. *Prog Neurobiol* 1999; 59: 469–508.
4. Autret A, Lucas B, Mondon K, et al. Sleep and brain lesions: a critical review of the literature and additional cases. *Neurophysiol Cliniq* 2001; 31: 356–375.
5. Lavie P. Sleep Disturbances in the Wake of Traumatic Events. *New Engl J Med* 2001; 345: 1825–1832.
6. The hypothalamus (Fig. 7) includes a large group of nerve nuclei which lie at the base of the midbrain in the floor and at the sides of the third ventricle.
    Sinton CM, McCarley RW. Neuroanatomical and neurophysiological aspects of sleep: basic science and clinical relevance. *Semin Clin Neuropsychiat* 2002; 5: 6–19.
7. 'Dominant' means that a child can inherit the condition even if only one parent has it.
8. Ebrahim IO, Howard RS, Kopelman MD, et al. The hypocretin/orexin system. *J Roy Soc Med* 2002; 95: 227–230.
9. Overeem S, Mignot E, Gert van Dijk J, Lammers GJ. Narcolepsy: clinical features, new pathophysiologic insights, and future perspectives. *J Clin Neurophysiol* 2002; 18:78–105.
10. Dickinson CJ (1965). *Neurogenic Hypertension*. Oxford: Blackwell Scientific Publications.
    Dickinson CJ. Neurogenic hypertension revisited. *Clin Sci* 1981; 60: 471–477.
    Dickinson CJ (1991). *Neurogenic Hypertension: A Synthesis and Review*. London: Chapman & Hall.
    Dickinson CJ. Reappraisal of the Cushing reflex: the most powerful neural blood pressure stabilizing system. *Clin Sci* 1990; 79: 543–550.
11. Crick F. Neural Networks and REM Sleep. *Biosci Rep* 1988; 8: 531–535.

Chapter 5 Psoriasis

1. Lebwohn M. Psoriasis. *Lancet* 2003; 361: 1197–1204.
2. Wrone-Smith T, Nickoloff BJ. Dermal injection of immunocytes induces psoriasis. *J Clin Invest* 1996; 98: 1878–1887.
3. Sayama K, Midorikawa K, Hanakawa Y, et al. Superantigen production by Staphylococcus aureus in psoriasis. *Dermatology* 1998; 196: 194–198.

Chapter 6 Thyroid disorders

1. Thyroglobulin is a unique protein because it can accommodate iodine atoms in its tyrosine residues. Tyrosine is technically an aromatic amino-acid, i.e. one containing a ring structure of six carbon atoms. Some tyrosine residues in the appropriately folded protein can exchange either one or two hydrogen atoms in their benzene rings for iodine atoms selectively accumulated from the diet and concentrated in the thyroid gland, thus making mono- and di-iodotyrosine. These remain part of the parent protein and are stored in this form. Later two of these molecules are split off and joined together by coupling enzymes to make the thyroid hormones triiodothyronine (T3) and tetraiodothyronine (T4). The latter is also known as thyroxine. T3 and T4 are stored, mostly combined with specialised binding proteins, in the follicles of the thyroid gland, from which the hormone can be released as required.

2. 'Amino-acids' all contain a nitrogen ('amino-') component linked to an acidic chemical group, as the name suggests. A 'peptide' contains two or more amino-acids strung together; a tripeptide contains three. The precise number of amino-acids which make up a 'polypeptide' is undefined, but when the number gets above about 30 a polypeptide is then described as a 'protein'. A small chemical molecule such as the hormone insulin (deficiency of which causes diabetes) can be described either as a large polypeptide or as a small protein.

3. Dayan CM. Interpretation of thyroid function tests. *Lancet* 2001; 357: 619–624.

4. Dickinson CJ. Cysticercosis and hypopituitarism. *Proc Roy Soc Med* 1955; 48: 892–893.

5. Weetman AP. Graves' Disease. *New Engl J Med* 2000; 343: 1236–1248.

6. Feliciano DV. Everything you wanted to know about Graves' disease. *Am J Surg* 1992; 164: 404–411.

Chapter 7 Blood supply of tumours

1. Dickinson CJ (1984). Cardiovascular system. In: *The Encyclopaedia of Medical Ignorance*, pp. 107–115 (eds Duncan R, Weston-Smith M). Oxford: Pergamon Press.

2. Olson TA, Mohanraj D, Roy S, Ramakrishnan S. Targeting the tumor vasculature: inhibition of tumor growth by a vascular endothelial growth factor-toxin conjugate. *Int J Cancer* 1997; 73: 865–870.

3. O'Reilly MS, Holmgren L, Shing Y, et al. Angiostatin: A novel angio-genesis inhibitor that mediates the suppression of metastases by a Lewis lung carcinoma. *Cell* 1994; 79: 315–328.

4. Sage EH. Pieces of 8 – bioactive fragments of extracellular proteins as regulators of angiogenesis. *Trend Cell Biol* 1997; 7: 182–186.

5. Ferrara N, et al. Discovery and development of Bevacizumab, an anti-

VEGF antibody for treating cancer. *Nat Rev Drug Discv* 2004; 3: 391–400.

Yang JC, Haworth L, Sherry RM, et al. A Randomized Trial of Bevacizumab, and Anti-Vascular Endothelial Growth Factor Antibody, for Metastatic Renal Cancer. *New Eng J Med* 2003; 349: 427–434.

6. Oberbauer R. Not nonsense but antisense – applications of antisense oligonucleotides in different fields of medicine. *Wien Klin Wochenschr* 1997; 109: 40–46.

Chapter 8 Osteoarthritis

1. Fitzgerald GA, Patrono C. The Coxibs, Selective Inhibitors of Cyclooxygenase-2. *New Engl J Med* 2001; 345: 433–442.
2. Reginster JY, Deroisy R, Rovati LC, et al. Long-term effects of glucosamine sulphate on ostoarthritis progression: a randomised, placebo-controlled clinical trial. *Lancet* 2001; 357: 251–256.
3. Evans CH, Georgescu HI. Observations on the senescence of cells derived from articular cartilage. *Mech Ageing Dev* 1983; 22: 179–191.
4. Niethard FU. Pathogenesis of osteoarthritis – approaches to specific therapy. *Am J Orthop* 1999; 28: 8–10.
5. Bailey AJ, Mansell JP. Do subchondral bone changes exacerbate or precede articular cartilage destruction in osteoarthritis of the elderly? *Gerontol* 1997; 43: 296–304.
6. Gaffney K, Williams RB, Jolliffe VA, Blake DR. Intra-articular pressure changes in rheumatoid and normal peripheral joints. *Ann Rheum Dis* 1995; 54: 670–673.
7. Iles JF, Stokes M, Young A. Reflex actions of knee joint afferents during contraction of the human quadriceps. *Clin Physiol* 1990; 10: 489–500.
8. Jawed S, Gaffney K, Blake DR. Intra-articular pressure profile of the knee joint in a spectrum of inflammatory arthropathies. *Ann Rheum Dis* 1997; 56: 686–689.
9. Peterson RO. Increased osteoarthritis in moose from Isle Royale. *J Wild Dis* 1988; 24: 461–466.
10. Spector TD, Hart DJ, Nandra D, et al. Low-level increases in serum C-reactive protein are present in early osteoarthritis of the knee and predict progressive disease. *Arthritis Rheum* 1997; 40: 723–727.

Chapter 9 Rheumatoid arthritis

1. Moore TL, Dorner RW. Rheumatoid factors. *Clin Biochem* 1993; 26: 75–84.
Technically speaking, auto-antibody reactions occur with the 'fragment crystallisable' (Fc) part of immunoglobulin G.

2. Kirschfink M. Controlling the complement system in inflammation. *Immunopharmacology* 1997; 38: 51–62.
3. Gaston JSH. Role of T-cells in the development of arthritis. *Clin Sci* 1998; 95: 19–31.
4. Klareskog L, Van der Heijde D, Gough A, et al. Therapeutic effect of the combination of etanercept and methotrexate compared with each treatment alone in patients with rheumatoid arthritis: double-blind randomised controlled trial. *Lancet* 2004; 363: 675–681.
5. Depraetere V, Golstein P. Dismantling in cell death: molecular mechanisms and relationship to caspase activation. *Scand J Immunol* 1998; 47: 523–531.
6. Casciola-Rosen L, Rosen A. Ultraviolet light-induced keratinocyte apoptosis: a potential mechanism for the induction of skin lesions and autoantibody production in LE. *Lupus* 1997; 6: 175–180.
7. Svendsen AJ, Holm NV, Kyvik K, et al. Relative importance of genetic effects in rheumatoid arthritis: historical cohort study of Danish nationwide twin population. *Br Med J* 2002; 324: 264–266.
8. Krause A, Kamradt T, Burmester GR. Potential infectious agents in the induction of arthritides. *Curr Opin Rheumatol* 1996; 8: 203–209.
9. Altschuler EL. Parvovirus B19 and the pathogenesis of rheumatoid arthritis: a case for historical reasoning. *Lancet* 1999; 354: 1026–1027.
10. Silman A, Bankhead C, Rowlingson B, et al. Do new cases of rheumatoid arthritis cluster in time or in space? *Int J Epidemiol* 1997; 26: 628–634.

Chapter 10 Duodenal and stomach ulcers

1. A 'strong' acid has all its constituent hydrogen atoms (protons) freely available in solution as positively charged hydrogen ions. Technically it is described as fully 'dissociated' into ions. Aqueous hydrochloric acid comprises H+ (proton) and Cl– (chloride) ions. By contrast, 'weak' acids like carbonic acid (produced when the waste gas, carbon dioxide, dissolves in water) and acetic acid (the main constituent of vinegar) are only partly dissociated into electrically charged ions. They are far less reactive.
2. Gastrin hormones are small polypeptides. The larger one comprises 34 amino-acids, the smaller one has 17.
3. Calam J, Baron JH. Pathophysiology of duodenal and gastric ulcer and gastric cancer. *Br Med J* 2001; 323: 980–985.
4. Historically, secretin is interesting because it was the first hormone to be identified. It was discovered in 1901, by Bayliss and Starling, who were working at University College in London. Today, some 50 hormones are known.
5. Seager JM, Hawkey CJ. Indigestion and non-steroidal anti-inflammatory drugs. *Br Med J* 2001; 323: 1236–1239.

6. 'H' stands for histamine, a natural chemical which plays a part in allergic reactions in the lungs and in the skin through stimulating 'H1' receptors. When histamine combines with 'H2' receptors in the lining cells of the stomach it makes the stomach secrete acid. The so-called 'anti-histamine' drugs, which are used to combat hay fever and other allergic conditions, block the H1 receptors and ameliorate allergic reactions but have minimal effects on stomach acid secretion. It was Black's investigation of the possibility of selectively blocking the 'H2' effects of histamine which led to the introduction into clinical medicine of an important new class of drugs – and to his Nobel prize.

7. Warren JR, Marshall BJ. Unidentified curved bacilli in gastric epithelium in active chronic gastritis. *Lancet* 1983; i: 1273–1275.

8. Hawkey CJ. Eradication of *Helicobacter pylori* should be pivotal in managing peptic ulceration. *Br Med J* 1994; 309: 1570–1572.
Suerbaum S, Michetti P. Helicobacter pylori infection. *New Engl J Med* 2002; 347: 1175–1186.

9. Harris A, Misiewicz JJ. Management of *Helicobacter pylori* infection. *Br Med J* 2001; 323: 1047–1050.

Chapter 11 Bile and gall bladder disorders

1. Johnson CD. Upper abdominal pain: Gall bladder. *Br Med J* 2001; 323: 1170–1173.

2. Misciagna G, Guerra V, Di Leo A, et al. Insulin and gall stones: a population case control study in southern Italy. *Gut* 2002; 47: 144–147.

3. Neuberger J. Primary biliary cirrhosis. *Lancet* 1997; 350: 875–879.

4. Haydon GH, Neuberger J. PBC: an infectious disease? *Gut* 2000; 47: 586–588.

Chapter 12 Pancreatitis

1. 'Exocrine': description of a gland whose secreted chemical product is delivered by a duct system to a specific site away from the gland itself (from Greek: *exo* = out of; *krino* = to separate). On the other hand, 'endocrine' (Greek: *endon* = within) describes a gland whose secretion (a hormone) is delivered into the bloodstream. It can therefore act anywhere in the body.

2. Munoz A, Katerndahl DA. Diagnosis and management of acute pancreatitis. *Am Fam Physicn* 2002; 62: 164–174.

3. Sakorafas GH, Tsiotos GG, Sarr MG. Ischemia/Reperfusion-Induced. Pancreatitis. *Digest Surg* 2002; 17: 3–14.

4. Dassopoulos T, Ehrenpreis ED. Acute pancreatitis in human immunodeficiency virus-infected patients: a review. *Am J Med* 1999; 107: 78–84.

5. Kukor Z, Mayerle J, Kruger B, et al. Presence of cathepsin B in the

479

human pancreatic secretory pathway and its role in trypsinogen activation during hereditary pancreatitis. *J Biol Chem* 2002; 277: 21389–21396.

Chapter 13 Migraine

1. The laws of heredity were discovered in the nineteenth century by Gregor Mendel, an Austrian monk of the Augustinian order who became Abbot of Brünn. Working methodically in the monastery garden with both edible and sweet peas, he recognised two types of inheritance to which he gave the names 'dominant' and 'recessive'. He also recognised in cross-pollinated ('hybrid') peas that their offspring showed different characters in well-defined mathematical proportions. His observations passed unnoticed for many years, but he is now recognised as the father of modern genetics. He was an original scientist who ranks with the very greatest.
2. Ophoff RA, Terwindt GM, Vergouwe MN, et al. Familial hemiplegic migraine and episodic ataxia type-2 are caused by mutations in the Ca2+ channel CACN gene L1A4. *Cell* 1996; 87: 543–552.
3. Silberstein SD. Migraine. *Lancet* 2004; 363: 381–391.
4. Schmidt C. Migraine and cerebral blood flow during centrifugation. *Lancet* 1997; 350: 1145.
5. Goadsby PJ, Lipton RB, Ferrari MD. Migraine – Current Understandings and Treatment. *New Engl J Med* 2002; 346: 257–270.
   Chang BS, Lowenstein DH. Epilepsy. *New Engl J Med* 2003; 349: 1257–1266.

Chapter 14 Diabetes Type 1

1. This is caused by the kidneys' inability to absorb water properly from the fluid filtered through the glomeruli. This can be due either to lack of the hormone vasopressin (secreted from part of the pituitary gland in the centre of the brain) or to a (usually inherited) disease of the kidney tubules. In neither case is there any sugar in the urine, nor any excess of sugar in the blood.
2. Traditionally it is said that the high concentration of glucose causes an 'osmotic diuresis'. I have never felt much enthusiasm for this concept, physiologically. During glomerular filtration the relevant non-colloid osmotic pressures of plasma and glomerular filtrate are the same. My suggestion instead is that perhaps the passage of glomerular filtrate along the proximal kidney tubules is so fast that there is simply not enough time for the specialised processes absorbing glucose, other solutes and water to go to completion. This concept – which may, of course, be wrong – explains in a very simple way why hyperglycaemia can lead to excessive loss of salt as well as of glucose through the kidneys.

3. Chiarelli F, Pomilio M, Mohn S, et al. Serum angiogenin concentrations in young patients with diabetes mellitus. *Europ J Clin Invest* 2002; 32: 110–114.
4. The international 'unit' of insulin was defined before its chemical structure and molecular weight were known. Eventually we shall all doubtless learn to think of insulin dosage in milligrams or millimoles.
5. Van den Berghe G, Wouters P, Weekers F, et al. Intensive insulin therapy in critically ill patients. *New Engl J Med* 2001; 345: 1359–1367.
6. 'Autonomic' implies that this part of the central nervous system is automatic and virtually outside the control of the will. Most of the control centres are in the brain stem and midbrain, though higher brain centres also connect with the brain stem. The two main components of the system are the 'sympathetic' (mainly constricting blood vessels and increasing the heart rate and force of contraction) and the 'parasympathetic' (slowing down heart rate via the vagus nerves and dilating some blood vessels). A reader who has not encountered these terms needs to understand that 'sympathetic' in this context is a purely technical term: there is no other name for this system of nerves. It has no emotional significance!
7. Dickinson CJ (1991). *Neurogenic Hypertension*. London: Chapman & Hall (Fig. 8.5, p. 122).
8. The blood and body fluids outside cells are normally slightly on the alkaline side of neutrality, with a 'pH' (an inverse logarithmic measure of hydrogen ion activity) of about 7.4. The pH of blood can be measured instantaneously with an electronic pH meter. Physicians looking after sick patients with diabetic keto-acidosis pay as much attention to blood pH as they do to the level of glucose in the blood.
9. Atkinson MA. The $64000 question in diabetes continues. *Lancet* 2000; 35: 4–6.
10. Martin S, Wolf-Eichbaum D, Duinkerken G, et al. Development of Type 1 Diabetes despite Severe Hereditary B-Cell Deficiency. *New Engl J Med* 2001; 345: 1036–1040.
11. Lohmann T, Hawa M, Leslie RDG, et al. Immune reactivity to glutamic acid decarboxylase 65 in stiff-man syndrome and Type 1 diabetes mellitus. *Lancet* 2000; 356: 31–35.
12. Emilien G, Ponchon M, Caldas C, et al. Impact of genomics on drug discovery and clinical medicine. *Quart J Med* 2000; 93: 391–423.
13. Zavattari P, Lampis R, Motzo C, et al. Conditional linkage disequilibrium analysis of a complex disease superlocus, IDDM1 in the HLA region, reveals the presence of independent modifying gene effects influencing the Type 1 diabetes risk encoded by the major HLA-DQB1, -DRB1 disease loci. *Hum Mol Genet* 2001; 10: 881–889.
14. Riedler J, Braun-Fahrländer C, Eder W, et al. Exposure to farming in early life and development of asthma and allergy: a cross-sectional survey. *Lancet* 2001; 358: 1129–1133.
15. Raz I, Elias D, Avron A, et al. Beta-cell function in new-onset Type 1

diabetes and immunomodulation with a heat shock protein peptide (DiaPep277): a randomised, double-blind, phase II trial. *Lancet* 2001; 358: 1749–1753.

16. Atkinson MA, Eisenbarth GS. Type 1 diabetes: new perspectives on disease pathogenesis and treatment. *Lancet* 2001; 358: 221–229.

Chapter 15 Diabetes Type 2

1. Hu FB, Manson JE, Stampfer MJ, et al. Diet, lifestyle, and the risk of type 2 diabetes mellitus in women. *New Engl J Med* 2001; 345: 790–797.
2. Facchini FS, Stoohs RA, Reaven GM. Enhanced sympathetic nervous system activity. The linchpin between insulin resistance, hyperinsulinemia, and heart rate. *Am J Hypertens* 1996; 9: 1013–1017.
3. Sentinelli F, Romeo S, Arca M, et al. Human resistin gene, obesity, and type 2 diabetes: mutation analysis and population study. *Diabetes* 2002; 51: 860–862.
4. Schrezenmeir J, Jagla A. Milk and diabetes. *J Am Coll Nutrit* 2001; 19(Suppl): 176S-190S.
5. Goran MI. Metabolic precursors and effects of obesity in children: a decade of progress, 1990–1999. *Am J Clin Nutrit* 2001; 73: 158–171.
6. Baier LJ, Permana PA, Yang X, et al. A calpain-10 gene polymorphism is associated with reduced muscle mRNA levels and insulin resistance. *J Clin Invest* 2001; 106: R69–R73.
7. Kim JH, Nishina PM, Naggert JK. Genetic models for non-insulin-dependent diabetes mellitus in rodents. *J Bas Clin Physiol Pharmacol* 1998; 9: 325–345.
8. Fajans SS, Bell GI, Polonsky KS. Molecular Mechanisms and Clinical Pathophysiology of Maturity-Onset Diabetes of the Young. *New Engl J Med* 2001; 345: 971–980.
9. Gale EAM, Clark A. A drug on the market? *Lancet* 2000; 355: 61–63.
10. Shuldiner AR, Yang R, Gong D-W. Resistin, Obesity, and Insulin Resistance – The Emerging Role of the Adipocyte as an Endocrine Organ. *New Engl J Med* 2001; 345: 1345–1346.
11. Angulo P. Nonalcoholic fatty liver disease. *New Engl J Med* 2002; 346: 1221–1231.

Chapter 16 Obesity

1. Yanovski SZ, Yanovski JA. Obesity. *New Engl J Med* 2002; 346: 591–602.
2. Arterburn D, Noël PH. Obesity. *Br Med J* 2001; 322: 1406–1409.
3. Sharma AM, Grassi G. Obesity and hypertension: cause or consequence? *J Hypertens* 2001; 19: 2125–2126.
4. Pinel JP, Assanand S, Lehman DR. Hunger, eating, and ill health. *Am Psychol* 2002; 55: 1105–1116.
5. Vickers MH, Breier BH, Cutfield WS, et al. Fetal origins of hyperphagia,

obesity, and hypertension and postnatal amplification by hypercaloric nutrition. *Am J Physiol – Endocrin Metab* 2002; 279: E83–E87.

6. Zucker LM, Zucker TF. Fatty, a new mutation in the rat. *J Heredit* 1961; 52: 275–278.

7. 'Autosomal' means that the gene concerned is not on one of the chromosomes which determine sex. 'Recessive' means that inheriting one copy of the gene concerned (i.e. one from either parent) will have little or no effect on the recipient. The effect (or defect) will only appear when the gene is inherited from both parents.

8. Janeckova R. The role of leptin in human physiology and pathophysiology. *Physiol Rev* 2002; 50: 443–459.
   Rosenbaum M, Leibel RL. The Role of Leptin in Human Physiology. *New Engl J Med* 1999; 341: 913–915.

9. Mammès O, Aubert R, Betoulle D, et al. LEPR gene polymorphisms: associations with overweight, fat mass and response to diet in women. *Europ J Clin Invest* 2001; 31: 398–404.

10. Kawai K, Sugimoto K, Nakashima K, et al. Leptin as a modulator of sweet taste sensitivity in mice. *Proc Nat Acad Sci USA* 2000; 97: 1104–1109.

11. Batterham HL, Cohen MA, Ellis SM, et al. Inhibition of Food Intake in Obese Subjects by Peptide YY_{3-36}. *New Eng J Med* 2003; 349: 941–948.

12. Sadaf Farooqi I, Keogh JM, Yeo GSH, et al. Clinical Spectrum of Obesity and Mutations in the Melanocortin 4 Receptor Gene. *New Engl J Med* 2003; 348: 1085–1095.

13. Pinkney J, Williams G. Ghrelin gets hungry. *Lancet* 2002; 359: 1360–1361.

14. Kliewer SA, Xu HE, Lambert MH, Willson TM. Peroxisome proliferator-activated receptors: from genes to physiology. *Rec Prog Horm Res* 2001; 56: 239–263.

15. Martinez JA. Body-weight regulation: causes of obesity. *Proc Nutrit Soc* 2002; 59: 337–345.

16. Dickinson CJ. (1950). *Electrophysiological Technique*. London: Morgan Bros.

17. Hickey MS, Calsbeek DJ. Plasma leptin and exercise: recent findings. *Sport Med* 2002; 31: 583–589.

18. Finer N, James WP, Kopelman PG, et al. One-year treatment of obesity: a randomized, double-blind, placebo-controlled, multicentre study of orlistat, a gastrointestinal lipase inhibitor. *Int J Obes metab Dis* 2000; 24: 306–313.

Chapter 17 Endometriosis

1. Child TJ, Tan SL. Endometriosis: aetiology, pathogenesis and treatment. *Drugs* 2001; 61: 1735–1750.

2. Kasule J, Chimbira THK. Endometriosis in African Women. *Cent Afric J Med* 1987; 33: 157–159.
3. 'Polywogs' in the USA
4. Thomas EJ. Endometriosis, 1995 – confusion or sense? *Int J Gynaecol Obstet* 1995; 48: 149–155.
5. Koninckx PR, Ide P, Vandenbroucke W, Brosens IA. New aspects of the pathophysiology of endometriosis and associated infertility. *J Reprod Med* 1980; 24: 257–260.
6. Darrow SL, Vena JE, Batt RE, et al. Menstrual cycle characteristics and the risk of endometriosis. *Epidemiology* 1993; 4: 135–142.
7. D'Hooghe TM. Clinical relevance of the baboon as a model for the study of endometriosis. *Fertil Steril* 1997; 68: 613–625.
8. Dickinson CJ. Could tight garments cause endometriosis? *Br J Obst Gynec* 1999; 106: 1003–1005.
9. D'Hooghe TM, Mwenda JM, Hill JA (eds). The Baboon as a Non-human Primate Model for The Study of Human Reproduction. *Gynec Obstet Invest* 2004; 57: 1–57.
10. Giudice LC, Kao LC. Endometriosis. *Lancet* 2004; 364: 1789–1799.
11. The reasons for this are complicated and difficult to explain briefly. The negative interstitial pressure is generated by the 'osmotic' pressure exerted by the proteins in the blood plasma, tending all the time to suck fluid out of the interstitial space and into the bloodstream.

Chapter 18 Glaucoma

1. Wax MB, Ridley ME, Magargal LE. Reversal of retinal and optic disc ischemia in a patient with sickle cell trait and glaucoma secondary to traumatic hyphema. *Ophthalmology* 1982; 89: 845–851.
2. Teng C, Gurses-Ozden R, Liebmann JM, et al. Effect of a tight necktie on intraocular pressures. *Br J Ophthalmol* 2003; 87: 946–948.
3. Rozsa FW, Shimizu S, Lichter PR, et al. GLC1A mutations point to regions of potential functional importance on the TIGR/MYOC protein. *Mol Vis* 1998; 4: 20.
4. Damji KF, Bains HS, Stefansson E, et al. Is pseudoexfoliation syndrome inherited? A review of genetic and nongenetic factors and a new observation. *Ophthal Genet* 1998; 19: 175–185.
5. De Vivero C, O'Brien C, Lanigan L, Hitchings R. Diurnal intraocular pressure variation in low-tension glaucoma. *Eye* 1994; 8: 521–523.
6. Pena JD, Netland PA, Vidal I, et al. Elastosis of the lamina cribrosa in glaucomatous optic neuropathy. *Exp Eye Res* 1998; 67: 517 524.
7. Steely HT, Jr, English-Wright SL, Clark AF. The similarity of protein expression in trabecular meshwork and lamina cribrosa: implications for glaucoma. *Exp Eye Res* 2000; 70:17–30.
8. They include the general categories of prostaglandin analogues,

topical carbonic anhydrase inhibitors, beta-blockers and α–adrenergic agonists.

Chapter 19 Alzheimer's disease

1. The localisation of different types of memory has been derived by comparing different diseases or injuries affecting various parts of the brain with the memory disorders that each has been consistently found to produce. Localisation of different functions has also been confirmed by recording the chemical (metabolic) activity of different parts of the brain while different memory tasks are being attempted and different nerve cells activated. This can be done from outside the brain by techniques (PET) which can measure local blood flow and local rate of consumption of glucose by brain cells. In addition, another technique (SPECT) allows the rates of blood flow in different parts of the brain to be compared. Yet another technique (fMRI) allows measurement of the local oxygen content of different brain areas.
2. Salehi A, Ravid R, Gonatas NK, Swaab DF. Decreased activity of hippocampal neurons in Alzheimer's disease is not related to the presence of neurofibrillary tangles. *J Neuropathol Exp Neurol* 1995; 54: 704–709.
3. All body cells contain in their nucleus and cytoplasm large multi-subunit protein complexes called 'proteasomes'. The 26S proteasome collects within it unwanted proteins which have been marked out for degradation and removal by being tagged with the protein ubiquitin (Latin: *ubique* = everywhere). Inside the proteasome the proteins are unfolded, then split into their component peptides. These can then either be reused for new protein synthesis or removed from the cell.
4. Hendriksen JVRB, Nottet HSLM, Smits HA. Secretases as targets for drug design in Alzheimer's disease. *Europ J Clin Invest* 2002; 32: 60–68.
5. Hsiao K, Chapman P, Nilsen S, et al. Correlative memory deficits, Abeta elevation, and amyloid plaques in transgenic mice. *Science* 1996; 274: 99–102.
6. Forloni G, Tagliavini F, Bugiani O, Salmona M. Amyloid in Alzheimer's disease and prion-related encephalopathies: studies with synthetic peptides. *Prog Neurobiol* 1996; 49: 287–315.
7. Bucciantini M, Giannoni E, Chiti F, et al. Inherent toxicity of aggregates implies a common mechanism for protein misfolding diseases. *Nature* 2002; 416: 507–511.
8. Schmidt ML, Lee VM, Forman M, et al. Monoclonal antibodies to a 100–kd protein reveal abundant A beta-negative plaques throughout gray matter of Alzheimer's disease brains. *Am J Pathol* 1997; 151: 69–80.
9. Thome J, Kornhuber J, Munch G, et al. New hypothesis on etiopathogenesis of Alzheimer syndrome. Advanced glycation end products (AGEs) [in German]. *Nervenarzt* 1996; 67: 924–929.

10. Armstrong RA, Winsper SJ, Blair JA. Aluminium and Alzheimer's disease: review of possible pathogenic mechanisms. *Dementia* 1996; 7: 1–9.
11. Seshadri S, Beiser A, Selhub J, et al. Plasma homocysteine as a risk factor for dementia and Alzheimer's disease. *New Engl J Med* 2002; 346: 476–483.
12. Snowdon DA, Kemper SJ, Mortimer JA, et al. Linguistic ability in early life and cognitive function and Alzheimer's disease in late life. Findings from the Nun Study. *J Am Med Ass* 1996; 2: 528–532.
13. Stern Y, Gurland B, Tatemichi TK, et al. Influence of education and occupation on the incidence of Alzheimer's disease. *J Am Med Ass* 1994; 271: 1004–1010.
14. Whalley LJ, Thomas BM, McGonigal G, et al. Epidemiology of presenile Alzheimer's disease in Scotland (1974–88). I. Non-random geographical variation. *Br J Psychiat* 1995; 167: 728–731.
15. A neurotransmitter is a chemical released locally from a nerve ending which modifies the receptive state of another adjacent excitable nerve cell. More than 40 different ones have been recognised.
16. Edland SD, Silverman JM, Peskind ER, et al. Increased risk of dementia in mothers of Alzheimer's disease cases: evidence for maternal inheritance. *Neurology* 1996; 47: 254–256.

Chapter 20 Coronary heart disease: Atheroma

1. A clot comprises a 'polymer' (Greek: 'many parts') of the protein fibrin, which is made from a soluble circulating blood protein (fibrinogen). As the protein condenses into a polymer it traps red blood cells and other debris in the clot.
2. Boersma E, Mercado N, Poldermans D, et al. Acute myocardial infarction. *Lancet* 2003; 361: 847–858.
3. Zimetbaum PJ, Josephson ME. Use of the Electrocardiogram in Acute Myocardial Infarction. *New Engl J Med* 2003; 348: 933–940.
4. A traditional so-called 'Mediterranean' diet is characterised by a high intake of vegetables, peas, beans, fruits, unrefined cereals and olive oil, with a moderately high intake of available fish, a regular but moderate intake of wine with meals, a low-to-moderate intake of dairy products (preferably as cheese or yoghourt), and a low intake of meat, poultry and saturated fat. The long term benefits of a Mediterranean diet are difficult to prove conclusively because of the many confounding factors, but there is highly suggestive recent evidence that it can improve long term survival. See: Trichopoulos A, Costacou T, Barnia C, Trichopoulos D. Adherence to a Mediterranean diet and survival in a Greek population. *New Engl J Med* 2003; 348: 2599–2608.
5. Heart Protection Study Collaborative Group. MRC/BHF Heart Protection Study of cholesterol lowering with simvastatin in 20536 high-risk

individuals: a randomised placebo-controlled trial. *Lancet* 2002; 360: 7–22.

6. Day INM, Wilson DI. Genetics and cardiovascular risk. *Br Med J* 2001; 23: 1409–1412.

7. Hill JM, Zalos G, Halcox JPJ, et al. Circulating Endothelial Progenitor Cells, Vascular Function, and Cardiovascular risk. *New Engl J Med* 2003; 348: 593–600.

8. Corder R, Douthwaite JA, Lees DM, et al. Endothelin-1 Synthesis by Red Reduced Wine. *Nature* 2001; 414: 863–866.

9. Dickinson CJ. Does folic acid harm people with vitamin B12 deficiency? *Quart J Med* 1995; 88: 357–364.

10. Mattila KJ, Valtonen VV, Nieminen MS, Asikainen S. Role of infection as a risk factor for atherosclerosis, myocardial infarction, and stroke. *Clin Infect Dis* 1998; 26: 719–734.

11. Ridker PM, Buring JE, Cook NR, Rifai N. C reactive protein, the metabolic syndrome, and risk of incident cardiovascular events: an 8–year follow-up of 14719 American women. *Circulation* 2003; 107: 391–397.
Koenig W. Heart disease and the inflammatory response. *Br Med J* 2000; 321: 187–188.

12. Buffon A, Biasucci LM, Liuzzo G, et al. Widespread coronary inflammation in unstable angina. *New Engl J Med* 2002; 347: 5–12.

13. Ishizaka N, Ishizaka Y, Takahashi E, et al. Association between hepatitis C virus seropositivity, carotid-artery plaque, and intima-media thickening. *Lancet* 2002; 359: 133–135.

14. Grimes DS, Hindle E, Dyer T. Respiratory infection and coronary heart disease: progression of a paradigm. *Quart J Med* 2000; 93: 375–383.

15. Nichol KL, Nordin J, Mullooly J, et al. Influenza Vaccination and Reduction in Hospitalizations for Cardiac Disease and Stroke among the elderly. *New Engl J Med* 2003; 348: 1322–1332.

16. Smith GD, Ebrahim S. 'Mendelian randomisation': can genetic epidemiology contribute to understanding environmental determinants of disease? *Int J Epidemiol* 2003; 32: 1–22.

17. Fatty acids are just what their name suggests. They incorporate an acid end of their molecule and a string of carbon atoms joined together in a chain. 'Saturated' means that each carbon atom making up the chain has all its four available chemical bonds either joined up to other carbon atoms or to hydrogen atoms. If two adjacent carbon atoms are joined by a double bond, leaving a potential combining site (bond) unfilled, the compound is 'unsaturated'. A molecule containing two or more double bonds is described as 'polyunsaturated'. The position of the double bond closest to the methyl end of the chain defines two main families of fatty acids: n-3 (ω-3), and n-6 (ω-6). Fish oils contain predominantly n-3 fatty acids. Many vegetable oils comprise mainly n-6 fatty acids. These are believed to be less protective than the n-3 group.

18. Thies F, Garry JMC, Yaqoob P, et al. Association of n-3 polyunsatu-

rated fatty acids with stability of atherosclerotic plaques: a randomised controlled trial. *Lancet* 2003; 361: 477–485.

19. Heptinstall S. The importance of platelet aggregation in coronary heart disease. *Br J Cardiol* 2000; 7(Suppl 1): S27–S30.

20. Lenfant C. Clinical Research to Clinical Practice – Lost in Translation? *New Engl J Med* 2003; 349: 868–874.

21. Varma C, Brecker SJD. Predictors of mortality in acute myocardial infarction. *Lancet* 2001; 358: 1473–1474.

Chapter 21 Heart failure

1. Called 'epinephrine' in the USA because of patent rights in the name 'adrenaline' at the time that the hormone was discovered.

2. Blood volume can be measured during life by injecting into a vein a known quantity of some labelled material, e.g. chemically or radioactively tagged red blood cells, or radioactively labelled albumin, which will stay in the bloodstream for at least a few minutes. Then a sample of blood is withdrawn and the concentration of the labelled material measured. The lower the concentration, the greater the volume of circulating blood.

3. Starr I. Role of the 'static blood pressure' in abnormal increments of venous pressure, especially in heart failure. II. Clinical and Experimental Studies. *Am J med Sci* 1940; 199: 40–55.

4. Named by Paintal (see note 5 below) 'J' receptors, because they are 'juxta-capillary' and lie between lung capillaries and the alveoli (the terminal air sacs of the lungs). They can be stimulated by lung congestion and also by carbon dioxide. Nerve fibres coming from these receptors join the vagus nerves on each side. These run up to the brain in the neck, alongside the internal carotid arteries.

5. Dickinson CJ, Paintal AS. Stimulation of pulmonary type-J receptors by carbon dioxide. *Clin Sci* 1970; 38: 33P.

6. Fox KF, Cowie MR, Wood DA, et al. Coronary artery disease as the cause of incident heart failure in the population. *Europ Heart J* 2001; 22: 228–236.

7. Cleland JGF, McGowan J, Clark A, Freemantle N. The evidence for β-blockers in heart failure. *Br Med J* 1999; 318: 824–825.

8. Stevenson LW. Beta-Blockers for Stable Heart Failure. *New Engl J Med* 2002; 346: 1346–1347.

9. Jessup M, Brozena S. Heart failure. *New Engl J Med* 2003; 348: 2007–2018.

10. Lenfant C. Clinical Research to Clinical Practice – Lost in Translation? *New Engl J Med* 2003; 349: 868–874.

Chapter 22 Clubbing of the fingers

1. Stoller JK, Moodie D, Schiavone WA, et al. Reduction of Intrapulmonary Shunt and Resolution of Digital Clubbing Associated with Primary Biliary Cirrhosis after Liver Transplantation. *Hepatology* 1990; 11: 54–58.
2. Dickinson CJ. The aetiology of clubbing and hypertrophic osteoarthropathy. *Europ J Clin Invest* 1993; 23: 330–338.
3. Dickinson CJ, Martin JF. Megakaryocytes and platelet clumps as the cause of finger clubbing. *Lancet* 1987; ii: 1434–1435.

   I chanced upon John Martin's fascinating work and calculations when I was browsing around posters at a meeting of the British Medical Research Society. Posters are a popular way of communicating new scientific information at meetings. The poster I saw was provocatively headed 'Platelets are made in the lungs'. I had always believed that platelets were made in the bone marrow. It took me ten minutes' careful study to realise what John and his colleagues were getting at, and to the realisation that particulate rather than dissolved matter might perhaps account for clubbing. Our meeting led directly to our original publication. It's always worth looking at posters at scientific meetings!
4. Fox SB, Day CA, Gatter KC. Association between platelet microthrombi and finger clubbing. *Lancet* 1991; 338: 313–314.
5. Wood WG (1982). Developmental haemopoiesis. In: *Blood and its disorders* (eds Hardisty RM, Weatherall DJ). Oxford: Blackwell.

Chapter 23 Hepatitis

1. Simpson KJ, Henderson NC, Bone-Larson CL, et al. Chemokines in the pathogenesis of liver disease: so many players with poorly defined roles. *Clin Sci* 2003; 104: 47–63.
2. Fathalla SE, Al-Jama AA, Al-Sheikh IH, Islam SI. Seroprevalence of hepatitis A virus markers in Eastern Saudi Arabia. *Saudi Med* J 2000; 21: 945–949.
3. Gregorio GV, Choudhuri K, Ma Y, et al. Mimicry between the hepatitis B virus DNA polymerase and the antigenic targets of nuclear and smooth muscle antibodies in chronic hepatitis B virus infection. *J Immunol* 1999; 162: 1802–1810.
4. Application of the technique of molecular cloning has allowed the development of specific tests for this virus being developed without the virus ever having been cultured.
5. Harris HE, Ramsay ME, Andrews N, et al. Clinical course of hepatitis C virus during the first decade of infection: cohort study. *Br Med J* 2002; 324: 450–453.
6. Thomas DL, Astemborski J, Rai RM, et al. The natural history of

hepatitis C virus infection: host, viral, and environmental factors. *J Am Med Ass* 2001; 284:450–456.

7. Kjaergard LL, Krogsgaard K, Glaud C. Interferon alfa with or without ribavirin for chronic hepatitis C: systematic review of randomised trials. *Br Med J* 2001; 323: 1151–1155.

8. He J, Binn LN, Tsarev SA, et al. Molecular characterization of a hepatitis E virus isolate from Namibia. *J Biomed Sci* 2001; 7: 334–338.

9. Romano L, Fabris P, Tanzi E, et al. GBV-C/hepatitis G virus in acute nonA-E hepatitis and in acute hepatitis of defined aetiology in Italy. *J Med Virol* 2001; 61: 59–64.

10. Rigas B, Hasan I, Rehman R, et al. Effect of treatment outcome of coinfection with SEN viruses in patients with hepatitis C. *Lancet* 2001; 358: 1961–1964.

11. Perrillo RP. Acute flares in chronic hepatitis B: the natural and unnatural history of an immunologically mediated liver disease. *Gastroenterology* 2001; 120: 1009–1022.

12. Mehta SH, Cox A, Hoover DR, et al. Protection against persistence of hepatitis C. *Lancet* 2002; 359: 1478–1483.

Chapter 24 Irritable bowel syndrome

1. Fida R, Lyster DJ, Bywater RA, Taylor GS. Colonic migrating motor complexes (CMMCs) in the isolated mouse colon. *Neurogastroent Motil* 1997; 9: 99–107.

2. Bell IR, Schwartz GE, Peterson JM, Amend D. Symptom and personality profiles of young adults from a college student population with self-reported illness from foods and chemicals. *J Am Coll Nutr* 1993; 12: 693–702.

3. Kingham JG, Dawson AM. Origin of chronic right upper quadrant pain. *Gut* 1985; 26: 783–788.
    Orr WC, Crowell MD, Lin B, et al. Sleep and gastric function in irritable bowel syndrome: derailing the brain-gut axis. Gut 1997; 41: 390–393.

4. Farthing MJG. Treatment of irritable bowel syndrome. *Br Med J* 2005; 330: 429–430.

5. Bindslev-Jensen C. Food allergy. *Br Med J* 1998; 316: 1299–1302.

6. Tornblom H, Lindberg G, Nyberg H, Veress B. Full-thickness biopsy of the jejunum reveals inflammation and enteric neuropathy in irritable bowel syndrome. *Gastroenterology* 2002; 123: 2144–2147.

Chapter 25 Ulcerative colitis and Crohn's disease

1. Farrell RJ, Peppercorn MA. Ulcerative colitis. *Lancet* 2002; 359: 331–340.

2. Shanahan F. Crohn's disease. *Lancet* 2002; 359: 62–69.

3. Von Andrian UH, Engelhardt B. α4 Integrins as Therapeutic Targets in Autoimmune Disease. *New Engl J Med* 2003; 348: 68–72.
4. Anonymous. A case-control study of ulcerative colitis in relation to dietary and other factors in Japan. The Epidemiology Group of the Research Committee of Inflammatory Bowel Disease in Japan. *J Gastroenterol* 1995; 30(Suppl 8); 9–12.

Chapter 26 Haemochromatosis: Disorders involving iron

1. Gutierrez JA, Yu J, Wessling-Resnick M. Characterization and chromosomal mapping of the human gene for SFT, a stimulator of Fe transport. *Biochem Biophys Res Commun* 1998; 253: 739–742.
   Barton JC, Edwards CQ (eds) (2000). *Hemochromatosis: genetics, pathophysiology, diagnosis, and treatment.* Cambridge: CUP.
2. Thalassaemia (Greek: *thalassa* = sea: i.e. a blood disease found around the Mediterranean sea) is a genetic condition in which the bone marrow is not able to make enough of one of the component parts of the oxygen-carrying protein haemoglobin. This causes a type of anaemia which is classified as a 'haemoglobinopathy'. Although thalassaemia is clinically and chemically different from sickle-cell disease – another haemoglobinopathy – some genetic predisposition to either of these defects may give some protection against locally prevalent diseases, especially malaria.
3. Davies PJ. Was Beethoven's cirrhosis due to hemochromatosis? *Ren Fail* 1995; 17: 77–86.
4. Hetet G, Elbaz A, Gariepy J, et al. Association studies between haemochromatosis gene mutations and the risk of cardiovascular diseases. *Europ J Clin Invest* 2001; 31: 382–388.
5. Beutler E, Felitti VJ, Koziol JA, et al. Penetrance of 845G-A (C282Y) HFE hereditary haemochromatosis mutation in the USA. *Lancet* 2002; 359: 211–218.
   Bomford A. Genetics of haemochromatosis. *Lancet* 2002; 360: 1673–1681.
6. Townsend A, Drakesmith H. Role of HFE in iron metabolism, hereditary haemochromatosis, anaemia of chronic disease, and secondary iron overload. *Lancet* 2002; 369: 780–790.
7. Griffiths WJH, Kelly AL, Smith SJ, Cox TM. Localization of iron transport and regulatory proteins in human cells. *Quart J Med* 2000; 93: 575–587.
8. Stewart SF, Day CP. Liver disorder and the HFE locus. *Quart J Med* 2001; 94: 453–456.
9. Seamark CJ, Hutchinson M. Should asymptomatic haemochromatosis be treated? *Br Med J* 2000; 320: 1314–1317.

Chapter 27 Folic acid and neural tube defects

1. Reynolds EH. Folic acid, ageing, depression, and dementia. *Br Med J* 2002; 324: 1512–1515.
2. Botez MI, Cadotte M, Beaulieu R, et al. Neurologic disorders responsive to folic acid therapy. *Canad Med Ass J* 1976; 115: 217–223.
3. Kamei T, Kohno T, Ohwada H, et al. Experimental study of the therapeutic effects of folate, vitamin A, and vitamin B12 on squamous metaplasia of the bronchial epithelium. *Cancer* 1993; 71: 2477–2483.
4. MRC Vitamin Study Research Group. Prevention of neural tube defects: results of the Medical Research Council Vitamin Study. *Lancet* 1991; 338: 131–137.
5. Wild J, Schorah CJ, Sheldon TA, Smithells RW. Investigation of factors influencing folate status in women who have had a neural tube defect-affected infant. *Br J Obst Gynaec* 1993; 100: 546–549.
6. Dickinson CJ. Does folic acid harm people with vitamin B12 deficiency? *Quart J Med* 1995; 88: 357–364.
7. Bailey LB (ed) (1995). *Folate in health and disease.* New York: Marcel Dekker.
8. Oakley GP. Folic Acid – Preventable Spina Bifida and Anencephaly. *J Am med Ass* 1993; 269: 1292–1293.
9. A rare but very dangerous pre-malignant condition of the colon which often comes to light by causing anaemia.

Chapter 28 Parkinson's disease

1. Lang AE, Lozano AM. Parkinson's disease. *New Engl J Med* 1998; 339: 1044–1053 & 1130–1143 (2 parts).
2. Galvin JE, Lee VM, Baba M, et al. Monoclonal antibodies to purified cortical Lewy bodies recognize the mid-size neurofilament subunit. *Ann Neurol* 1997; 42: 595–603.
3. Schrag A, Ben-Shlomo Y, Quinn NP. Cross-sectional prevalence survey of idiopathic Parkinson's disease and parkinsonism in London. *Br Med J* 2000; 321: 21–22.
4. Shimura H, Schlossmacher MG, Hartori N, et al. Ubiquitination of a new form of alpha-synuclein by parkin from human brain: implications for Parkinson's disease. *Science* 2001; 293: 263–269.
5. Mizuno Y, Hattori N, Mori H. Genetics of Parkinson's disease. *Biomed Pharmacother* 1999; 53: 109–116.
6. Charlett A, Dobbs RJ, Dobbs SM, et al. Parkinsonism: siblings share *Helicobacter pylori* seropositivity and facets of syndrome. *Acta Neurol Scand* 1999; 99: 26–35.
7. Rascol O, Brooks DJ, Korczyn AD, et al. A five-year study of the incidence of dyskinesia in patients with early Parkinson's disease who

were treated with ropinirole or levodopa. *New Engl J Med* 2000; 342: 1481–1491.

8. Prusiner SB. Shattuck Lecture – Neurodegenerative diseases and prions. *New Engl J Med* 2001; 344: 1516–1526.

Chapter 29 Paget's disease of bone

1. Kanis JA (1998). *Pathophysiology and treatment of Paget's disease of bone*. London: Dunitz.
2. Good DA, Busfield F, Fletcher BH, et al. Linkage of Paget disease of bone to a novel region on human chromosome 18q23. *Am J Hum Genet* 2002; 70: 517–525.
3. Hocking LJ, Herbert CA, Nicholls RK, et al. Genomewide search in familial Paget disease of bone shows evidence of genetic heterogeneity with candidate loci on chromosomes 2q36, 10p13, and 5q35. *Am J Hum Genet* 2002; 69: 1055–1061.
4. Ebersole JL, Taubman MA, Smith DJ, et al. Human immune responses to oral microorganisms. II. Serum antibody responses to antigens from *Actinobacillus actinomycetemcomitans* and the correlation with localized juvenile periodontitis. *J Clin Immunol* 1983; 3: 321–331.
5. Zafiropoulos GG, Flores-de-Jacoby L, Hungerer KD, Nisengard RJ. Humoral antibody responses in periodontal disease. *J Periodontol* 1992; 63: 80–86.
6. Dickinson CJ. The possible role of osteoclastogenic oral bacteria products in etiology of Paget's disease. *Bone* 2000; 26: 101–102.
7. Blix IJ, Hars R, Preus HR, Helgeland K. Entrance of *Actinobacillus actinomycetemcomitans* into HEp-2 cells in vitro. *J Periodontol* 1992; 63: 723–728.
8. Renier J-C, Audran M. Progression in length and width of Pagetic lesions, and estimation of age at disease onset. *Rev Rhum* 1997; 64: 35–43.
9. Wheeler TT, Alberts MA, Dolan TA, McGorray SP. Dental, visual, auditory and olfactory complications in Paget's disease of bone. *J Am Geriatr Soc* 1995; 43: 1384–1391.
10. Barry HC (1969). *Paget's disease of bone*. Edinburgh: Livingstone.

Chapter 30 Osteoporosis

1. Hydroxyapatite has the chemical formula $3(Ca_3(PO_4)_2)Ca(OH)_2$.
2. Cummings SR, Black DM, Nevitt MC, et al. Bone density at various sites for prediction of hip fractures. *Lancet* 1993; 341: 72–75.
3. Cummings SR, Melton LJ. Epidemiology and outcomes of osteoporotic fractures. *Lancet* 2002; 359: 1761–1767.

4. Delmas PD. Treatment of postmenopausal osteoporosis. *Lancet* 2002; 359: 2018–2026.
5. Boyden LM, Mao J, Belsky J, et al. High bone density due to a mutation in LDL-receptor-related protein 5. *New Engl J Med* 2002; 346: 1513–1521.
6. For complex reasons, one of which is that kidney failure allows the build up of protein waste products, some of which combine strongly with calcium and reduce the effective calcium concentration.
7. Eastell R, Reid DM, Compston J, et al. Secondary prevention of osteoporosis: when should a non-vertebral fracture be a trigger for action? *Quart J Med* 2001; 94: 575–597.

Chapter 31 High blood pressure: 'Essential hypertension'

1. Dickinson CJ (1965). *Neurogenic Hypertension*. Oxford: Blackwell Scientific Publs.
   Dickinson CJ (1991). *Neurogenic Hypertension*. London: Chapman & Hall.
2. Mann A. Hypertension: psychological aspects and diagnostic impact in a clinical trial. *Psychol Med* 1984; Monograph Suppl 5.
3. Huxley R, Neil A, Collins R. Unravelling the fetal origins hypothesis: is there really an inverse association between birthweight and subsequent blood pressure? *Lancet* 2002; 360: 659–665.
4. Medical Research Council Working Party. Course of blood pressure in mild hypertensives after withdrawal of long-term antihypertensive treatment. *Br Med J* 1986; 293: 988–992.
5. Swales JD (ed) (1994). *Textbook of Hypertension*. Oxford: Blackwell Scientific Publs.

Chapter 32 Hypertension from the kidneys

1. Thompson JMA, Dickinson CJ. The relation between the excretion of sodium and water and the perfusion pressure in the isolated, blood-perfused, rabbit kidney, with special reference to the changes occurring in clip-hypertension. *Clin Sci Mol Med* 1976; 50: 223–236.
2. Guyton AC, Coleman TG, Granger HJ. Circulation: Overall regulation. *Ann Rev Physiol* 1972; 34: 13–46.
3. Dickinson CJ, Lawrence JR. A slowly developing pressor response to small concentrations of angiotensin: its bearing on the pathogenesis of chronic renal hypertension. *Lancet* 1963; i: 1354–1356.
4. Dickinson CJ, Yu R. Mechanisms Involved in the Progressive Pressor Response to Very Small Amounts of Angiotensin in Conscious Rabbits. *Circulat Res* 1967; 20/21(Suppl II): II-157–II-163.
5. Yu R, Dickinson CJ. Neurogenic effects of angiotensin. *Lancet* 1965; ii: 1276–1277.

6. Boehm M, Nabel EG. Angiotensin-converting enzyme 2 – a new cardiac regulator *New Engl J Med* 2002; 347: 1295–1297.
7. Muirhead EE. Renal vasodepressor mechanisms: the medullipin system. *J Hypertens* 1993; 11(Suppl 5): S53–S58.

Chapter 33 Kidney failure: Chronic glomerulonephritis

1. *Two Lives: Death Odyssey of Transplant Surgeon, by O.M. Beleil, M.D., in conversation with Cliff Osmond.* Published and distributed in 1973 by Precision Printers, Inc., 5261 West Jefferson Boulevard, Los Angeles, California 90016, USA.
2. Dialysis (the Greek word means 'separation') is a good description of the movement of water and salts through the semi-permeable membrane lining the abdominal cavity. Some soluble waste products like urea (the major breakdown product of proteins) simply move by diffusion across the concentration gradient from their high concentration in body fluids to zero concentration in the dialysing fluid. To extract additional water, as in Omer's case, it is necessary to use a dialysing fluid with a high 'osmotic' pressure which can in effect suck large volumes of fluid out of the bloodstream.
3. Brenner BM, Meyer TW, Hostetter TH. Dietary protein intake and the progressive nature of kidney disease: the role of hemodynamically mediated glomerular injury in the pathogenesis of progressive glomerular sclerosis in aging, renal ablation, and intrinsic renal disease. *New Engl J Med* 1982; 307: 652–659.
   Anderson S, Brenner BM. The role of intraglomerular pressure in the initiation and progression of renal disease. *J Hypertens* 1986; 4 (Suppl): S236–S238.
4. Apperloo AJ, de Zeeuw D, de Jong PE. A short-term antihypertensive treatment-induced fall in glomerular filtration rate predicts long-term stability of renal function. *Kidn Internat* 1997; 51: 793–797.
5. Fored CM, Ejerblad E, Lindblad P, et al. Acetaminophen, aspirin, and chronic renal failure. *New Engl J Med* 2001; 345: 1801–1808.
6. Field M. Tumour necrosis factor polymorphisms in rheumatic diseases. *Quart J Med* 2001; 94: 237–246.
7. Nakamura A, Yuasa T, Ujike A, et al. Fcgamma receptor IIB-deficient mice develop Goodpasture's syndrome upon immunization with type IV collagen: a novel murine model for autoimmune glomerular basement membrane disease. *J Exp Med* 2000; 191: 899–906.
8. Mostoslavsky G, Fischel R, Yachimovich N, et al. Lupus anti-DNA autoantibodies cross-react with a glomerular structural protein: a case for tissue injury by molecular mimicry. *Europ J Immunol* 2001; 31: 1221–1227.
9. Donadio JV, Grande JP. IgA Nephropathy. *New Engl J Med* 2002; 347: 738–748.

10. Hsu SI, Ramirez SB, Winn MP, et al. Evidence for genetic factors in the development and progression of IgA nephropathy. *Kidn Internat* 2001; 57: 1818–1835.
11. Suzuki S, Gejyo F, Arakawa M. Pathogenesis of IgA nephropathy: role of outer membranes of *Haemophilus parainfluenzae* antigens [in Japanese]. *Nippon Rinsho* 1997; 55: 1580–1587.
12. Jefferson JA, Johnson RJ. Treatment of hepatitis C-associated glomerular disease. *Sem Nephrol* 2001; 20: 286–292.
13. Jessen RH, Emancipator SN, Jacobs GH, Nedrud JG. Experimental IgA-IgG nephropathy induced by a viral respiratory pathogen. Dependence on antigen form and immune status. *Lab Invest* 1992; 67: 379–386.
14. Ravnskov U. Hydrocarbon exposure may cause glomerulonephritis and worsen renal function: evidence based on Hill's criteria for causality. *QJMed* 2001; 93: 551–556.
15. Dagher L, Moore K. The hepatorenal syndrome. *Gut* 2001; 49: 729–737.

Chapter 34 Strokes and high blood pressure

1. PROGRESS MC. Progress Management Committee: Blood pressure lowering for the secondary prevention of stroke: rationale and design for progress. *J Hypertens* 1996; 14 (Suppl 2): S41–S46.
2. Challa VR, Moody DM, Bell MA. The Charcot-Bouchard aneurysms controversy: impact of a new histologic technique. *J Neuropath Exper Neurol* 1992; 51: 264–271.
3. Dickinson CJ. Why are strokes related to hypertension? Classic studies and hypotheses revisited. *J Hypertens* 2001; 19: 1515–1521.
4. Dickinson CJ, Thomson AD. High blood pressure and stroke: necropsy study of heart-weight and left ventricular hypertrophy. *Lancet* 1960; ii: 342–345.
5. Dickinson CJ, Thomson AD. A post mortem study of the main cerebral arteries with special reference to the cause of strokes. *Clin Sci* 1961; 20: 131–142.
6. Mohr JP, Thompson JLP, Lazar RM, et al. A comparison of warfarin and aspirin for the prevention of recurrent ischemic stroke. *New Engl J Med* 2001; 345: 1444–1451.
7. Powers WJ. Oral anticoagulant therapy for the prevention of stroke. *New Engl J Med* 2001; 345: 1493–1495.
8. Dickinson CJ. Strokes and their relationship to hypertension. *Curr Opin Nephrol Hypertens* 2003; 12: 91–96.
9. MacMahon S, Neal B. Differences between blood-pressure-lowering drugs. *Lancet* 2000; 356: 352–353.
10. Dickinson CJ. *Neurogenic Hypertension* (1965). Blackwell Scientific Publications. Fig 37: p.137.
11. Vaughan CJ, Delanty N. Neuroprotective properties of statins in cerebral ischemia and stroke. *Stroke* 1999; 30: 1969–1973.

Chapter 35 Pre-eclampsia: Pregnancy-induced high blood pressure

1. The placenta (commonly known as the 'afterbirth') is a large plate-shaped fleshy structure which by the end of pregnancy is about 8 inches in diameter and weighs a bit more than a pound. It is firmly attached to the inside wall of the womb (uterus) and connected to the fetus (the proper name for a child still in the womb) by the umbilical cord. The placenta is a filter. It keeps back the mother's blood cells, and also most proteins, but it lets through water, glucose and other nutrients, and removes waste products. The filtered blood also supplies oxygen to the fetus and removes carbon dioxide.

2. The main sign of the fetus being unwell is a fall in heart rate (below 110 beats/min), especially when accompanied by irregularity of rhythm. This usually reflects a poor placental blood supply and is what the midwife or doctor checks for with the ultrasonic fetal heart detector. An excessive rise of fetal heart rate (170 beats/min) may also occur with fetal distress, but is uncommon.

3. Levine RJ, Maynard SE, Qian C, et al. Circulating angiogenic factors and the risk of preeclampsia. *New Engl J Med* 2004; 350: 672–683.

4. Haller H, Hempel A, Homuth V, et al. Endothelial-cell permeability and protein kinase C in pre-eclampsia. *Lancet* 1998; 351: 945–949.

5. Schobel HP, Fischer T, Heuszer K, et al. Preeclampsia – state of sympathetic overactivity. *New Engl J Med* 1996; 335: 1480–1485.

6. Smarason AK, Sargent IL, Redman CW. Endothelial cell proliferation is suppressed by plasma but not serum from women with preeclampsia. *Am J Obstet Gynecol* 1996; 174: 787–793.

7. Poston L. Leptin and preeclampsia. *Semin Reprod Med* 2002; 20: 131–138.

8. Brown MA. The physiology of pre-eclampsia. *Clin Exp Pharmacol Physiol* 1995; 22: 781–791.

9. Taylor RN. Review: immunobiology of preeclampsia. *Am J Reprod Immunol* 1997; 37: 79–86.

10. Robillard PY, Hulsey TC, Perianin J, et al. Association of pregnancy-induced hypertension with duration of sexual cohabitation before conception. *Lancet* 1994; 344: 973–975.

11. Skjaerven R, Wilcox AJ, Lie RT. The interval between pregnancies and the risk of preeclampsia. *New Engl J Med* 2002; 346: 33–38.

12. Chappell LC, Seed PT, Briley AL, et al. Effect of antioxidants on the occurrence of pre-eclampsia in women at increased risk: a randomised trial. *Lancet* 1999; 354: 810–815.

Chapter 36 Pulmonary hypertension

1. Giaid A, Yanagisawa M, Langleben D, et al. Expression of endothelin-1 in the lungs of patients with pulmonary hypertension. *New Engl J Med* 1993; 328: 1732–1739.

2. Rubin LJ, Badesch BD, Barst RJ, et al. Bosentan therapy for pulmonary arterial hypertension. *New Engl J Med* 2002; 346: 896–903.
3. Morse JH, Jones AC, Barst RJ, et al. Mapping of familial primary pulmonary hypertension locus (PPH1) to chromosome 2q31–q32. *Circulation* 1997; 95: 2603–2606.
4. Du L, Sullivan CC, Chu D, et al. Signaling molecules in Nonfamilial Pulmonary Hypertension. *New Engl J Med* 2003; 348: 500–509.
5. Cool CD, Pradeep RR, Yeager ME, et al. Expression of Human Herpesvirus 8 in Primary Pulmonary Hypertension. *New Engl J Med* 2003; 349: 1113–1122.

Chapter 37 Polycystic ovary syndrome

1. Lockwood GM, Muttukrishna S, Groome NP, et al. Mid-follicular phase pulses of inhibin B are absent in polycystic ovarian syndrome and are initiated by successful laparoscopic ovarian diathermy: a possible mechanism regulating emergence of the dominant follicle. *J Clin Endocrinol Metab* 1998; 83: 1730–1735.
2. LH (lueinising hormone) is so called because its secretion creates the yellow body (corpus luteum, from Latin: *luteus* = yellow) in the bed of the egg which has just been released from the ovary. LH promotes the secretion of oestrogens. If the egg is not fertilised, the corpus luteum shrinks and disappears after about 2 weeks. In the male the identical hormone is called 'interstitial-cell stimulating hormone' (ICSH) which promotes the secretion of testosterone by the testes.
3. Dickinson CJ (1977). *A Computer Model of Human Respiration.* Lancaster: MTP Press Ltd.
4. Hopkinson ZEC, Sattar N, Fleming R, Greer IA. Polycystic ovarian syndrome: the metabolic syndrome comes to gynaecology. *Br Med J* 1998; 317: 329–332.
5. Ciampelli M, Lanzone A. Insulin and polycystic ovary syndrome: a new look at an old subject. *Gynecol Endocrinol* 1998; 12: 277 -292.
6. Sills ES, Perloe M, Palermo GD. Correction of hyperinsulinemia in oligoovulatory women with clomiphene-resistant polycystic ovary syndrome: a review of therapeutic rationale and reproductive outcomes. *Europ J Obstet Gynecol Reprod Biol* 2000; 91: 135–141.
7. Franks S, Gharani N, Gilling-Smith C. Polycystic ovary syndrome: evidence for a primary disorder of ovarian steroidogenesis. *J Steroid Biochem Mol Biol* 1999; 69: 269–272.
8. Sozen I, Arici A. Hyperinsulinism and its interaction with hyperandrogenism in polycystic ovary syndrome. *Obstet Gynecol Surv* 2001; 55: 321–328.
9. Harborne L, Fleming R, Lyall H, et al. Descriptive review of the evidence for the use of metformin in polycystic ovary syndrome. *Lancet* 2003; 361: 1894–1900.

10. Jacobs HS, Conway GS. Leptin, polycystic ovaries and polycystic ovary syndrome. *Hum Reprod Updat* 1999; 5: 166–171.
11. Fénichel P, Gobert B, Carré Y, et al. Polycystic ovary syndrome in autoimmune disease. *Lancet* 1999; 353: 2210.

Chapter 38 Chronic fatigue syndrome: So-called 'ME'

1. White PD, Grover SA, Kangro HO, et al. The validity and reliability of the fatigue syndrome that follows glandular fever. *Psychol Med* 1995; 25: 917–924.
2. Ayres JG, Flint N, Smith EG, et al. Post-infection fatigue syndrome following Q fever. *Quart J Med* 1998; 91: 105–123.
3. Pearn JH. Chronic fatigue syndrome: chronic ciguatera poisoning. *Med J Aust* 1997; 166: 309–310.
4. Abbey SE, Garfinkel PE. Neurasthenia and chronic fatigue syndrome: the role of culture in the making of a diagnosis. *Am J Psychiat* 1991; 148: 1638–1646.
5. Ichise M, Salit IE, Abbey SE, et al. Assessment of regional cerebral perfusion by 99Tcm-HMPAO SPECT in chronic fatigue syndrome. *Nucl Med Commun* 1992; 13: 767–772.
6. Costa DC, Tannock C, Brostoff J. Brainstem perfusion is impaired in chronic fatigue syndrome. *Quart J Med* 1995; 88: 767–773.
7. Schwartz RB, Garada BM, Komaroff AL, et al. Detection of intracranial abnormalities in patients with chronic fatigue syndrome: comparison of MR imaging and SPECT. *Am J Roentgenol* 1994; 162: 935–941.
8. Cope H, Pernet A, Kendall B, David A. Cognitive functioning and magnetic resonance imaging in chronic fatigue. *Br J Psychiat* 1995; 167: 86–94.
9. Georgiades E, Behan WMH, Kilduff LP, et al. Chronic fatigue syndrome: new evidence for a central fatigue disorder. *Clin Sci* 2003; 105: 213–218.
10. Hess CW, Bassetti C. Neurology of consciousness and of consciousness disorders [in German]. *Schweiz Rund Med Praxis* 1994; 83: 212–219.
11. Tirelli U, Chierichetti F, Tavio M, et al. Brain positron emission tomography (PET) in chronic fatigue syndrome: preliminary data. *Am J Med* 1998; 105: 54S-58S.
12. Bruno RL, Frick NM, Cohen J. Polioencephalitis, stress, and the etiology of post-polio sequelae. *Orthopedics* 1991; 14: 1269–1276.
13. Dickinson CJ. Chronic fatigue syndrome – aetiological aspects. *Europ J Clin Invest* 1997; 27: 257–267.

Chapter 39 Vasculitis: Temporal arteritis and allied conditions

1. Salvarani C, Cantini F, Boiardi L, Hundr GG. Polymyalgia Rheumatica and Giant-cell arteritis. *New Engl J Med* 2002; 347: 261–271.

Weyand CM, Goronzy JJ. Medium- and Large-Vessel Vasculitis. *New Engl J Med* 2003; 349: 160–169.
2. Ralston DR, Marsh CB, Lowe MP, Wewers MD. Antineutrophil cytoplasmic antibodies induce monocyte IL-8 release. Role of surface proteinase-3, alpha 1–antitrypsin, and Fcgamma receptors. *J Clin Invest* 1997; 100: 1416–1424.

Chapter 40 Schizophrenia

1. Mortensen PB, Pedersen CB, Westergaard T, et al. Effects of family history and place and season of birth on the risk of schizophrenia. *New Engl J Med* 1999; 340: 603–608.
2. Hoge EA, Friedman L, Schulz SC. Meta-analysis of brain size in bipolar disorder. *Schizophr Res* 1999; 37: 177–181.
3. Halliday GM. A review of the neuropathology of schizophrenia. *Clin Exper Pharmacol Physiol* 2001; 28: 64–65.
4. Torrey EF. Are we overestimating the genetic contribution to schizophrenia? *Schizophr Bull* 1992; 18: 159–170.
5. Brzustowicz LM, Hodgkinson KA, Chow EW, et al. Location of a major susceptibility locus for familial schizophrenia on chromosome 1q21–q22. *Science* 2001; 288: 678–682.
6. Milunsky J, Huang XL, Wyandt HE, Milunsky A. Schizophrenia susceptibility gene locus at Xp22.3. *Clin Genet* 1999; 55: 455–460.
7. Bailer U, Leisch F, Meszaros K, et al. Genome scan for susceptibility loci for schizophrenia. *Neuropsychobiol* 2001; 42: 175–182.
   Harrison PJ, Owen MJ. Genes for schizophrenia? Recent findings and their pathophysiological implications. *Lancet* 2003; 361: 417–419.
8. Pallast EG, Jongbloet PH, Straatman HM, Zielhuis GA. Excess seasonality of births among patients with schizophrenia and seasonal ovopathy. *Schizophr Bull* 1994; 20: 269–276.
9. Huttunen MO, Machon RA, Mednick SA. Prenatal factors in the pathogenesis of schizophrenia. *Br J Psychiat* 1994; Suppl: 15–19.
10. Cannon TD, Rosso IM, Hollister JM, et al. A prospective cohort study of genetic and perinatal influences in the etiology of schizophrenia. *Schizophr Bull* 2001; 26: 351–366.
11. Lillehoj EP, Ford GM, Bachmann S, et al. Serum antibodies reactive with non-human primate retroviruses identified in acute onset schizophrenia. *J Neurovirol* 2001; 6: 492–497.
    Karlsson H, Bachmann S, Schroder J, et al. Retroviral RNA identified in the cerebrospinal fluids and brains of individuals with schizophrenia. *Proc Nat Acad Sci USA* 2001; 98: 4634–4639.
12. Lipkin WI, Schneemann A, Solbrig MV. Borna disease virus: implications for human neuropsychiatric illness. *Trend Microbiol* 1995; 3: 64–69
13. Pantelis C, Velakoulis D, McGorry PD, et al. Neuroanatomical abnorm-

alities before and after onset of psychosis: a cross-sectional and longitudinal MRI comparison. *Lancet* 2003; 361: 281–288.
14. Pinker S (2002). *The Blank Slate: The modern denial of human nature.* London: Allen Lane.

Chapter 41 Fainting

1. Hainsworth R (1996). Physiology and pathophysiology of syncope. In: *Syncope in the older patient* (ed Kenny RA), pp.15–32. London: Chapman & Hall.
2. Henry JP. On the Triggering Mechanism of Vasovagal Syncope. *Psychosom Med* 1984; 46: 91–93.
3. Öberg B, Thorén P. Increased Activity in Left Ventricular Receptors during Hemorrhage or Occlusion of Caval Veins in the Cat. A Possible Cause of the Vasovagal Reaction. *Acta Physiol Scand* 1972; 85: 164–172.
4. Hainsworth R. Reflexes From the Heart. *Physiol Rev* 1991; 71: 617–658.
5. Scherrer U, Vissing S, Morgan BJ, et al. Vasovagal syncope after infusion of a vasodilator in a heart-transplant patient. *New Engl J Med* 19 90; 322: 602–604.
6. Dickinson CJ. Fainting precipitated by collapse-firing of venous baroreceptors. *Lancet* 1993; 342: 970–972.
7. Pearce JW, Henry JP. Changes in cardiac afferent nerve-fiber discharges induced by hemorrhage and adrenaline. *Am J Physiol* 1955; 183: 650 (abstract).

Chapter 42 Motor neurone disease

1. Shaw PJ. Science,medicine, and the future. *Br Med J* 1999; 318: 1118–1121.
2. This particular Greek mouthful is descriptive: *a* = without; *myo* = muscle; *troph* = nourishment (implying that the muscles become wasted); 'lateral sclerosis' = the side parts of the spinal cord which become hard or thickened from disease.
3. 'Autosomal' refers to inheritance which is independent of the sex of the affected person; 'dominant' is defined elsewhere (p. 475). The obverse of 'autosomal' is 'sex-linked'. As its name suggests, this involves the sex chromosomes. Colour blindness and haemophilia are sex-linked, and only occur in males.
4. Strong MJ, Grace GM, Orange JB, Leeper HA. Cognition, language, and speech in amyotrophic lateral sclerosis: a review. *J Clin Exp Neuropsychol* 1996; 18: 291–303.
5. Kurtzke JF. Epidemiology of amyotrophic lateral sclerosis. *Adv Neurol* 1982; 36: 281–302.

6. Riggs JE. Trauma, axonal injury, and amyotrophic lateral sclerosis: a clinical correlate of a neuropharmacologic model. *Clin Neuropharmacol* 1995; 18: 273–276.
   Rowland LP. Controversies about amyotrophic lateral sclerosis. *Neurologia* 1996; 11 (Suppl 5): 72–74.
   Longstreth WT, Nelson LM, Koepsell TD, van Belle G. Hypotheses to explain the association between vigorous physical activity and amyotrophic lateral sclerosis. *Med Hypoth* 1991; 34: 144–148.
7. Mizusawa H, Nakamura H, Wakayama I, et al. Skein-like inclusions in the anterior horn cells in motor neuron disease. *J Neurol Sci* 1991; 105: 14–21.
   Delisle MB, Carpenter S. Neurofibrillary axonal swellings and amyotrophic lateral sclerosis. *J Neurol Sci* 1984; 63: 241–250.
8. Migheli A, Attanasio A, Schiffer D. Ubiquitin and neurofilament expression in anterior horn cells in amyotrophic lateral sclerosis: possible clues to the pathogenesis. *Neuropathol Appl Neurobiol* 1994; 20: 282–289.
9. Leigh PN, Whitwell H, Garofalo O, et al. Ubiquitin-immunoreactive intraneuronal inclusions in amyotrophic lateral sclerosis. Morphology, distribution, and specificity. *Brain* 1991; 14: 775–788.
10. Okamoto K, Hirai S, Amari M, et al. Bunina bodies in amyotrophic lateral sclerosis immunostained with rabbit anti-cystatin C serum. *Neurosci Lett* 1993; 162: 125–128.
11. Scherzinger E, Lurz R, Turmaine M, et al. Huntingtin-encoded polyglutamine expansions form amyloid-like protein aggregates in vitro and in vivo. *Cell* 1997; 90: 549–558.
12. Yoshida S, Mitani K, Wakayama I, et al. Bunina body formation in amyotrophic lateral sclerosis: a morphometric-statistical and trace element study featuring aluminum. *J Neurol Sci* 1995; 130: 88–94.
    Takahashi H, Ohama E, Ikuta F. Are bunina bodies of endoplasmic reticulum origin? An ultrastructural study of subthalamic eosinophilic inclusions in a case of atypical motor neuron disease. *Acta Pathol Jpn* 1991; 41: 889–894.
13. Shaw PJ, Ince PG, Falkous G, Mantle D. Cytoplasmic, lysosomal and matrix protease activities in spinal cord tissue from amyotrophic lateral sclerosis (AL) and control patients. *J Neurol Sci* 1996; 139 (Suppl): 71–75.
14. Martin LJ, Al-Abdulla NA, Brambrink AM, et al. Neurodegeneration in excitotoxicity, global cerebral ischemia, and target deprivation: A perspective on the contributions of apoptosis and necrosis. *Brain Res Bull* 1998; 46: 281–309.
15. Williams LR. Oxidative stress, age-related neurodegeneration, and the potential for neurotrophic treatment. *Cerebrovasc Brain Metab Rev* 1995; 7: 55–73.
    Gorman AM, McGowan A, O'Neill C, Cotter T. Oxidative stress and apoptosis in neurodegeneration. *J Neurol Sci* 1996; 139 (Suppl): 45–52.
16. Eki T, Abe M, Furuya K, et al. A long-range physical map of human

chromosome 21q22.1 band from the YAC continuum. *Mamm Genom* 19; 7: 303–311.

17. Andersen PM, Forsgren L, Binzer M, et al. Autosomal recessive adult-onset amyotrophic lateral sclerosis associated with homozygosity for Asp90Ala CuZn-superoxide dismutase mutation. A clinical and genealogical study of 36 patients. *Brain* 1996; 119: 1153–1172.

18. Lyons TJ, Liu H, Goto JJ, et al. Mutations in copper-zinc superoxide dismutase that cause amyotrophic lateral sclerosis alter the zinc binding site and redox behavior of the protein. *Proc Natl Acad Sci USA* 1996; 93: 12240–12244.

19. Cote F, Collard JF, Julien JP. Progressive neuronopathy in transgenic mice expressing the human neurofilament heavy gene: a mouse model of amyotrophic lateral sclerosis. *Cell* 1993; 73: 35–46.

20. Price DL, Koliatsos VE, Wong PC, et al. Motor neuron disease and model systems: aetiologies, mechanisms and therapies. *Ciba Foundation Symposium* 1996; pp 3–13.

21. de la Rua-Domenech R, Wiedmann M, Mohammed HO, et al. Equine motor neuron disease is not linked to Cu/Zn superoxide dismutase mutations: sequence analysis of the equine Cu/Zn superoxide dismutase cDNA. *Gene* 1996; 178: 83–88.

22. Shaw PJ, Tomkins J, Slade JY, et al. CNS tissue Cu/Zn superoxide dismutase (SOD1) mutations in motor neurone disease (MND). *Neuroreport* 1997; 8: 3923–3927.

23. Oyanagi K, Makifuchi T, Ohtoh T, et al. Amyotrophic lateral sclerosis of Guam: the nature of the neuropathological findings. *Acta Neuropathol (Berl)* 1994; 88: 405–412.

24. Troost D, van den Oord JJ, de Jong JM, Swaab DF. Lymphocytic infiltration in the spinal cord of patients with amyotrophic lateral sclerosis. *Clin Neuropathol* 1989; 8: 289–294.

25. Smith RG, Engelhardt JI, Tajti J, Appel SH. Experimental immune-mediated motor neuron diseases: models for human ALS. *Brain Res Bull* 1993; 30: 373–380.

26. Appel SH, Smith RG, Engelhardt JI, Stefani E. Evidence for autoimmunity in amyotrophic lateral sclerosis. *J Neurol Sci* 1994; 124 (Suppl): 14–19.

27. Jaspert A, Claus D, Grehl H, Neundorfer B. Multifocal motor neuropathy: clinical and electrophysiological findings. *J Neurol* 1996; 243: 684–692.

28. Swanson NR, Fox SA, Mastaglia FL. Search for persistent infection with poliovirus or other enteroviruses in amyotrophic lateral sclerosis-motor neurone disease. *Neuromuscul Disord* 1995; 5: 457–465.

29. Muller WK, Schaltenbrand G. Attempts to reproduce amyotrophic lateral sclerosis in laboratory animals by inoculation of Schu virus isolated from a patient with apparent amyotrophic lateral sclerosis. *J Neurol* 1979; 220: 1–19.

30. Gardner MB, Rasheed S, Klement V, et al. Lower motor neuron disease

in wild mice caused by indigenous type C virus and search for a similar etiology in human amyotrophic lateral sclerosis. *UCLA For Med Sci* 1976; 217–234.

31. Hughes RA, O'Leary PD. Neurotrophic factors and the development of drugs to promote motoneuron survival. *Clin Exp Pharmacol Physiol* 1996; 23: 965–969.

32. Ono S, Imai T, Shimizu N, et al. Ciliary neurotropic factor in skin biopsies of patients with amyotrophic lateral sclerosis. *Lancet* 1998; 352: 958–959.

33. Pamphlett R, Waley P. Motor neuron uptake of low dose inorganic mercury. *J Neurol Sci* 1996; 135: 63–67.

34. Perl DP. Relationship of aluminum to Alzheimer's disease. *Environ Health Perspect* 1985; 63: 149–153.

35. Plato CC, Garruto RM, Fox KM, Gajdusek DC. Amyotrophic lateral sclerosis and parkinsonism-dementia on Guam: a 25–year prospective case-control study. *Am J Epidemiol* 1986; 124: 643–656.

36. Tosi L, Righetti C, Adami L, Zanette G. October 1942: a strange epidemic paralysis in Saval, Verona, Italy. Revision and diagnosis 50 years later of tri-ortho-cresyl phosphate poisoning. *J Neurol Neurosurg Psychiat* 1994; 57: 810–813.

37. Hansen JC, Danscher G. Organic mercury: an environmental threat to the health of dietary-exposed societies? *Rev Environ Health* 1997; 12: 107–116.

38. Nagashima K. A review of experimental methylmercury toxicity in rats: neuropathology and evidence for apoptosis. *Toxicol Pathol* 1997; 25: 624–631.

39. Shaw PJ. Excitotoxity and motor neurone disease: a review of the evidence. *J Neurol Sci* 1994; 124 (Suppl); 6–13.

40. Bensimon G, Lacomblez L, Meininger V. A controlled trial of riluzole in amyotrophic lateral sclerosis. ALS/Riluzole Study Group. *New Engl J Med* 1994; 330: 585–591.

41. Hirayama B, Hazama A, Loo DF, et al. Transport of cycasin by the intestinal Na+/glucose cotransporter. *Biochim Biophys Acta* 1994; 1193: 151– 154.

42. Abbott NJ. Astrocyte-endothelial interactions and blood-brain barrier permeability. *J Anat* 2002; 200: 629–638.

43. Dickinson CJ. Cerebral oxidative metabolism in essential hypertension: A meta-analysis. *J Hypertens* 1995; 13: 653–658.

44. Harno K, Rissanen A, Palo J. Glucose tolerance in amyotrophic lateral sclerosis. *Acta Neurol Scand* 1984; 70: 451–455.

45. Dalakas MC, Hatazawa J, Brooks RA, Di Chiro G. Lowered cerebral glucose utilization in amyotrophic lateral sclerosis. *Ann Neurol* 1987; 22: 580–586.

46. Mathe JF, Feve JR, Labat JJ, et al. Ischemia of the anterior horn of the spinal cord [in French]. *Rev Neurol (Paris)* 1989; 145: 60–64.

47. Fraser H, Behan W, Chree A, et al. Mouse inoculation studies reveal no

transmissible agent in amyotrophic lateral sclerosis. *Brain Pathol* 1996; 6: 89–99.

48. Horwich AL, Weissman JS. Deadly conformations – protein misfolding in prion disease. *Cell* 1997; 89: 499–510.

49. Bucciantini M, Giannoni E, Chiti F, et al. Inherent toxicity of aggregates implies a common mechanism for protein misfolding diseases. *Nature* 2002; 416: 507–511.

50. Martin JB. Molecular Basis of the Neurodegenerative Disorders. *New Engl J Med* 1999; 340: 1970–1980.

51. Bruijn LI, Becher MW, Lee MK, et al. ALS-linked SOD1 mutant G85R mediates damage to astrocytes and promotes rapidly progressive disease with S1–containing inclusions. *Neuron* 1997; 18: 327–338.

52. Martin J, Hartl FU. Chaperone-assisted protein folding. *Curr Opin Struct Biol* 1997; 7: 41–52.

53. Melnick J, Argon Y. Molecular chaperones and the biosynthesis of antigen receptors. *Immunol Today* 1995; 16: 243–250.

54. Tomkins J, Usher P, Slade JY, et al. Novel insertion in the KSP region of the neurofilament heavy gene in amyotrophic lateral sclerosis (ALS). *Neuroreport* 1998; 9: 3967–3970.

INDEX

Bunina bodies
  Alzheimer's disease, 204
  motor neurone disease, 454
C-reactive protein, 92, 221, 426
Caesarean section, 342
caffeine, 305, 324
calcium
  bone, 321
  pancreatitis, 130
calpain-10, 160
cancer
  blood supply necessity, 73
  liver, 255
  lung, clubbing association, 245
  obesity, 167
cannabis, 438
cantharidic acid, 110
carbon dioxide, 5
  asthma, 25
  effects resembing insulin, 159, 340
  ventilation, 5
carbon tetrachloride, 251
cardiac, see heart
cardiomyopathies, 231
carotid arteries, 344, 379
cartilage, 83
  metabolism, 87, 89
  osteoarthritis, 83
  rheumatoid arthritis, 94
cassavism, 460
CAT brain scan, 438
cataplexy, 49
cells
  division rate, 74, 77
  survival, 74
cerebellum, multiple sclerosis, 32
cerebral, see brain
cervix, uterine, 192
chaperone proteins, 466
chelation, of iron, 287
chest muscles, 8
Cheyne-Stokes breathing, 412
chlamydial infection, 24, 430
  arthritides, 99
  heart attacks, 222
cholecalciferol, 328
cholecystectomy, 120
cholecystokinin, 107
cholera, 265
cholesterol, 119
  atheroma, 218

familial hypercholesterolaemia, 218
chondrocytes, 88
chromosomes, 472
  replication, 74, 206
chronic fatigue syndrome (CFS), 417
chronic obstructive pulmonary disease
    (COPD), 7, 18
ciguatera poisoning, 418
cilia, 12
ciliary body, 194
circadian rhythms, 46
circulation, anatomy, 331
cirrhosis, 254
  clubbing, 239
  primary biliary, 123
clopidogrel, 217
clotting, blood, 214, 222
clubbing of fingers, 239
  causes, 241
  disease associations, 243
coffee, sleep, 47
cognitive behaviour therapy, 423
colitis, ulcerative, 271
collagen, 56, 88, 219, 323
collapse-firing, venous baroreceptors, 449
complement system, 95
copper-zinc superoxide dismutase, 138,
    456
cornea, 193
coronary heart disease, 213
cortex, sleep, 44
cortisol, see steroids
coxibs (type 2), 85
Coxiella burneti, 418
creatinine, 365
cretinism, 62
Crohn's disease, 271
  T-lymphocytes, 38
Cushing response, 343
cyanosis, pulmonary embolism, 402
cycasin, 460, 462
cyclophosphamide, 428
cyclosporin, 278, 281
cystic duct, 122
cysticercosis, 67
cytokines, 18, 77, 91, 96
cytoplasm, 23
DDAH, 221
dementia
  Alzheimer's disease, 201
  Parkinson's disease, 302

509

demyelination, multiple sclerosis, 34, **38**
deoxyribosenucleic acid (DNA), 23
   repair, 73
   viruses, 254
depression, 420
desferrioxamine, 287
diabetes
   tropical, 154
   Type 1, 145
   Type 2, 157
diaphragm of lungs, 7
diarrhoea, 265
diclofenac, 85
diesel smoke, 24
diffusion, molecular rates, 75
digestion, 104
diplopia, multiple sclerosis, 32
diuresis, osmotic, 146, **480**
diuretic drugs, heart failure, 235
divalent metal transporter-1 (DMT-1),
   285
dopamine
   Parkinson's disease, 302, 420
   schizophrenia, 438
Down's syndrome, 206
dreaming, REM sleep, 41
dropsy, see oedema
duodenal ulcer, 113
duodenum, 103
   iron absorption, 285
dyspnoea, asthma, 17
ECG, 216
eclampsia, 392
EGCG treatment, haemochromatosis, 287
elastin
   eye, 197
   lung, 10
elastosis, lamina cribrosa, 199
electrocardiography (ECG), 216
electroencephalography (EEG), 41
embolism, 215
   pulmonary, 401
emphysema, 5
empyema, clubbing, 240
encephalitis lethargica, 305
endocarditis, clubbing, 240
endometriosis, 179, 181
endometrium, 80, 179, 410
endostatin, 78
endothelin, 348, 383, 401
endothelium, vascular, 77, 220

diabetes, 220
   permeability, preeclampsia, 397
enterokinase, 128
eosinophils, asthma, 24
epidemiology, see topics
epidermis, psoriasis, 54
epilepsy/migraine association, 141
epinephrine, see adrenaline
epithelium, 273
Epstein-Barr (E-B) virus, 36, 124, 280,
   418
erythrocyte sedimentation rate (ESR), 58,
   426
erythropoietin, 367
essential hypertension, see hypertension
Escherichia coli, 145
etanercept, 58
excitotoxic theory (MND), 461
exercise
   blood pressure effects, 336,
   bone density, 324
   cardiac effects, 225
   obesity, 169
   pulmonary artery pressure, 401
   Type 2 diabetes protection, 158
   ventilation, 5
exophthalmos, thyrotoxicosis, 66
expiration, 7
eye disease, diabetes, 147
eye movements, multiple sclerosis, 34
fainting, 441
fallopian tubes, 182
familial hemiplegic migraine, 138
fat
   absorption, 129
   digestion, 129
   metabolism, diabetes, 149
fatigue
   chronic fatigue syndrome, 417
   iron deficiency, 286
   thyroid disorders, 64
fatty acids, 223
feedback, negative, 342
femoral arteries, 346
femur, avascular necrosis of head, 323
ferritin, 285
ferroportin, 288
fertility, PCOS, 412
festination, Parkinsonism, 301
fetal
   distress, 392

platelet immaturity, 247
programming, 169
fibrillation, ventricular, 213
fibrinogen, 222
fibroblast growth factor, 75
finger blood flow, clubbing, 240
fish oils, 223
flavivirus, 99
foam cells, arterial wall, 221
folding, proteins, 466
folic acid, 291
  food fortification, 296
  homocysteine, 208
  ill effects, 294
  preventing neural tube defects, 296
  protection against arterial disease, 220
food fortification, 296
forced expired volume, 8
free radicals, 456
GABA, 308
gall bladder, 119, **121**
gamma amino butyric acid (GABA),
  308
gastric inhibitory polypeptide (GIP), 174
gastric ulcer, 115
gastrin, 105
gastroscopy, 109
genetics, see individual topics
ghrelin, 173
glandular feve, see Epstein-Barr virus
glaucoma, 191
glial cells, 463
glitazones, 162
glomeruli
  filtration rate (GFR), 366
  hypertension, 146, 371
  systemic hypertension, 371
glomerulonephritis, 315, 365
glucagon, 129, 149
glucosamine, 85
glucose
  brain, 463
  cerebral, 203
  diabetes, 145
  diffusion rate, 75
  metabolism, 203
  steroid effects, 22
  urine, 145
glucocorticoids, see steroids
glutamate, Alzheimer's disease, 203
glutamine repeats, 454

glutamic acid decarboxylase (GAD), 153,
  160
gluten, intolerance, 266
glycogen, 149
goitre, 65
gonioscopy, 197
Goodpasture's syndrome, 373
granulomata, 425
Graves' disease, 66, 69
gravity, effects on bone, 324
growth factors, 44, 62, 76, 243
gut
  nerve plexus, 263
  contraction waves, 263
H2-blocking drugs, 110
haematemesis, 110
haemochromatosis, **154**, 283, 287
haemoglobin, 284
  glycosylated, 147
haemophilus infection, 374
haemorrhage
  intracerebral, 377
  subarachnoid, 378
heart
  atria, 445, 448
  attack, 412
  cyanotic disease, clubbing, 240, 403
  failure, 225
  output, 225
  thyrotoxicosis, 64
  transplantation, 225, 445
  valves, 225
  ventricular receptors, 445
  weight, 386
heat regulation, thyroid hormones, 63
heat-shock proteins, 466
Heberden's nodes, 88
Helicobacter pylori, 111
Henoch-Schönlein purpura, 374, 425, 432
hepatitis, 251
  A, 252
  B, 254
  C, 256, 374
  D, E, G, 258
  SEN, 258
hepatorenal syndrome, 375
herpes simplex virus, 205
HFE glycoprotein, 288
hip
  fractures, 90
  osteoarthritis, 85

511

jejunum, 104
Johne's disease, 279
joints
  fluid, 84
  pain, 84
  pressures, 89
  proprioceptors, 85
Kaposi's sarcoma, 405
ketosis, diabetic, 151
kidney
  afferent arterioles, 146
  anatomy, 353
  arterioles, 371
  artery stenosis, 356
  artificial, 368
  biopsy, 367
  excretion rate perfusion relation, 234
  failure, 365, 369
  hypertension causation, 234, 338, 355
  proteinuria, 146
  sodium depletion, 370
kilopascals, pressure measurement, 334
knee joint, 86, 94
knuckles, rheumatoid arthritis, 94
lactobacilli, 265
lamina cribrosa, 195
lamivudine, 255
laparoscopy, 120, 180, 183
Laplace's law, 381
larynx, 5
lathyrism, 460
legionnaires' disease, 28
lens, 193
leptin, 169, 413
  receptors, 170
  source, 170
leukotriene antagonists, 26
levodopa, 308
Lewy bodies, 204, 304
lipase, orlistat, 176
lipocortin, see annexins
lipohyalinosis, cerebral arteries, 382
lipoproteins, 158, 218
liquorice, causing hypertension, 358
lithium, 57, 419
liver
  cancer, 255
  disease causing clubbing, 241, 244
  failure, 252
  inflmmation (hepatitis), 254
  viruses, 251

long-acting thyroid stimulator (LATS), 68
low-pressure glaucoma, 198
lung
  abscess, 244
  asthma, 17
  chronic obstructive disease, 5
  circulation, 244, 333
  infections, 5
  macrophages, 12
  ventilation, 8
  volume, 8
  X-rays, emphysema, 8
lyme disease, 99
lymphocytes
  B-cells, 23, 68, 95
  helper cells, 38
  T-cells, 23, 37, 56, 96, 153, **474**
lymphoma, stomach, 115
macula, 191
magnesium, preeclampsia, 396
magnetic resonance imaging (MRI), 33, 138, 202
  functional, 138
magnetic brain stimulation, 141
malabsorption, 266
malaria, 14
mannose-binding protein, 96
mast cells, 24, 97
matrix-degrading metalloproteinases (MMPs), 75
'ME' (chronic fatigue syndrome), 417
measles virus, 276, 314
  MMR vaccination, 276
mediterranean diet, 217
megakaryocytes, clubbing, 242
melanocortins, 173
melanocyte stimulating hormone (MSH), 173
melatonin, 46
membrane attack complex (MAC), 96
memory, 201
Mendelian inheritance, 480
meningitis, 96
menstruation
  baboons, 411
  cyclical, 410
  retrograde, 183
mercury
  manometer, 333
  poisoning, 461

513